D0930090

Micronutrient Deficiencies during the Weaning Period and the First Years of Life

Nestlé Nutrition Workshop Series
Pediatric Program, Vol. 54

Micronutrient Deficiencies during the Weaning Period and the First Years of Life

Editors

J. M. Pettifor, Johannesburg, South Africa
S. Zlotkin, Toronto, Canada

KARGER

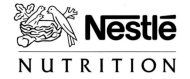

Nestec Ltd., 55 Avenue Nestlé, CH–1800 Vevey (Switzerland)
S. Karger AG, P.O. Box, CH–4009 Basel (Switzerland)   www.karger.com

Printed in Switzerland on acid-free paper by Reinhardt Druck, Basel
ISBN 3–8055–7720–6
ISSN 0742–2806

Library of Congress Cataloging-in-Publication Data

Nestlé Nutrition Workshop (54th : 2003 : Sao Paulo, Brazil)
    Micronutrient deficiencies during the weaning period and the first years of life / editors,
J.M. Pettifor, S. Zlotkin.
        p. ; cm. – (Nestlé Nutrition workshop series, ISSN 0742–2806 ; v. 54. Paediatric Programme)
    Includes bibliographical references and index.
    ISBN 3–8055–7720–6
    1. Trace element deficiency diseases in children–Congresses. 2. Nutrition disorders in
children–Congresses. 3. Nutrition disorders in infants–Congresses. 4. Trace elements in
nutrition–Congresses. I. Pettifor, John M. II. Zlotkin, Stanley. III. Title. IV. Nestlé
Nutrition workshop series ; v. 54. V. Nestlé Nutrition workshop series. Paediatric –
Programme.
        [DNLM: 1. Deficiency Diseases–Child, Preschool–Congresses. 2. Deficiency
Diseases–Infant–Congresses. 3. Micronutrients–deficiency–Child,
Preschool–Congresses. 4. Micronutrients–deficiency–Infant–Congresses. WD 105
N468ma 2004]
    RJ399.T7N37 2003
    618.92′39–dc22

2004046609

Contents

VII Preface

IX Foreword

XI Contributors

1 Role for Micronutrient Interactions in the Epidemiology
of Micronutrient Deficiencies: Interactions of Iron, Iodine
and Vitamin A
Hurrell, R.F.; Hess, S.Y. (Zurich)

21 The Epidemiology of Vitamin D and Calcium Deficiency
Pettifor, J.M. (Johannesburg)

37 Epidemiology of Micronutrient Deficiencies in Developing
and Developed Countries, Specifically Zinc, Copper,
Selenium and Iodine
Castillo-Duran, C.; Ruz, M. (Santiago)

53 Stable Isotope Methods in Micronutrient Research
Abrams, S.A. (Houston, Tex.)

67 Interactions between Micronutrients: Synergies and
Antagonisms
Lönnerdal, B. (Davis, Calif.)

83 Influence of Food Intake, Composition and Bioavailability
on Micronutrient Deficiencies of Infants during the Weaning
Period and the First Year of Life
Gibson, R.S. (Dunedin); Hotz, C. (Cuemavaca); Perlas, L.A.
(Metro Manila)

Contents

105 Micronutrient Malnutrition and Poverty
Bloem, M.W.; de Pee, S. (Singapore)

**119 Impact of Micronutrient Deficiencies on Behavior and
Development**
Lozoff, B. (Ann Arbor, Mich.); Black, M.M. (Baltimore, Md.)

137 Impact of Micronutrient Deficiencies on Immune Function
Semba, R.D. (Baltimore, Md.)

**153 Impact of Micronutrient Deficiencies on Bone Growth and
Mineralization**
Specker, B. (Brookings, S. Dak.)

**173 Impact of Infections on Micronutrient Deficiencies in
Developing Countries**
Bhutta, Z.A. (Karachi)

187 The Economic Impact of Micronutrient Deficiencies
Horton, S. (Toronto, Ont.)

**203 Practical Considerations for Improving Micronutrient
Status in the First Two Years of Life**
Parvanta, I.; Knowles, J. (Atlanta, Ga.)

**213 Specific Strategies to Address Micronutrient Deficiencies
in the Young Child: Targeted Fortification**
Neufeld, L.M. (Morelos); Ramakrishnan, U. (Atlanta, Ga.)

**233 Specific Strategies to Address Micronutrient Deficiencies in
the Young Child: Supplementation and Home Fortification**
Zlotkin, S.; Tondeur, M. (Toronto, Ont.)

249 Crystal Ball Gazing: Micronutrients for All by 2015
Mannar, M.G.V. (Ottawa, Ont.)

263 Conclusions

269 Subject Index

Preface

In economically advanced countries, mineral and vitamin deficiencies have virtually been eliminated over the past 50 years through a combination of national legislation mandating the fortification of some staple foods and voluntary fortification of foods typically sold in grocery stores. The iodization of salt is perhaps the best example of mandated fortification, while ready-to-eat breakfast cereals are a typical example of the voluntary fortification of a commonly eaten food. Historically, the problem of anemia in children largely disappeared in North America and Western Europe only after the introduction and social marketing of highly fortified foods targeted to children. Although pockets of infants and children remain at risk, including infants born prematurely, those living in poverty, new immigrants and some aboriginal groups, generally the eradication of micronutrient deficiencies in the West is recognized as a successful public health accomplishment. The same cannot be said for most developing countries. In developing countries, fortified infant cereals are often unavailable or beyond the reach of financially impoverished communities, and recommendations to use formula are inappropriate, since it competes with breast-feeding.

Iron deficiency is the most common preventable nutritional deficiency in the world despite global goals for its reduction. In the developing world it is estimated that more than 50% of children less than 4 years of age are anemic primarily due to a diet inadequate in bioavailable iron. In some African and South Asian countries, the prevalence of iron-deficiency anemia is as high as 80% of young children. Among the many risk factors that contribute to iron-deficiency anemia in children are low birth weight, early cord clamping, maternal anemia, high rates of infectious disease including malaria, *Helicobacter pylori*, and helminth infections, poverty, poor access to iron-rich foods, and other nutritional deficiencies which impede the incorporation of iron into hemoglobin.

The present volume reviews current knowledge of micronutrient deficiencies during the critical weaning period and first years of life, and follows on a highly successful workshop held a year previously, which looked at micronutrient deficiencies in the first months of life. The workshop provided a logical chronology of the issues and challenges associated with micronutrient deficiencies during this critical later phase of infant and toddler development. To understand the extent of the problem, the first speakers explored the epidemiology of micronutrient deficiencies including state-of-the-art discussions on the use of stable isotopic methods to investigate factors affecting the absorption and interactions of micronutrients. Following directly on the epidemiology was a session on the various etiological factors which predispose 'at risk' populations of infants and young children to micronutrient deficiencies. The Workshop was updated on the more traditional factors like food composition and infectious diseases that would be expected to influence micronutrient status, but in addition, socio- and geopolitical factors like poverty, globalization, and natural disasters were also considered in a thoughtful presentation and panel discussion. In the third session, the health and economic implications of micronutrient deficiencies were considered. Presenters, who are world experts in the field, emphasized the cognitive, intellectual, and social-emotional impairments that may not be reversible in children under 2 years of age with iron-deficiency anemia compared to those without iron deficiency anemia. These children have reduced learning capacity and school achievement and as adults decreased wages and work capacity. Although most in attendance were aware of the health implications of micronutrient deficiencies, it was less well known that its burden results in a reduction of 4.5% of GDP through reduced learning and ultimately poorer paying jobs.

The final session was devoted to a wide-ranging discussion on strategies for the prevention of micronutrient deficiencies. Despite the widely acknowledged lack of success of current public health interventions to prevent micronutrient deficiencies, the presentations and discussion were markedly upbeat and positive. Speakers emphasized that through a combination of food diversification, general supplementation, targeted fortification and 'home fortification' the problem could be addressed. By developing partnerships between the private and public sector and through the initiatives of governments and nongovernmental organizations, the prevention of micronutrient deficiencies was deemed by the Workshop to be a real possibility.

What distinguishes the Nestlé Workshops from others is the format of short presentations followed by long discussions. This thoughtful format allows the speakers and audience to actively interact for more than the usual 5 minutes of questions. As the reader will come to understand, the inclusion of the questions, cross-discussion and debate during the question period is a highlight of the Workshop. Thus the proceedings do more than present state-of-the-art information, they provide a thoughtful and hopefully useful discourse on this important topic.

J.M. Pettifor and S. Zlotkin

Foreword

For this 54th Nestlé Pediatric Nutrition Workshop, which took place in October 2003 in Sao Paulo, the topic 'Micronutrient Deficiencies during the Weaning Period and the First Years of Life' was chosen as a follow-up to the 52nd workshop on 'Micronutrient Deficiencies in the First Months of Life'.

We were interested in the epidemiology of micronutrient deficiencies and the interactions between the various micronutrients, the appropriate methods in micronutrient research, the influence of food intake and bio-availability on micronutrient deficiencies, the relation between micronutrient malnutrition and poverty, the effect of micronutrient deficiencies on behavior and development, immune functions as well as on bone growth and miner-alization, the influence of infections on micronutrient deficiencies in developing countries, the economic impact of micronutrient deficiencies, and finally strategies for the prevention of micronutrient deficiencies in the young child. In order to answer these questions we sought the knowledge of various experts to clarify the pathogenesis of micronutrient deficiencies in the young child and to develop preventive strategies.

I would like to thank the two chairmen, Prof. John Pettifor and Prof. Stanley Zlotkin, who are well-known experts in this field, for putting the program together and inviting as speakers the opinion leaders in the field of micronutrients in health and various disease conditions. Pediatricians invited from 14 countries contributed to the discussions that are published in this book. Mr. João Oliveira and his team from Nestlé Brazil provided all logistical support, so that participants gained an appreciation of the Brazilian hospitality. Dr. Denis Barclay from the Nestlé Research Center in Lausanne, Switzerland, was responsible for the scientific coordination. His cooperation with the chairpersons was essential for the success of this workshop.

Prof. Wolf Endres, MD

Vice-President
Nestec Ltd., Lausanne, Switzerland

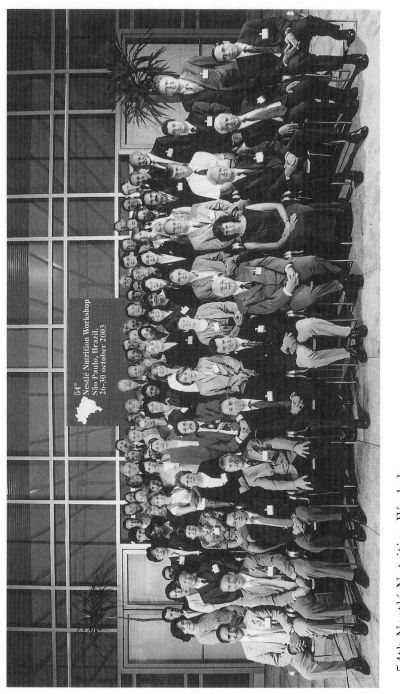

54th Nestlé Nutrition Workshop
Pediatric Program
São Paulo, October 26–30, 2003

Contributors

Chairpersons & Speakers

Prof. Steven A. Abrams

Children's Nutrition Research Center
1100 Bates, Suite 7066
Houston, TX 77030
USA
Tel.: +1 713 798 7124
Fax: +1 713 798 7119
E-Mail: sabrams@bcm.tmc.edu

Prof. Zulfiqar Bhutta

Department of Paediatrics
The Aga Khan University
Stadium Road
P.O. Box 3500, Karachi 74800
Pakistan
Tel.: +92 21 4930 051 (ext. 4721)
Fax: +92 21 4934 294/4932 095
E-Mail: zulfiqar.bhutta@aku.edu

Dr. Martin W. Bloem

Helen Keller Worldwide
#02–13 China Court
China Square Central
20 Cross Street
Singapore 048422
Tel.: +65 62361973
E-Mail: mwbloem@compuserve.com

Prof. Carlos A. Castillo-Durán

Instituto de Nutrición y Tecnología de los Alimentos (INTA)
Universidad de Chile
Macul 5540, Macul, Santiago
Chile
Tel.: +56 2 678 1503
Fax: +56 2 221 4030
E-Mail: ccastd@uec.inta.uchile.cl

Prof. Rosalind S. Gibson

Department of Human Nutrition
University of Otago
P.O. Box 56, Dunedin 9015
New Zealand
Tel.: +64 3 479 7955
Fax: +64 3 479 7958
E-Mail: Rosalind.Gibson@stonebow.otago.ac.nz

Prof. Susan Horton

Munk Center for International Studies
University of Toronto
1, Devonshire Place
Toronto M5S 3K7
Canada
Tel.: +1 416 287 7129/416 946 8947
Fax: +1 416 287 7029/416 946 8915
E-Mail: horton@chass.utoronto.ca

Prof. Richard F. Hurrell

Laboratory of Human Nutrition
Swiss Federal Institute of Technology (ETH)
P.O. Box 474
8803 Rüschlikon
Switzerland
Tel.: +41 1 704 57 01
Fax: +41 1 704 57 10
E-Mail: richard.hurrell@ilw.agrl.ethz.ch

Contributors

Prof. Bo Lönnerdal

Department of Nutrition
University of California
One Shields Ave
Davis, CA 95616
USA
Tel.: +1 530 752 8347
Fax: +1 530 752 3564
E-Mail: bllonnerdal@ucdavis.edu

Dr. Betsy Lozoff

Center for Human Growth and
Development
University of Michigan
300 N. Ingalls
Ann Arbor, MI 48109 0406
USA
Tel.: +1 734 764 2443
Fax: +1 734 936 9288
E-Mail: blozoff@umich.edu

Mr. Marthi Venkatesh Mannar

Micronutrient Initiative
P.O. Box 56127
250 Albert Street
Ottawa, Ontario K1R 7Z1
Canada
Tel.: +1 613 782 6814
Fax: +1 613 782 6838
E-Mail: vmannar@micronutrient.org

Dr. Lynnette Marie Neufeld

Instituto Nacional de Salud Pública
Av. Universidad 655
Santa Maria Ahuacatitlan
Cuernavaca, Morelos, 62508
Mexico
Tel./Fax: +52 777 329 3016
E-Mail: lneufeld@correo.insp.mx

Mr. Ibrahim Parvanta

Centers for Disease Control and
Prevention
Division of Nutrition and Physical
Activity
Mailstop K25
4770 Buford Hwy., N.E.
Atlanta, GA 30341
USA
Tel.: +1 770 488 5865
Fax: +1 770 488 5369
E-Mail: iparvanta@cdc.gov

Prof. John M. Pettifor

Chris Hani Baragwanath Hospital
Department of Paediatrics
P.O. Bertsham 2013
Johannesburg
South Africa
Tel.: +27 11 933 1530
Fax: +27 11 938 9074
E-Mail: pettiforjm@
medicine.wits.ac.za

Dr. Richard Semba

Department of Ophtalmology
John Hopkins University School of
Medicine
500 N. Broadway, Suite 700
Baltimore, MD 21205
USA
Tel.: +1 410 955 3572
Fax: +1 410 955 0629
E-Mail: rdsemba@jhmi.edu

Prof. Bonny Specker

South Dakota State University
Box 2204, EAM Building
Brookings, SD 57007
USA
Tel.: +1 605 688 4645
Fax: +1 605 688 4220
E-Mail: bonny_specker@sdstate.edu

Dr. Stanley Zlotkin

The Hospital for Sick Children
Division of Gastroenterology and
Nutrition
University Avenue
Toronto, Ontario M5G 1X8
Canada
Tel.: +1 416 813 6171
Fax: +1 416 813 4972
E-Mail: szlotkin@sickkids.ca

Moderators

Prof. Marco Antônio Barbieri

Department of Child Care and
Paediatrics
São Paulo University (USP) –
Ribeirão Preto
Av. Bandeirantes, 3900
Ribeirão Preto, SP
Brazil
Cep: 14049–900
Tel.: +55 16 602 2573, 602 3316/17
Fax: +55 16 602 2700
E-Mail: mabarbie@fmrp.usp.br

Prof. Artur Delgado

São Paulo University
Department of Paediatrics
Av. Jacutinga, 352 – apto 81
São Paulo, SP
Brazil
Cep: 04515–030
Tel.: +55 11 505 130 96
Fax: +55 11 503 161 17
E-Mail: arturfd@aol.com

Prof. Fernando José De Nóbrega

Albert Einstein Hospital
Rua Traipu, 1251
São Paulo, SP
Brazil
CEP: 01235–000
Tel.: +55 11 91923313, 3872 1804
Fax: +55 11 3872 1001
E-Mail: fjnobrega@sti.com.br

Prof. Hugo Da Costa Ribeiro Júnior

Unidade Metabólica Fima Lifshitz
Federal University of Bahia
Rua Padre Feijó S/N
Salvador, BA
Brazil
Cep: 40110–170
Tel.: +55 71 3312027, 91199892
Fax: +55 71 3312027
E-Mail: hugocrj@ufba.br

Invited attendees

Prof. Maria Luiza Aléssio / Brazil
Prof. Carlos Alberto Nogueira De Almeida / Brazil
Prof. Olga Maria Silverio Amancio / Brazil
Prof. Teresa Negreira Navarro Barbosa / Brazil
Dr. Ciro Bertoli / Brazil
Dr. Anne Lise Dias Brasil / Brazil
Prof. Antonio Celso Calçado / Brazil
Prof. Ary Lopes Cardoso / Brazil
Dr. Adriano De Castro Filho / Brazil
Prof. Silvia M.F. Cozzolino / Brazil
Dr. Maria Arlete Meil Schimith Escrivão / Brazil
Dr. Jocemara Gurmini / Brazil
Prof. Yu Kar Ling Koda / Brazil
Prof. Christiane Araújo Chaves Leite / Brazil
Dr. Luiz Anderson Lopes / Brazil
Prof. Fábio Ancona Lopez / Brazil
Prof. Ângela Mattos / Brazil
Dr. Elza Daniel De Mello / Brazil
Prof. Mauro Batista De Morais / Brazil
Prof. Rocksane De Carvalho Norton / Brazil
Prof. Naylor Alves De Oliveira / Brazil
Dr. Fernanda Luisa Ceragioli Oliveira / Brazil
Prof. Domingos Palma / Brazil
Prof. Sheila Percope / Brazil
Prof. Hélio Fernandes Da Rocha / Brazil
Dr. Roseli Sacardo Sarni / Brazil
Prof. Luciana Rodrigues Silva / Brazil
Prof. Marilisa Stenghel Froes Souza / Brazil
Prof. José Augusto Taddei / Brazil
Dr. Rosana Tumas / Brazil
Dr. Mario Vieira / Brazil
Prof. Zongyi Ding / China
Prof. Shian Yin / China

Contributors

Prof. Parampalli Padmanabha Maiya / India
Dr. Jose Rizal Latief Batubara / Indonesia
Dr. Husein Albar / Indonesia
Dr. Riza Iriani Nasution / Indonesia
Prof. Marcelo Assumma / Italy
Dr. Rinaldo Zanini / Italy
Dr. Noorizan Abdul Majid / Malaysia
Prof. Swee Fong Tang / Malaysia
Dr. Salvador Villalpando-Carrión / Mexico
Dr. Edgar Vasquez Garibay / Mexico
Dr. Hassan Afilal / Morocco
Dr. Abdesselam Nbou / Morocco
Dr. Jules Tolboom / Netherlands
Dr. Benjamín Sablan Jr. / Philippines
Dr. Carla Maria Barreto Silva Souza Rego / Portugal
Prof. Mehari Gebre-Medhin / Sweden
Prof. Khanh Nguyen Gia / Vietnam
Dr. Hoa Nguyen Thi / Vietnam

Nestlé participants

Mr. Paulo Castro / Brazil
Dr. Aderson Damião / Brazil
Mr. João Henrique Oliveira / Brazil
Mrs. Valéria Oliveira / Brazil
Ms. Lesley Scharf / Canada
Ms. Patricia Mogrovejo / Ecuador
Mrs. Mieke Beemsterboer / Netherlands
Dr. Denis Barclay / Switzerland
Prof. Wolf Endres / Switzerland
Dr. Pierre Guesry / Switzerland

Pettifor JM, Zlotkin S (eds): Micronutrient Deficiencies during the Weaning Period and the
First Years of Life. Nestlé Nutrition Workshop Series Pediatric Program, vol 54, pp 1–19,
Nestec Ltd., Vevey/S. Karger AG, Basel, © 2004.

Role for Micronutrient Interactions in the Epidemiology of Micronutrient Deficiencies: Interactions of Iron, Iodine and Vitamin A

Richard F. Hurrell and Sonja Y. Hess

Institute of Food Science and Nutrition,
Swiss Federal Institute of Technology, Zurich, Switzerland

Introduction

Iron, iodine and vitamin A are the most common micronutrient deficiencies and affect one third or more of the world's population. It is estimated that 2 billion people are anemic based on low hemoglobin (Hb) levels, that 1.9 billion have inadequate iodine nutrition based on low urinary iodine levels, and that 250 million preschool children are vitamin A-deficient based on low serum retinol concentrations [1]. The prevalence of anemia due solely to iron deficiency is less certain because anemia has several different causes including the deficiency of iron, the deficiency of other micronutrients, infections and malaria. It has been suggested, based on the findings of Asobayire et al. [2], that the prevalence of iron-deficiency anemia (IDA) can be estimated as approximately half of the prevalence of anemia per se [1], and additionally that there are a similar number of people who have iron deficiency (no iron stores) without anemia as have iron deficiency with anemia. Thus it can be estimated that about 2 billion people are iron deficient, of which about 1 billion have IDA.

It has been common practice to evaluate the epidemiology of micronutrient deficiencies separately for each micronutrient and to develop individual strategies for their prevention or treatment. Simple logic, however, would tell us that single micronutrient deficiencies rarely occur in isolation, especially in infants, children and women from the poorer socioeconomic groups in the developing world. Growing children and pregnant and lactating women have a higher requirement for all nutrients, and economically poor populations typically consume nutritionally poor diets based on cereals and legumes, with

1

little animal-source foods, fruits and vegetables. It is well accepted that such diets are low in bioavailable iron and vitamin A. Low iron bioavailability is a major factor in the etiology of iron deficiency [3], together with parasitic infections [4] and high menstrual blood losses in women of child-bearing age [5]. Low dietary retinol and low intake and poor bioavailability of pro-vitamin A carotenoids are likewise the major factor in the etiology of vitamin A deficiency [6]. Plant-based diets, however, would also be expected to be low in zinc, riboflavin, vitamin B_6 and vitamin B_{12}, and, if little fruit and vegetables are consumed, also low in vitamin C and folate. Deficiencies of these micronutrients, although rarely measured, could also coexist with iron and vitamin A deficiencies and, in addition, if the soils are low in iodine [7] or selenium [8], deficiencies in iodine and selenium may also be present.

As multiple micronutrient deficiencies coexist, it is therefore possible that a deficiency of one micronutrient influences the etiology, prevention or treatment of another micronutrient deficiency. Table 1 shows the prevalence data reported for iron, iodine and/or vitamin A deficiencies in the same individual [9–17]. Clearly many interactions between micronutrients are possible but recent attention has focused on interactions influencing the etiology of anemia, including IDA, and interactions influencing iodine deficiency. In addition to iron, low intakes of vitamin A [18], riboflavin [19], folic acid, vitamins B_{12}, B_6 and C [20] could all influence the etiology of anemia. Similarly, in addition to low iodine intake [7] and intake of goitrogens [21], poor iron status [12], vitamin A status [22] or selenium status [23] may influence the etiology of iodine deficiency, and may reduce the efficacy of the strategies used for its prevention or treatment [14, 24].

This review focuses on the possible interactions of iron and vitamin A in the etiology of anemia and the possible interactions of iron and iodine in the etiology of iodine deficiency.

Interaction of Vitamin A with Iron in the Etiology of Anemia

The link between vitamin A deficiency and anemia has been known for many years. What is still not known is the mechanism by which vitamin A exerts its effect. An interaction of vitamin A in iron metabolism is the most likely explanation and several mechanisms have been proposed [25]. In tropical countries, the high prevalence of infectious diseases might also play a role as vitamin A deficiency can decrease immune function, due to a modulation of hematopoiesis [26], and thus increase the anemia of infection [27].

In the classic study of Hodges et al. [28], 8 middle-aged men were fed a combination of 3 different vitamin A-deficient diets together with mineral and vitamin supplements for 360–770 days. The intake of all nutrients, except vitamin A, was judged adequate. However, despite a daily intake of 18–19 mg iron, the men developed mild anemia after about 6 months. As plasma retinol levels fell from what was described as plentiful ($>30 \mu g/dl$) to adequate ($20–30 \mu g/dl$) and on to low ($<20 \mu g/dl$), the mean Hb values fell from 15.6 to 12.9 g/dl and onto 11.9 g/dl. The anemia was not responsive to iron therapy until the subjects were repleted with vitamin A.

Cross-Sectional Studies

Despite the influence of other nutritional factors and infectious diseases on both vitamin A and iron status, many cross-sectional studies in developing countries have reported a positive correlation between serum retinol and Hb concentration. The correlation becomes more apparent with lower vitamin A status [20].

Possible Interactions of Vitamin A in Iron Metabolism

Iron metabolism can be described as a closed loop representing primarily the formation and destruction of red cells. Small amounts of iron enter this loop via the absorption of dietary iron and, in balance, an equivalent amount of iron exits in the loop as losses from blood and tissues (fig. 1). Vitamin A deficiency has been proposed to influence iron metabolism either via a decrease in erythropoiesis with less iron incorporated into red blood cells [25] or indirectly by improving immune function and decreasing the anemia of infection [26]. In addition, dietary vitamin A has been reported to increase iron absorption [29]. Proving these theories, as well as confirming the effect of vitamin A, on iron absorption has been difficult, and the exact mechanism of the vitamin A/iron interaction still remains to be established.

In rats, vitamin A deficiency reduces the incorporation of radioactive iron into erythrocytes by almost 50% [30], alters red blood cell morphology [31], produces mild anemia [32, 33], lowers plasma total iron-binding capacity and percent transferrin saturation [33–35], but not circulating transferrin concentrations [35], and causes an accumulation of iron in the liver [30, 36], spleen [30, 33, 34] and bone [33, 34]. Vitamin A deficiency in rats, in addition, appears to increase iron absorption from the gut [30, 32, 33].

Based on these studies Roodenburg et al. [34] hypothesized that vitamin A deficiency impairs erythropoiesis so that mild anemia with malformed cells develops. The abnormal erythrocytes would be broken down by the macrophages of the reticuloendothelial system at an increased rate and so help explain the accumulation of iron in the spleen. In vitro studies would indicate that retinoids influence erythropoiesis but that the influence is complex, depending on the stage of erythrocyte development [37], and may involve a direct effect on erythropoietin formation [38]. However, Roodenburg et al. [25] could find no evidence in rats that vitamin A deficiency effects erythropoiesis and speculated that iron accumulation in the spleen may be related to a reduced iron transport due to an inhibition of transferrin synthesis, although Mejia and Arroyave [35] found no decrease in circulating

Table 1. Epidemiological studies of anemia, iron, vitamin A and iodine deficiencies and co-occurrence

Subjects	Year	Location	Prevalence of single deficiency			Prevalence of multiple deficiencies				Ref.
			iron	vitamin A	iodine	iron and vitamin A	iron and iodine	vitamin A and iodine	iron and vitamin A and iodine	
Infants 6–12 months (n = 98)	1998	South Africa	39% IDA; Hb <110 g/l, SF <10 µg/l	13% VAD; serum retinol <0.7 µmol/l		7% ID and VAD				9
Children 1–5 years (n = 919)	1995	Republic of Marshall Islands	24% IDA; 54% ID; Hb <110 g/l, SF <12 µg/l	60% VAD; serum retinol <0.7 µmol/l		33% ID and VAD				10
Children 1–5 years (n = 1,243)	1996	Honduras	29% anemia; Hb <110 g/l	14% VAD; serum retinol <0.7 µmol/l; 45% low vitamin A stores; serum retinol <1.05 µmol/l		16% anemia and low vitamin A stores				11
Children 6–12 years (n = 419)	1997	Côte d'Ivoire	27% IDA; Hb <110 g/l and SF <12 µg/l or TfR >8.5 mg/l and ZPP >40 µmol/mol heme		45% goiter by palpation		19% IDA and goiter			12
Children 6–15 years (n = 329)	1999	Côte d'Ivoire	17% IDA; 35% ID; Hb <115 g/l, SF <12 µg/l or TfR >8.5 mg/l and ZPP >40 µmol/mol heme	45% VAD; serum retinol <0.7 µmol/l	74% goiter by ultrasound using provisional WHO/ICCIDD reference values[1]	10% IDA and VAD; 18% ID and VAD	12% IDA and goiter, 26% ID and goiter	32% VAD and goiter	10% IDA, VAD and goiter; 14% ID, VAD and goiter	13

Group	Year	Country	Iron status	Vitamin A	Iodine/goiter	Combined deficiency	Ref
Children 6–15 years (n = 377)	2001	Morocco	36% IDA; 51% ID; Hb <115 g/l, SF <12 μg/l or TfR >8.5 mg/l and ZPP >40 μmol/mol heme		71% goiter by ultrasound using provisional WHO/ICCIDD reference values[1]	35% IDA and goiter; 50% ID and goiter	14
Pregnant women 16–19 years (n = 151)	2000	India	46% anemia; Hb <110 g/l	16% night blindness	15% goiter by palpation	2% anemia, night blindness and goiter	15
Pregnant women 15–40 years (n = 336)	1994–1997	Nepal	64% IDA; 81% ID; Hb <110 g/l, SF <10 μg/l and/or ZPP >70 μmol/mol heme	54% low vitamin A stores; serum retinol <1.05 μmol/l		38% SF <10 μg/l and serum retinol <1.05 μmol/l	16
Anemic pregnant women (n = 150)		Malawi	55% IDA; Hb <105 g/l and SF <30 μg/l	39% VAD; serum retinol <1.05 μmol/l		17% IDA and VAD	17

Hb = Hemoglobin; ID = iron deficiency; IDA = iron deficiency anemia; SF = serum ferritin; TfR = transferrin receptor; VAD = vitamin A deficiency; ZPP = zinc protoporphyrin.

[1]Zimmermann MB, Molinari L, Spehl M, et al: Updated provisional WHO/ICCIDD reference values for sonographic thyroid volume in iodine-replete school-age children. IDD Newslett 2001;17:12.

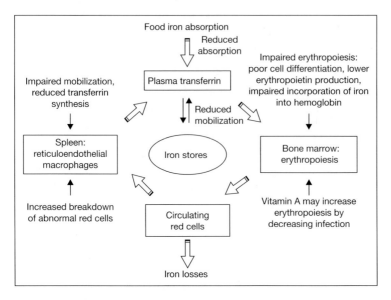

Fig. 1. Possible influence of vitamin A deficiency on iron metabolism.

transferrin concentrations in vitamin A-deficient rats. Nevertheless, it is possible that vitamin A is involved somehow in the release of iron from the spleen or the liver stores, or perhaps directly in the incorporation of iron into Hb. Some evidence for an influence of vitamin A on the mobilization of liver and spleen iron comes from the study of van Stuijvenberg et al. [39]. Children receiving an iron-fortified soup increased serum iron levels and transferrin saturation to a greater extent when plasma retinol levels were >40 μg/dl as compared to <20 μg/dl.

Infection

Although it seems reasonable to speculate that vitamin A enhances immunity, reduces infection and thus the anemia of infection, there are little data available to support this directly [40].

Absorption

Human studies investigating the influence of vitamin A on iron absorption have produced contradictory results. One group has reported an increase in iron absorption by Venezuelan subjects from iron-fortified bread meals in the presence vitamin A or β-carotene [29, 41] (fig. 2). The other group reported no effect of vitamin A on iron absorption when similar meals were fed to Swiss and Swedish students [42] and an inhibition of iron absorption when vitamin A was added to a maize meal fed to vitamin A-deficient children in the

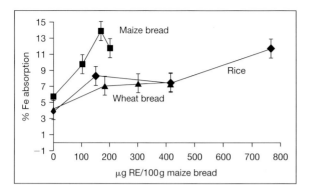

Fig. 2. Influence of vitamin A and β-carotene on iron absorption (including both iron absorption and iron incorporation into hemoglobin) from maize bread, wheat bread and rice meals [41]. Maize flour and wheat flour were fortified with 5 and 2 mg Fe, respectively, as ferrous fumarate and fed as bread with margarine and cheese. Rice was unfortified and fed with margarine.

Côte d'Ivoire [43]. In the same children, there was no effect on iron absorption of vitamin A 3 weeks after they had been supplemented with a high dose of vitamin A. The methods used to estimate iron absorption in all studies were similar and based on erythrocyte incorporation of either stable or radioactive isotopes. This methodology quantifies iron that is first absorbed and then incorporated into Hb. Any effect of vitamin A could be on either the absorption stage, or on the subsequent incorporation of iron into Hb, or on both the absorption and utilization.

It is difficult to explain these contradictory results. Small differences in methodology seem an unlikely explanation. It seems more probable that differences in the nutritional status of the study subjects or their disease state at the time of the absorption study could explain their different responses to dietary vitamin A. Erythropoiesis, including the incorporation of iron into Hb, can be influenced by factors other than iron and vitamin A nutrition. Riboflavin [19], folic acid, vitamin B_{12} and vitamin B_6 status [20] can all influence red cell formation, as can chronic infections [44]. A detailed nutritional status evaluation of the study subjects from Venezuela and the Côte d'Ivoire was not made. Previous studies in the Côte d'Ivoire have reported that chronic infections, malaria, and intestinal parasites are common in school-aged children from similar populations [2]. These combined results from Venezuela, Côte d'Ivoire and Europe thus indicate the complexity of the interaction of vitamin A status, dietary vitamin A and iron metabolism and emphasize the difficulty in extrapolating results from an industrialized to a developing country, and even extrapolating from one developing country to another developing country where diet and lifestyle are different.

Interventions

Many intervention studies have shown that vitamin A supplements, or foods fortified with vitamin A, improve blood Hb concentrations in children and pregnant or lactating women [40]. In addition, some studies have shown that dual supplementation of iron with vitamin A have a greater impact on Hb concentrations than iron alone, in both children [45] and pregnant women [18]. However, some studies have shown no significant effect of vitamin A on Hb concentrations [46], which might be expected especially if vitamin A status is adequate [47].

From these studies, it can be concluded that both vitamin A and iron are required for normal red cell production. The exact nature of the interaction, however, is not known, but vitamin A could be needed for erythropoiesis, including the incorporation of iron into Hb, and may be needed for mobilization of iron from spleen or the liver stores. Alternatively, the positive influence of vitamin A on the immune system may influence erythropoiesis via an influence on the anemia of infection. Because other nutritional factors and disease factors can influence erythropoiesis, it is not possible to generalize on the additional beneficial effect on anemia prevention or treatment of providing both iron and vitamin A. Where vitamin A nutrition is marginal and iron deficiency common, dual fortification or supplementation can be recommended. Where other micronutrients may be lacking in the diet, then multiple micronutrient fortification together with iron may be necessary to get the maximum impact on iron status.

Interactions of Iron and Iodine Metabolism

Extensive data from animal studies indicate that iron deficiency, with or without anemia, impairs thyroid metabolism. Weanling rats fed iron-deficient diets have significantly lower plasma triiodothyronine (T_3) and thyroxine (T_4) concentrations and blunted thyrotropin (TSH) responses compared to rats fed adequate iron [48]. Rats with iron deficiency have reduced peripheral conversion of T_4 to T_3 [49] and significantly lower hepatic 5'-deiodinase activity than controls [50]. However, a limitation to these earlier studies is the lack of pair-feeding, as some of the observed effects of anemia could be explained by reduced food intake and thus caloric restriction. A widely recognized effect of thyroid hormones is their influence over energy metabolism [51]. As food intake is reduced in anemia, the lower thyroid hormone concentration may be in part a physiologic adaptation. This has been confirmed by reduced thyroid hormone concentrations in modified fasting of rats [52].

A few studies in humans also showed that IDA decreases the thyroid hormone concentration. However, the results are not consistent. Beard et al. [53] reported a significant difference in T_3 concentration between anemic

(Hb <110 g/l) and non-anemic women although TSH was in the normal range. On the other hand, there was a nonsignificant 10% lower T_3 concentration in severely anemic (Hb 75 g/l) Venezuelan subjects [54] and no difference in T_3, T_4 and TSH in iron-deficient anemic American women [55]. Although, in the latter study, when the women were subjected to cold exposure, T_3, T_4 and TSH increased to a lesser extent than in the non-anemic women.

Cross-Sectional Studies

Data from the few available cross-sectional studies, which have investigated the correlation between iodine deficiency and IDA, are equivocal. A survey in Ethiopian children found no correlation in goiter rate or thyroid hormone levels and iron status [56]. However, in severely vitamin A-deficient Ethiopian children, low levels of T_3 were associated with low serum iron and low transferrin saturation [57]. A national screening in 2,917 children in Iran has reported a highly significant difference in goiter rates by palpation between children with low and normal serum ferritin (SF) levels [58]. Goiter was 3.8 times more prevalent in schoolchildren with low SF levels than in children with normal SF concentrations. Moreover, Zimmermann et al. [12] in 1997 assessed iron status and goiter rate by palpation in 419 children aged 6–15 years in two villages in western Côte d'Ivoire and found a relative risk of 1.9 (confidence interval 1.5–2.3) for goiter for children with IDA.

Possible Mechanisms of the Iodine and Iron Interaction

It is not clear how iron deficiency exerts its effects on thyroid and iodine metabolism. There are several theories in the literature as to the possible interactions of iodine and iron metabolism. These include alterations in the thyroid hormone feedback system, a reduced syntheses of thyroid hormones in the thyroid, a lower transformation of T_4 to T_3 in the peripheral tissue, and nonspecific alterations due to hypoxic stress (lack of oxygen). Beard et al. [59] suggest that IDA induces changes in thyroid metabolism through alterations in central nervous system control resulting in an altered feedback system. Under normal conditions, thyroid hormones inhibit the synthesis of TSH directly at the pituitary level and indirectly via a decrease in the secretion of thyrotropin-releasing hormone at the hypothalamic level.

In the periphery, the lowered $[^{125}I]T_3$ binding to hepatic nuclei shown in rats could also be a contributory mechanism [60]. In addition, IDA leads to a decreased hepatic 5'-deiodinase activity, which catalyzes the conversion of T_4 to T_3 [50, 61, 62]. The depression of 5'-deiodinase activity is greater in more severely iron-deficient anemic rats (72%) than in the less severely anemic rats (25%) [61]. Although the lowered hepatic 5'-deiodinase activity observed in iron deficiency may be at least partially attributed to low plasma T_4 concentrations, normalizing plasma T_4 did not normalize hepatic 5'-deiodinase activity. These observations suggest that the mechanisms that control hepatic 5'-deiodinase activity (e.g. enzyme synthesis, allosteric regulation of enzyme activity) are directly affected by iron deficiency, regardless of thyroid hormone status [61]. According to Beard et al. [59], however, the effect of iron deficiency on either the hepatic 5'-deiodinase or the brown fat deiodinase II observed in rats is rather minimal. Moreover, using an in vitro method, outer ring deiodinase activity is not affected by either ferric or ferrous iron [63]. It should be noted that this enzyme is also selenium-dependent [23]. Presumably, in iron-deficient anemic rats, a smaller portion of T_4 is converted to T_3 and a larger portion is converted to reverse T_3, a physiologically inactive metabolite, which indicates that iron-deficient rats are functionally hypothyroid, with a tendency toward thyroid hormone inactivation versus activation [64].

Another potential mechanism for reduced thyroid hormone concentration in IDA is impairment of thyroid peroxidase (TPO) activity. TPO is a glycosylated, heme enzyme bound to the apical membrane of the thyrocytes [65]. It plays a key role in thyroid hormone synthesis as it catalyzes the two initial steps, iodination of the thyroglobulin and coupling of the iodotyrosine residues [66]. We have recently shown that TPO activity is significantly reduced in IDA [67]. Male weanling Sprague-Dawley rats ($n = 84$) were assigned to 7 groups. Three groups (ID-3, ID-7, ID-11) were fed iron-deficient diets containing 3, 7 and 11 μg iron/g diet. An iron-sufficient diet was fed to 3 pair-fed groups, whereas it was consumed ad libitum by 1 control group. After 4 weeks, Hb, T_3 and T_4 were significantly lower in the iron-deficient groups than in the control group ($p < 0.001$). TPO activity (by both guaiacol and iodide assays) was markedly reduced by iron deficiency ($p < 0.05$). Compared to the ad libitum control group, TPO activity per total thyroid determined by the guaiacol assay in the ID-3, ID-7 and ID-11 groups was decreased by 56, 45 and 33%, respectively ($p < 0.05$).

Thyroid metabolism could also be impaired nonspecifically by iron deficiency through anemia and lowered oxygen transport, similar to the thyroid impairment of hypoxia found in animals [68]. Thyroid impairment was also found in chronically hypoxic children, who had not only increased levels of reverse T_3, but also decreased concentrations of T_4 and T_3, whereas in acutely hypoxic children, mean serum T_4 and T_3 concentrations were not altered, but the mean serum reverse T_3 concentration was significantly elevated [69]. However, in healthy subjects hypoxic stress led to marked elevations in plasma T_4 and T_3 within 4 h and the increased levels were maintained during the entire period of exposure [70, 71]. This indicates that in a healthy subject, hypoxia cannot entirely explain hypothyroidism associated with IDA.

Evidence from Intervention Studies

In a first study in 1997, Zimmermann et al. [12] investigated the effect of a 200-mg oral dose of iodine as iodized oil in non-anemic ($n = 51$) and iron-deficient anemic ($n = 53$) children with goiter in western Côte d'Ivoire.

At 15 and 30 weeks the thyroid volume was significantly reduced in the non-anemic group compared to the IDA group ($p < 0.001$). A clear difference in goiter prevalence was apparent at 15 and 30 weeks, when goiter rates were 62 and 64% in the IDA group and only 31 and 12% in the non-anemic group, respectively. After 30 weeks, the TSH and T_4 concentrations improved significantly in the non-anemic group compared to the IDA group. Beginning at 30 weeks, the children with IDA were given 60 mg oral iron as ferrous sulfate 4 times/week for 12 weeks [72]. This resulted in an increase in Hb ($\pm$SD) from 97 ± 8 g/l at 30 weeks to 122 ± 8 g/l at 50 weeks. The change in thyroid volume, which had reached a plateau at weeks 10–30, began to fall again after iron supplementation. Consequently, goiter prevalence in the IDA group, which had remained at 62–64% from weeks 10 to 30, was reduced after iron supplementation to 31 and 20% at 50 and 65 weeks.

A randomized, double-blind, placebo-controlled trial in 5–14 years old children in Côte d'Ivoire confirmed that iron supplementation (60 mg iron/day, 4 days/week for 16 weeks) improves the efficacy of iodized salt in goitrous children with iron deficiency [24]. The mean reduction in thyroid volume in the iron-treated group was twice that in the placebo group: -22.8 ± 10.7 compared to -12.7 ± 10.1%. In a 9-month fortification trial in goitrous Moroccan children comparing dual-fortified salt containing iodine and iron with iodized salt alone [73], greater improvement in thyroid function was found in the group receiving the dual-fortified salt. The prevalence of goiter and hypothyroidism was significantly reduced in the dual-fortified salt group, compared to the iodized salt group. Overall, these results suggest that a high prevalence of iron deficiency among children in areas of endemic goiter may reduce the effectiveness of iodized salt programs and strongly support the current recommendations by the World Health Organization [74] for combined supplementation and fortification using multiple micronutrients.

References

1   Allen L, De Benoist B, Dary O, Hurrell R: Guidelines on Food Fortification. Geneva, WHO, 2004, in press.
2   Asobayire FS, Adou P, Davidsson L, et al: Prevalence of iron deficiency with and without concurrent anemia in population groups with high prevalences of malaria and other infections: A study in Côte d'Ivoire. Am J Clin Nutr 2001;74:776–782.
3   Taylor PG, Mendez-Castellanos H, Martinez-Torres C, et al: Iron bioavailability from diets consumed by different socioeconomic strata of the Venezuelan population. J Nutr 1995;125: 1860–1868.
4   Stoltzfus RJ, Chwaya HM, Montresor A, et al: Malaria, hookworms and recent fever are related to anemia and iron status indicators in 0- to 5-year old Zanzibari children and these relationships change with age. J Nutr 2000;130:1724–1733.
5   Hallberg L, Rossander-Hulthén L: Iron requirements in menstruating women. Am J Clin Nutr 1991;54:1047–1058.
6   West CE, Eilander A, van Lieshout M: Consequences of revised estimates of carotenoid bioefficacy for dietary control of vitamin A deficiency in developing countries. J Nutr 2002; 132:2920S–2926S.

7 Delange F: Iodine deficiency; in Braverman LE, Utiger RD (eds): The Thyroid: A Fundamental and Clinical Text, ed 8. Philadelphia, Lippincott, 2000, pp 295–316.

8 Brown KM, Arthur JR: Selenium, selenoproteins and human health: A review. Public Health Nutr 2001;4:593–599.

9 Oelofse A, Van Raaij JM, Benade AJ, et al: Disadvantaged black and coloured infants in two urban communities in the Western Cape, South Africa differ in micronutrient status. Public Health Nutr 2002;5:289–294.

10 Palafox NA, Gamble MV, Dancheck B, et al: Vitamin A deficiency, iron deficiency, and anemia among preschool children in the Republic of the Marshall Islands. Nutrition 2003;19:405–408.

11 Albalak R, Ramakrishnan U, Stein AD, et al: Co-occurrence of nutrition problems in Honduran children. J Nutr 2000;130:2271–2273.

12 Zimmermann M, Adou P, Torresani T, et al: Persistence of goiter despite oral iodine supplementation in goitrous children with iron deficiency anemia in Côte d'Ivoire. Am J Clin Nutr 2000;71:88–93.

13 Hess SY: Interactions between Iodine and Iron Deficiencies; ETH Diss No. 15002. Zürich, Swiss Federal Institute of Technology, 2003.

14 Zimmermann MB, Zeder C, Chaouki N, et al: Dual fortification of salt with iodine and micro-encapsulated iron: A randomized, double-blind, controlled trial in Moroccan schoolchildren. Am J Clin Nutr 2003;77:425–432.

15 Pathak P, Singh P, Kapil U, Raghuvanshi RS: Prevalence of iron, vitamin A, and iodine deficiencies amongst adolescent pregnant mothers. Indian J Pediatr 2003;70:299–301.

16 Dreyfuss ML, Stoltzfus RJ, Shrestha JB, et al: Hookworms, malaria and vitamin A deficiency contribute to anemia and iron deficiency among pregnant women in the plains of Nepal. J Nutr 2000;130:2527–2536.

17 van den Broek NR, Letsky EA: Etiology of anemia in pregnancy in south Malawi. Am J Clin Nutr 2000;72:247S–256S.

18 Suharno D, West CE, Muhilal, et al: Supplementation with vitamin A and iron for nutritional anaemia in pregnant women in West Java, Indonesia. Lancet 1993;342:1325–1328.

19 Powers HJ: Riboflavin-iron interactions with particular emphasis on the gastrointestinal tract. Proc Nutr Soc 1995;54:509–517.

20 Fishman SM, Christian P, West KP: The role of vitamins in the prevention and control of anaemia. Public Health Nutr 2000;3:125–150.

21 Gaitan E: Goitrogens in food and water. Annu Rev Nutr 1990;10:21–39.

22 Ingenbleek Y, De Visscher M: Hormonal and nutritional status: Critical conditions for endemic goiter epidemiology? Metabolism 1979;28:9–19.

23 Arthur JR, Beckett GJ, Mitchell JH: The interactions between selenium and iodine deficiencies in man and animals. Nutr Res Rev 1999;12:55–73.

24 Hess SY, Zimmermann MB, Adou P, et al: Treatment of iron deficiency in goitrous children improves the efficacy of iodized salt in Côte d'Ivoire. Am J Clin Nutr 2002;75:743–748.

25 Roodenburg AJ, West CE, Beguin Y, et al: Indicators of erythrocyte formation and degradation in rats with either vitamin A or iron deficiency. J Nutr Biochem 2000;11:223–230.

26 Thurnham DI: Vitamin A, iron, and haemopoiesis. Lancet 1993;342:1312–1313.

27 Means RT Jr: The anaemia of infection. Baillieres Best Pract Res Clin Haematol 2000;13:151–162.

28 Hodges RE, Sauberlich HE, Canham JE, et al: Hematopoietic studies in vitamin A deficiency. Am J Clin Nutr 1978;31:876–885.

29 Layrisse M, Garcia-Casal MN, Solano L, et al: The role of vitamin A on the inhibitors of non-heme iron absorption: Preliminary results. Nutr Biochem 1997;8:61–67.

30 Mejia LA, Hodges RE, Rucker RB: Clinical signs of anemia in vitamin A-deficient rats. Am J Clin Nutr 1979;32:1439–1444.

31 Mejia LA, Hodges RE, Rucker RB: Role of vitamin A in the absorption, retention and distribution of iron in the rat. J Nutr 1979;109:129–137.

32 Sijtsma KW, Van Den Berg GJ, Lemmens AG, et al: Iron status in rats fed on diets containing marginal amounts of vitamin A. Br J Nutr 1993;70:777–785.

33 Roodenburg AJ, West CE, Yu S, Beynen AC: Comparison between time-dependent changes in iron metabolism of rats as induced by marginal deficiency of either vitamin A or iron. Br J Nutr 1994;71:687–699.

34 Roodenburg AJ, West CE, Hovenier R, Beynen AC: Supplemental vitamin A enhances the recovery from iron deficiency in rats with chronic vitamin A deficiency. Br J Nutr 1996;75:623–636.

35 Mejia LA, Arroyave G: Lack of direct association between serum transferrin and serum biochemical indicators of vitamin A nutriture. Acta Vitaminol Enzymol 1983;5:179–184.
36 Staab DB, Hodges RE, Metcalf WK, Smith JL: Relationship between vitamin A and iron in the liver. J Nutr 1984;114:840–844.
37 Perrin MC, Blanchet JP, Mouchiroud G: Modulation of human and mouse erythropoiesis by thyroid hormone and retinoic acid: Evidence for specific effects at different steps of the erythroid pathway. Hematol Cell Ther 1997;39:19–26.
38 Semba RD, Kumwenda N, Taha TE, et al: Impact of vitamin A supplementation on anaemia and plasma erythropoietin concentrations in pregnant women: A controlled clinical trial. Eur J Haematol 2001;66:389–395.
39 van Stuijvenberg ME, Kruger M, Badenhorst CJ, et al: Response to an iron fortification programme in relation to vitamin A status in 6–12-year-old school children. Int J Food Sci Nutr 1997;48:41–49.
40 Semba RD, Bloem MW: The anemia of vitamin A deficiency: Epidemiology and pathogenesis. Eur J Clin Nutr 2002;56:271–281.
41 Garcia-Casal MN, Layrisse M, Solano L, et al: Vitamin A and beta-carotene can improve non-heme iron absorption from rice, wheat and corn by humans. J Nutr 1998;128:646–650.
42 Walczyk T, Davidsson L, Rossander-Hulthen L, et al: No enhancing effect of vitamin A on iron absorption in humans. Am J Clin Nutr 2003;77:144–149.
43 Davidsson L, Adou P, Zeder C, et al: The effect of retinyl palmitate added to iron-fortified maize porridge on erythrocyte incorporation of iron in African children with vitamin A deficiency. Br J Nutr 2003;90:337–343.
44 Jansson LT, Kling S, Dallman PR: Anemia in children with acute infections seen in a primary care pediatric outpatient clinic. Pediatr Infect Dis 1986;5:424–427.
45 Mwanri L, Worsley A, Ryan P, Masika J: Supplemental vitamin A improves anemia and growth in anemic school children in Tanzania. J Nutr 2000;130:2691–2696.
46 Villamor E, Mbise R, Spiegelman D, et al: Vitamin A supplementation and other predictors of anemia among children from Dar Es Salaam, Tanzania. Am J Trop Med Hyg 2000;62:590–597.
47 Kolsteren P, Rahman SR, Hilderbrand K, Diniz A: Treatment for iron deficiency anaemia with a combined supplementation of iron, vitamin A and zinc in women of Dinajpur, Bangladesh. Eur J Clin Nutr 1999;53:102–106.
48 Brigham D, Beard J: Iron and thermoregulation: A review. Crit Rev Food Sci Nutr 1996;36:747–763.
49 Dillman E, Gale C, Green W, et al: Hypothermia in iron deficiency due to altered triiodothyronine metabolism. Am J Physiol 1980;239:R377–R381.
50 Beard J, Tobin B, Green W: Evidence for thyroid hormone deficiency in iron-deficient anemic rats. J Nutr 1989;119:772–778.
51 Lanni A, Moreno M, Lombardi A, et al: Control of energy metabolism by iodothyronines. J Endocrinol Invest 2001;24:897–913.
52 Schröder-van der Elst JP, van der Heide D: Effects of streptozocin-induced diabetes and food restriction on quantities and source of T4 and T3 in rat tissues. Diabetes 1992;41:147–152.
53 Beard JL, Borel MJ, Derr J: Impaired thermoregulation and thyroid function in iron-deficiency anemia. Am J Clin Nutr 1990;52:813–819.
54 Martinez-Torres C, Cubeddu L, Dillmann E, et al: Effect of exposure to low temperature on normal and iron-deficient subjects. Am J Physiol 1984;246:R380–R383.
55 Lukaski HC, Hall CB, Nielsen FH: Thermogenesis and thermoregulatory function of iron-deficient women without anemia. Aviat Space Environ Med 1990;61:913–920.
56 Wolde-Gebriel Z, West CE, Gebru H, et al: Interrelationship between vitamin A, iodine and iron status in schoolchildren in Shoa Region, central Ethiopia. Br J Nutr 1993;70:593–607.
57 Wolde-Gebriel Z, Gebru H, Fisseha T, West CE: Severe vitamin A deficiency in a rural village in the Hararge region of Ethiopia. Eur J Clin Nutr 1993;47:104–114.
58 Azizi F, Mirmiran P, Sheikholeslam R, et al: The relation between serum ferritin and goiter, urinary iodine and thyroid hormone concentration. Int J Vitam Nutr Res 2002;72:296–299.
59 Beard JL, Brigham DE, Kelley SK, Green MH: Plasma thyroid hormone kinetics are altered in iron-deficient rats. J Nutr 1998;128:1401–1408.
60 Smith SM, Johnson PE, Lukaski HC: In vitro hepatic thyroid hormone deiodination in iron-deficient rats: Effect of dietary fat. Life Sci 1993;53:603–609.

61 Brigham DE, Beard JL: Effect of thyroid hormone replacement in iron-deficient rats. Am J Physiol 1995;269:R1140–R1147.
62 Smith SM, Deaver DR, Beard JL: Metabolic rate and thyroxine monodeiodinase activity in iron-deficient female Sprague-Dawley rats: Effects of the ovarian steroids. J Nutr Biochem 1992;3:461–466.
63 Kaplan MM, Utiger RD: Iodothyronine metabolism in rat liver homogenates. J Clin Invest 1978; 61:459–471.
64 Smith SM, Finley J, Johnson LK, Lukaski HC: Indices of in vivo and in vitro thyroid hormone metabolism in iron-deficient rats. Nutr Res 1994;14:729–739.
65 Taurog AM: Hormone synthesis: Thyroid iodine metabolism; in Braverman LE, Utiger RD (eds): The Thyroid: A Fundamental and Clinical Text, ed 8. Philadelphia, Lippincott, 2000, pp 61–85.
66 Dunn JT, Dunn AD: Update on intrathyroidal iodine metabolism. Thyroid 2001;11:407–414.
67 Hess SY, Zimmermann MB, Arnold M, et al: Iron deficiency anemia reduces thyroid peroxidase activity in rats. J Nutr 2002;132:1951–1955.
68 Surks MI: Effect of thyrotropin on thyroidal iodine metabolism during hypoxia. Am J Physiol 1969;216:436–439.
69 Moshang T Jr, Chance KH, Kaplan MM, et al: Effects of hypoxia on thyroid function tests. J Pediatr 1980;97:602–604.
70 Sawhney RC, Malhotra AS: Thyroid function in sojourners and acclimatised low landers at high altitude in man. Horm Metab Res 1991;23:81–84.
71 Basu M, Pal K, Malhotra AS, et al: Free and total thyroid hormones in humans at extreme altitude. Int J Biometeorol 1995;39:17–21.
72 Zimmermann M, Adou P, Torresani T, et al: Iron supplementation in goitrous, iron-deficient children improves their response to oral iodized oil. Eur J Endocrinol 2000;142:217–223.
73 Zimmermann MB, Zeder C, Chaouki N, et al: Addition of microencapsulated iron to iodized salt improves the efficacy of iodine in goitrous, iron-deficient children: A randomized, double-blind, controlled trial. Eur J Endocrinol 2002;147:747–753.
74 World Health Organization, United Nations Children's Fund, United Nations University: Iron Deficiency Anemia: Assessment, Prevention, and Control. Geneva, WHO, 2001, WHO/NHD/01.3.

Discussion

Dr. Guesry: What were the respective levels of phytic acid in the maize bread in Switzerland and Venezuela? In Switzerland flour is usually quite refined.

Dr. Hurrell: We used a maize flour from Migros, a local supermarket. The phytic acid content was found to be about 300 mg/100 g which is a fairly high phytic acid-containing maize flour and not so different from that used in Venezuela. We did not use a degermed maize flour, but if the germ is removed from maize you get a non-phytic acid-containing maize flour.

Dr. Pettifor: You showed a very small effect of vitamin A supplementation on iron status basically. Would you postulate then on whether you believe vitamin A plays as a major role? It is just one of the many aspects in the many different areas that could influence iron status.

Dr. Hurrell: The exact role of vitamin A has not been demonstrated, but one possible effect of vitamin A on iron bioavailability could be related to its influence on the incorporation of iron into the hemoglobin. During iron bioavailability studies, it is common practice to calculate iron absorption by assuming an 80% erythrocyte incorporation of absorbed iron in normal healthy individuals. This 80% value varies from 60 to 90%, so it is a rough approximation. We wondered whether the contradictory results obtained on the influence of vitamin A on iron absorption could be related to this incorporation factor being different in subjects with different vitamin A status. In the first 2 studies I presented iron absorption in a traditional way using an 80% incorporation factor. In the last study, which was recently published, Davidsson et al. [1] reported erythrocyte incorporation directly avoiding the use of an incorporation factor.

The group of Roodenburg et al. [2] made a series of rat studies about 10 years ago, and they suggested that one other major effect of vitamin A on iron metabolism might be the release or the mobilization of iron from the stores. The other possibility is that vitamin A is needed for the differentiation of the red blood cells.

Dr. Zlotkin: In your second slide on epidemiology, you showed estimated numbers on deficiencies of iodine, iron and vitamin A around the world. I was quite taken with the fact that the estimates are different depending on who is giving the lecture or whose article you have. The issue is important from an advocacy perspective because, when we go to policy makers, it is quite important that we can justify the numbers we use. How important do you think it is from an epidemiological perspective that we have some agreement on the definition of terms? For example, in your talk you didn't define your terms at all; the terms of how we define iron deficiency. We know in West Africa, for example, that much of the anemia is not from nutritional deficiencies but from malaria. That number may be lumped in with the total of 1 billion with iron deficiency. So again my question is, how important is it that we agree on the definition of terms?

Dr. Hurrell: This is extremely important, but it is a very difficult question. The prevalence estimates I presented came from the WHO and will be published next year in the Fortification Guidelines which I have been involved in putting together. One of the main problems in preparing this document was obtaining reliable prevalence values. I can speak only for iron because that is my main area. Normally the prevalence of iron deficiency is based on hemoglobin levels. The data I presented were also based on hemoglobin values and, in addition, we assumed that half of the people who were anemic had iron-deficiency anemia (IDA) and half had anemia of other causes. According to the WHO, there are 2 billion people who are anemic worldwide. The estimation that 50% of the anemic subjects have IDA was an average based on African studies which reported that 80% of the anemia in children was due to iron deficiency and some 30–40% in women. By taking a 50% average value we came up with 1 billion people worldwide with IDA. Again in some African studies about the same number of people have IDA as have iron deficiency without IDA. So the prevalence of iron deficiency without IDA is about the same as the prevalence of iron deficiency with IDA, so we get back to the 2 billion people with iron deficiency, half with anemia and half without. Recently we have been doing efficacy studies and needed cohorts of children or women with IDA. In some countries we have found it extremely difficult to find subjects with IDA, which led me to comment that the best way to cure IDA is to look for it. We had this problem recently in Thailand and in Morocco, and some other colleagues have reported the same difficulty. There should therefore be a major effort by the WHO to make prevalence data much more accurate so that we can advocate them with a clear conscience. This refers especially to iron prevalence data. I can't really say much about the prevalence data for vitamin A and iodine, which may be more accurate.

Dr. Mannar: In all of this, what is the influence of zinc and folic acid deficiencies on iron status and vice versa, and is this an important factor, especially during the early years? I wonder whether any work has been done?

Dr. Hurrell: I think that should be left to this afternoon because Dr. Lönnerdal is going to discuss zinc, and I have already taken one of his interactions. I wouldn't like to take another one.

Dr. Pettifor: To follow up on the issue that Dr. Zlotkin mentioned, the issue of prevalence. We are talking about micronutrient deficiencies, particularly in the weaning period. If you look at the values, particularly for IDA, the hemoglobin values which have been used vary from 10 to 10.5 to 11 as the cutoff points. What is the recommended cutoff point for IDA in this age group? In the weaning period, it alters prevalence significantly depending on which cutoff point is used.

Dr. Hurrell: I think Dr. Zlotkin can answer that one. He is the pediatrician.

Dr. Zlotkin: The WHO definition is that a hemoglobin under 110 would be defined as anemia in this age group. There is some question about the value or the meaning of this particular value because if anemia is defined based on functional outcomes, it is in my view, and we will have a discussion on this, that the functional impact of anemia is probably not apparent at 110 but it is at some value below that. So for research purposes anemia is defined based on hemoglobin of anywhere between 100 and 110, but the current official recommendation by the WHO is hemoglobin of <110 g/l, less than 11 mg/dl or 110 g/l.

Dr. Tolboom: Going back to Venezuela and then to the Côte d'Ivoire, you said that farmers in Venezuela could have been vitamin A-deficient and that could explain the possible effect of supplementation. What was the vitamin A status of the children in the Côte d'Ivoire? We know from the UNICEF program that there is seasonality in serum retinol levels. Perhaps malaria was already mentioned as an infection that has an influence on serum retinol levels. Could you comment on that?

Dr. Hurrell: The vitamin A status was not measured in the Venezuelan subjects, so we don't know what the vitamin A status was. It was just a shot in the dark really when we decided to look at vitamin A. In the Côte d'Ivoire all the children had low serum retinol levels, and I think about half of them had serum retinol levels below the cutoff for marginal deficiency, which is 0.7 μmol/l. We also performed this modified relative dose-response test by injecting the children with dehydroretinol and then measuring the retinol/dehydroretinol ratio. Using this methodology, which we did with Dr. Tarnumihardjo who is a specialist in this area, all the children had a low vitamin A status. These children lived in the north of the country, in an area which is now held by opposition rebel forces. The vitamin A intake was very low, and clearly these children were not getting vitamin A supplementation.

Dr. Lozoff: I want to go back to the hemoglobin question. In the literature in the last couple of years some researchers have proposed that the level of 110 is too high for infants and toddlers [3]. It is generally based on Swedish and Honduran studies that Dr. Lönnerdal might comment on. I want to urge anyone who has performed infant studies in which iron supplementation was well supervised, and ideally also included other vitamins, to analyze and publish their results. This would help to determine the level of hemoglobin after supplementation in this age group in various populations. For Costa Rica and Chile, where iron supplementation was very carefully supervised, the average value after supplementation was well above 11. In Costa Rica, of course, it was higher due to the slight elevation, but the mean was 135 g/l. In Chile the mean was above 120 g/l. These observations would not support the movement to reduce the cutoff. It seems as though we need more data before such a change is accepted.

Dr. Lönnerdal: I can respond first to you why we studied the lower cutoff. A colleague of mine did studies in Guatemala, at the same time we were doing studies in Sweden, where breast-feeding is common. When the infants start with weaning foods, they get iron-supplemented complementary foods, meats, and all kinds of iron sources. Their iron intake is quite good, but we found 33% anemia in Swedish infants by 6 months of age. We didn't quite believe that this was correct. This was similar to what was found in Guatemala, and that is why we wondered if the cutoff at that age is actually correct. Another thing that I would like to add and I will touch upon it from another angle this afternoon, is that Dr. Abrams and I, together with my Swedish colleagues, did a study in which we looked at iron absorption between 4 and 6 and 6 and 9 months of age [4]. Between 4 and 6 months of age the infant cannot homeostatically control iron absorption. If their iron status is excellent and you give them iron, they will make more and more hemoglobin. We know now from our animal studies that the regulatory machinery for iron absorption is just not there at a young age. They don't have a developed signaling system. After 6 months of age infants start regulating iron absorption. In Africa, this is the weaning period and that is another situation, but by using a fairly high cutoff for hemoglobin in the young infant, I think we are fooling ourselves.

Dr. Lozoff: This is a great reminder that even within the infant period, it is important to be very specific about the age periods. In Chile and Costa Rica, all the children were over 12 months of age. So one of the risks is that people are not careful enough about specifying what particular period they are talking about. This is just a warning to all of us.

Dr. Barclay: I would like to address the interaction of calcium and iron. Today we have more and more calcium with calcium-fortified products on the market. In the 1990s there were some short-term absorption studies showing that at high doses calcium decreased iron absorption [5, 6]. What is the current state of knowledge on the longer-term effects of calcium on iron nutrition?

Dr. Hurrell: I think the earlier studies on the effect of higher levels of calcium on iron absorption were single meal studies carried out mainly by Hallberg et al. [6] in Sweden. They showed quite clearly that as the level of calcium increased, iron absorption was reduced. Hallberg et al. [7] did one study on milk formulas with high calcium levels and a milk formula with the same calcium level as human milk, and showed quite a marked difference in iron absorption. From those single meal studies there has been some concern about the influence of calcium on iron absorption. Reddy and Cook [8] then did a multiple meal study in which they looked at the effect of calcium on iron absorption over a 14-day period with a United States-type diet, which contained many different foods. It was a very varied diet, and no effect of calcium was found. Part of the problem in comparing single meal studies with multiple meal studies is that the comparison is always made with the United States diet. People in developing countries do not have a varied diet, but a much simpler monotonous diet. So I am sure that, in a developing country, phytic acid, vitamin C, tea, or calcium could still influence iron absorption. Again the question is can we extrapolate from the United States and Europe to developing countries where the problems really are?

Dr. Gebre-Medhin: I very much enjoyed your presentation; this is evidently the way we should go ahead. Of course it raises a couple of things on which I would like to comment. First is the issue of epidemiology that Dr. Zlotkin has taken up, and I missed the special article by Wolde-Gebriel et al. [9] who did a remarkable study in Ethiopia which showed the prevalence of iron deficiency, vitamin A and iodine, to be at much higher figures than those presented here. I am convinced that if this were done in Nigeria or Egypt or South Africa, they would give more or less the same picture. So we need to do a little more homework on epidemiology. Second is the issue of anemia, iron deficiency and IDA. These three different issues are not always adequately described in the literature. I believe it is very important to always define these three entities. The last comment I have, and a question, is the issue of carrier proteins and their influence on metabolism and infection and protein energy status. In your presentation you did not mention anything about carrier proteins as major determinants and causes of variation. Would you like to comment on that: retinol-binding protein, prealbumin, and the lot?

Dr. Hurrell: I didn't really look much at carrier proteins in this review. For the interaction of iodine and vitamin A, retinol-binding protein and transthyretin have potential for interaction because retinol-binding protein, which transports vitamin A is almost entirely associated with transthyretin which transports the thyroid hormones. There are fewer studies looking at the vitamin A–iodine interaction, but there are beginning to be more. One other interesting area in relation to vitamin A and iodine is in relation to transcription of thyroid-stimulating hormone. This is blocked by thyroxine and retinoic acid, so retinoic acid also plays a role in regulating thyroid volume. There are some animal studies that found an increased thyroid volume with vitamin A deficiency, and this is one of the other possible interactions [10]. There are many studies in developing countries indicating other possible interaction, but it is difficult to sift through all of these studies. I only presented those studies which supported interactions of iron, iodine and vitamin A, but I could have looked through and found studies which show no effects. So I gave a general picture of what I believe is the direction of our understanding. But you are right, the binding to carrier proteins could also be a very important variable in these interactions because these proteins are used by many micronutrients.

Dr. Lönnerdal: I would like to come back to the question that Dr. Barclay raised: calcium supplementation and its effect on iron. First it is not easy to really review the literature in detail because the results from these studies are actually in the calcium field and we are looking at the effect on iron. Therefore a year ago we did a meta-analysis which hasn't been published yet. There have been studies on preterm infants, term infants, young children, school-age children, young women, pregnant women, postmenopausal women, and in all these studies generous levels of calcium were given for 3 months up to 1 year. None of these studies showed an effect on hemoglobin or serum ferritin when they were measured [11]. That is the observational response to the question. With regard to functional response, we have been working on iron transporters, and if a monolayer of human intestinal cells is made in culture to look at the same phenomenon by adding generous levels of calcium, immediately or very soon afterwards in these cells iron absorption and iron transport are impacted. But we have something wonderful in the human body called metabolic adaptation. The intestinal cell will realize that something is happening and take steps to modify this, and therefore up- and downregulation on the iron transport machinery occur soon after the start of calcium supplementation (this has also not been published but will be soon). It will make account of the high calcium and adapt, and therefore there is no long-term effect. Just as Dr. Hurrell said about the single meal studies, many of these are switch-over studies. If suddenly a generous dose of calcium is given, the intestinal cell is going to say 'what's happening now?', and this is when iron absorption is measured, and an effect is seen. But after 2 or 4 weeks the body will deal with this higher level and the intestinal cell is going to be less surprised and take it into account and adapt. I think this explains why very different results are seen when short-term studies are done as opposed to long-term studies.

Mr. Parvanta: Just coming back to the epidemiology issue. I appreciated the comments about defining when we are talking about anemia versus iron deficiency versus IDA, and a lot of people don't make those distinctions, especially in population-based data. Beyond this problem of not defining what we are talking about, our experience has been that there are a lot of projects that do surveys or assessments of populations, especially just simply doing hemoglobin. First of all a lot of different methods are used and even when the methods are similar, the methodology in training and the level of care that goes into collecting that information is quite variable. For example, right now the heme Q instrument is widely used and we at Centers for Disease Control (CDC) certainly believe in the utility of that instrument and use it quite a bit ourselves. But our experience has shown that because the instrument appears to be so easy to use that not enough care is taken in standardizing procedures and methods. A lot of the time we find differences in results just due to methodology rather than the real situation. I just want to point out that of course the difficulty with iron has been that there has been no agreement on what the indicator of choice is, especially for assessing our population's iron status or iron deficiency. I am happy to say that we at the CDC have funded the WHO to convene an expert working group or workshop to basically agree on some definitions so that we can perhaps move forward with what we have rather than being in this quandary of what is the indicator to use. A final comment, I feel that a lot of times we talk about the biggest problems in the world being in Africa, Asia and

South America, which is true, but there are other parts of the world. I would especially like to point out that in Central and Eastern Europe, the former Soviet Union, there is a tremendous problem, even in the Middle-East, with regard to iron deficiency, and now there is some evidence even with vitamin A deficiency. At some levels they are subclinical but fairly significant in some surveys we recently have been working on in Jordan for example, and there is some evidence of vitamin A deficiency. Certainly with iron deficiency, I think we just cannot forget that part of the world as another area that requires a lot of interventions.

Dr. Hurrell: I agree.

References

1 Davidsson L, Adou P, Zeder C, et al: The effect of retinyl palmitate added to iron-fortified maize porridge on erythrocyte incorporation of iron in African children with vitamin A deficiency. Br J Nutr 2003;90:337–343.
2 Roodenburg AJ, West CE, Beguin Y, et al: Indicators of erythrocyte formation and degradation in rats with either vitamin A or iron deficiency. J Nutr Biochem 2000;11:223–230.
3 Domellöf M, Cohen RJ, Dewey KG, et al: Iron supplementation of breast-fed Honduran and Swedish infants from 4 to 9 months of age. J Pediatr 2001;138:679–687.
4 Domellöf M, Lönnerdal B, Abrams SA, Hernell O: Iron absorption in breast-fed infants: Effects of age, iron status, iron supplements and complimentary foods. Am J Clin Nutr 2002;76:198–204.
5 Cook JD, Dassenko SA, Whittaker P: Calcium supplementation: Effect on iron absorption. Am J Clin Nutr 1991;53:106–111.
6 Hallberg L, Brune M, Erlandsson M, et al: Calcium: Effect of different amounts on nonheme- and heme-iron absorption in humans. Am J Clin Nutr 1991;53:112–119.
7 Hallberg L, Rossander-Hulten L, Brune M, Gleerup A: Bioavailability in man of iron in human milk and cow's milk in relation to their calcium contents. Pediatr Res 1992;31:524–527.
8 Reddy MB, Cook JD: Effect of calcium intake on nonheme-iron absorption from a complete diet. Am J Clin Nutr 1997;65:1820–1825.
9 Wolde-Gebriel Z, West CE, Gebru H, et al: Interrelationship between vitamin A, iodine and iron status in schoolchildren in Shoa Region, central Ethiopia. Br J Nutr 1993;70:593–607.
10 Nockels CF, Ewing DL, Phetteplace H, et al: Hypothyroidism: An early sign of vitamin A deficiency in chickens. J Nutr 1984;114:1733–1736.
11 Lönnerdal B: Does a high dietary intake of calcium adversely affect iron status in humans? Scand J Nutr 1999;2:82–84.

Pettifor JM, Zlotkin S (eds): Micronutrient Deficiencies during the Weaning Period and the First Years of Life. Nestlé Nutrition Workshop Series Pediatric Program, vol 54, pp 21–35, Nestec Ltd., Vevey/S. Karger AG, Basel, © 2004.

The Epidemiology of Vitamin D and Calcium Deficiency

John M. Pettifor

MRC Mineral Metabolism Research Unit, Department of Paediatrics, University of the Witwatersrand and Chris Hani Baragwanath Hospital, Johannesburg, South Africa

At the time of weaning, the infant's food and nutrient intake changes radically from that derived from breast-milk to that derived from complementary foods. In developing countries particularly, this change may have serious consequences for the provision of nutrients, especially for micronutrients and vitamins. Two nutrients of particular importance for bone health are calcium and vitamin D. At the 52nd Nestle Workshop on Micronutrient Deficiencies, I discussed the pathogenesis of rickets in young infants due to maternal and infant deficiencies. Here I will discuss the epidemiology of vitamin D and calcium deficiency in the infant older than 6 months of age and young children.

Vitamin D Deficiency

Although classified as a nutrient, vitamin D should rather be considered a prohormone, as the typical diet of most populations contains insufficient vitamin D to maintain vitamin D sufficiency unless foods are fortified with the vitamin. The vitamin D status of an individual is largely maintained through the conversion of 7-dehydrocholesterol to vitamin D in the skin under the influence of ultraviolet light.

Vitamin D is the generic term for a number of different compounds, the most important of which are vitamin D_2 or ergocalciferol and vitamin D_3 or cholecalciferol. Both forms are found in the circulation in humans, although the amounts of each are dependent on the diet and the amount of skin exposure to ultraviolet light. Vitamin D_2 is formed by the ultraviolet irradiation of the sterol, ergosterol, in plants and is ingested by humans mainly through the fortification of foods with vitamin D_2. Vitamin D_3 on the other hand is generally derived from its formation in the skin under the influence of ultraviolet light, although dietary intakes may contribute as there is a move towards the fortification of foods with vitamin D_3 rather than vitamin D_2, which was the custom in the past.

A number of factors influence the amount of vitamin D formed in the skin; these include the duration and intensity of ultraviolet light exposure, the surface area of skin exposed, the degree of melanin pigmentation in the skin, and the amount of substrate available in the skin for conversion to vitamin D.

The wavelength of ultraviolet-B radiation needed for the formation of vitamin D is between 290 and 315 nm. The amount that reaches the earth's surface is dependent on the zenith angle of the sun, the amount of atmospheric pollution and the degree of cloud cover. Thus the further one moves from the equator, the less UV radiation that is able to reach the earth. Consequently vitamin D formation is reduced in countries of high latitude, and during the winter months. This has been well shown, for example, in South Africa, where in Johannesburg at 26°S there is good vitamin D formation throughout the year, while in Cape Town at 32°S there is limited vitamin D formation during the winter months from April through September [1]. That study also highlighted the importance of the time of the day, with maximal vitamin D production occurring between 10.00 and 15.00 h in the summer months. Similar but more extreme results have been obtained from Boston at 42°N, where during the winter months of November through February no significant production of previtamin D occurred, and from Edmonton (52°N), where no vitamin D synthesis occurred between October and April [2].

Ozone pollution in the air of industrialized cities could have a significant impact on the amount of UV-B reaching the earth, as it effectively absorbs UV radiation. Thus it could reduce the amount of cutaneous synthesis of vitamin D. Although the size of this effect has not been quantified, it could increase the risk of vitamin D deficiency in young infants and the elderly living in the industrial cities of North America and Europe [3].

Melanin granules, which are produced by melanocytes within the stratum basale of the epidermis, very effectively absorb UV-B radiation in the range of 290–320 nm, thus reducing the amount of UV-B available for vitamin D synthesis [4]. Thus the darker the skin pigmentation is, the greater the amount of sunshine that is required to produce a given amount of vitamin D. This is the likely explanation for the higher incidence of vitamin D deficiency in African-American infants in North America and other countries at high latitudes.

Another factor that is of considerable importance in determining the cutaneous synthesis of vitamin D is the surface area of skin exposed to UV radiation. In adults, even light clothing (with arms and legs exposed) as might be worn in summer significantly reduces the amount of vitamin D formed, while autumn clothing (with arms and legs covered) almost completely prevents the expected rise in serum vitamin D in response to whole body UV irradiation [5].

Vitamin D Sufficiency, Vitamin D Insufficiency and Vitamin D Deficiency

The classical presentation of vitamin D deficiency in infants and young children is rickets. Clinical and radiological rickets may take several months to develop depending on the growth rate of the child, the degree of vitamin D deficiency and the calcium content of the diet, even though biochemical abnormalities, such as hypocalcemia, hypophosphatemia, and elevated alkaline phosphatase and parathyroid hormone concentrations, may occur much earlier.

A more accurate assessment of vitamin D status is the circulating level of 25-hydroxyvitamin D (25-OHD). It is generally accepted that levels of <12 ng/ml (30 nmol/l) in children are indicative of vitamin D deficiency, however in the adult literature particularly, there is considerable controversy around the level that constitutes vitamin D sufficiency as it is suggested that levels above 12 ng/ml (30 nmol/l) may be inadequate to maintain bone health and biochemical normality although manifestations of osteomalacia or hypocalcemia do not occur. The serum concentration of 25-OHD above vitamin D deficiency levels but below that which is needed to provide optimal health is termed vitamin D insufficiency [6]. In children, there is less discussion and little evidence to suggest that values above 12 ng/ml may be inadequate. Thus in the pediatric literature, there is no clear indication that a situation of vitamin D insufficiency occurs. Further it must be understood that levels within the vitamin D deficiency range may not be associated with clinical, radiological or biochemical abnormalities, particularly if they are of short duration, as may occur during the winter months in countries at high latitude.

Vitamin D Deficiency in Infants and Young Children

From the above discussion, it is clear that the vitamin D status of infants and young children is determined by the combination of the dietary intake of vitamin D and of that produced in the skin under the influence of UV light.

The natural dietary sources of vitamin D for the infant or young child are limited as few unfortified complementary foods contain significant quantities of the vitamin. For this reason, all infant milk formulas are fortified at a level of approximately 400 IU (10 μg)/l and a number of other foods designed for infant feeding, such as infant cereals, may also be fortified by manufacturers. In North America, liquid cow's milk is also fortified, but a study has found that the amount of vitamin D actually present in milk is very variable ranging from <5 to >120% of the stated amount on the package label [7]. Breast milk too has only a limited vitamin D content (between 20–60 IU/l) [8, 9], which is inadequate to maintain vitamin D sufficiency in the infant.

Thus, unless the infant is drinking reasonable quantities of infant milk formula or fortified cow's milk (approximately 500–600 ml/day), vitamin D sufficiency will not be ensured unless cutaneous synthesis of vitamin D supplements the dietary intake. Several factors may hasten the onset vitamin D deficiency in the young infant, these include: (1) the global recommendation that breast-feeding should be exclusive and the preferred method of feeding for the first 6 months of life, thus precluding the intake of vitamin D-fortified infant foods in the early months of life, and (2) a low vitamin D status in the mother at the time of birth, as the placental transfer of vitamin D, in particular 25-OHD, from a replete mother to the fetus helps protect the infant from vitamin D deficiency in the first couple of months [10].

It is thus apparent that many infants and young children are dependent on the cutaneous synthesis of vitamin D in order to maintain vitamin D sufficiency. This has been highlighted by a study in Cincinnati by Specker and Tsang [11] who showed that in breast-fed infants the serum concentrations of 25-OHD correlated with sunlight exposure rather than with the vitamin D content of maternal breast milk.

Globally, vitamin D deficiency is characteristically a disease of infants and young children. The reasons for this are apparent if one considers the importance of UV light exposure in maintaining vitamin D sufficiency. Deficiency occurs typically in countries at high latitudes, where winter months are cold, and in countries where for social and religious reasons children are precluded from sunlight. The peak incidence of vitamin D deficiency occurs between 6 and 18 months of age and has a strong seasonal variation with the disease being most common in the late winter and early spring months [12].

The prevalence of vitamin D deficiency has been greatly reduced in a number of countries from that occurring at the end of the 19th and beginning of the 20th centuries, when in northern Europe the disease was almost universal in young children [13]. This has been achieved through health education, the use of vitamin D supplements and the introduction of food fortification. However vitamin D deficiency remains a problem in a number of developing countries and there has been a resurgence in several developed nations. A number of studies over the past 20–30 years have highlighted the continued high prevalence of vitamin D deficiency among the Asian communities in the United Kingdom [14], and among young children in countries such as Turkey, Greece, Mongolia, Tibet, China, Ethiopia [15], Saudi Arabia [16], Iran, Kuwait, the United Arab Emirates, India [17], and Pakistan. Furthermore there have been an increasing number of reports of vitamin D deficiency in dark-skinned immigrant communities in Australia [18], New Zealand and Europe, and in African-American infants in the USA [19].

The reasons for vitamin D deficiency in countries, such as China, Mongolia and Tibet, are clearly related to the high latitude and long and cold winters reducing the UV light exposure of the skin. In the Middle East, however, other mechanisms have been shown to play major roles. These include religious and social customs, such as purdah and the tradition of veiling, which preclude the mother and young infant from sunlight, and prolonged breast-feeding without vitamin D supplementation [20]. In Ethiopia, vitamin D deficiency is associated with protein-energy malnutrition and the lack of sunlight exposure [15]. In the USA, rickets occurs characteristically in African-American infants who are breast-fed, thus melanin pigmentation and the lack of vitamin D in breast milk appear to be major factors, although recently DeLucia et al. [21] have suggested that low dietary calcium intakes associated with weaning may play a role. The reasons for the high prevalence of vitamin D deficiency and rickets in Asian children in the UK have been extensively researched. Melanin pigmentation, extensive skin coverage by clothing, and low calcium and vitamin D intakes associated with vegetarian diets have all been indicted. Clements [22], some 15 years ago, provided a convincing explanation by which the low calcium intakes and decreased bioavailability of calcium in the traditional vegetarian diets were responsible for exacerbating vitamin D deficiency in the Asian community. In rat studies, he showed that low calcium intakes increased the catabolism of 25-OHD to non-active metabolites, thereby increasing the requirements of vitamin D to maintain vitamin D sufficiency.

It is thus clear that vitamin D deficiency remains a global problem and that many infants and young children are at risk of the consequences of the disease, which is only now beginning to receive attention from international agencies.

Dietary Calcium Deficiency

The estimation of the dietary requirements for calcium is difficult in humans in general, but even more so in infants and young children. As deficiency syndromes are not clearly defined, there are no biochemical tests which indicate the nutritional status for calcium, and dietary requirement studies are notoriously difficult to conduct in children of this age. These difficulties are highlighted if one compares the recommended dietary intakes made by various national bodies (table 1).

In adults, dietary calcium requirements may be calculated from that which is required to maintain the calcium balance at zero, however in children this is not possible as growing children should be in a significantly positive balance to allow for bone growth in particular. Furthermore intestinal calcium absorption varies not only with the nature of diet, but also with the adaptation of the body to calcium requirements and dietary calcium content.

The exclusively breast-fed or formula-fed infant is assured of an adequate calcium intake to meet the requirements for growth, however once weaning occurs and the consumption of milk drops off, the reduction in calcium intake associated with this decline in milk intake must be made up by weaning foods.

Table 1. Recommended dietary intakes of calcium (mg/day) and vitamin D (μg/day) made by national committees in the United Kingdom and North America for children of various ages [23]

	0–6 months		7–12 months		1–3 years		4–6 years	
	Ca	D	Ca	D	Ca	D	Ca	D
UK reference nutrient intake	525	8.5	525	7	350	7	450	0
USA/Canadian adequate intake	210–375	5	270	5	500	5	800	5

In developed countries, where dairy products are readily available, calcium intakes are generally maintained and there is little evidence of dietary calcium deficiency in the infant and young child populations. In the United Kingdom and the USA, it is estimated that dairy products provide over 60% of the calcium intake in young children [23, 24] and total calcium intakes exceed 600 mg/day.

In developing countries, the situation is often very different; the weaning diet is mainly cereal based and is often high in phytates, dairy products are frequently scarce and priced out of the reach of the average family, and the diet lacks variety. These factors coupled with frequent bouts of diarrhea and intestinal infections result in calcium intakes being low and possibly poorly absorbed. In a study of calcium intakes in toddlers in Egypt, Kenya and Mexico, mean daily intakes of 218, 210 and 735 mg, respectively, were obtained [25]. The reason for the higher intake in Mexican toddlers was because of the addition of lime to tortillas during their manufacture. Intakes similar to those in Egypt and Kenya have been found in young children in Nigeria [26] and South Africa [27]. In The Gambia [28], India and China intakes of around 300 mg/day are not unusual.

Thus calcium intakes of infants and young children differ markedly between developed and developing countries, yet is there any evidence that the low calcium content of the diets in developing countries is detrimental to health? This question has not been answered with certainty, and will be discussed in more detail elsewhere, however there is evidence to suggest that very low calcium intakes in growing children are responsible for rickets in the face of vitamin D sufficiency.

In the 1970s several isolated case reports appeared of infants developing rickets after having been placed on very restricted calcium intakes for the treatment of chronic diarrhea [29, 30]. In the same decade, we suggested that rickets in older children living in rural areas of South Africa might be due to dietary calcium lack as all had normal circulating levels of 25-OHD and elevated 1,25-$(OH)_2$D concentrations, and all responded to an improvement in calcium intake. Their calcium intakes were estimated to be between 150 and 200 mg/day, their diet being mainly corn based with no dairy products whatsoever [31]. Since then, a number of reports from Nigeria have indicated that low dietary calcium intakes might be associated with rickets in that country [32–34], and a similar etiology has been postulated as being responsible for rickets in Bangladesh [35]. In all of these studies, calcium intakes of approximately 200 mg/day have been measured. It is highly likely that low dietary calcium intakes are primarily responsible for the development of the bone disease, however other factors such as phytates, which influence the bioavailability of dietary calcium, might exacerbate its development, as no difference was found in calcium intakes between children with and without rickets in one case-controlled study.

An interesting report originating from the east coast of the USA has recently suggested that dietary calcium deficiency may play a role in the pathogenesis of rickets, particularly in African-American infants and toddlers [21]. Although calcium intakes were not measured, they were reported as being low with many of the children being weaned onto diets which contained little or no dairy products after prolonged breast-feeding.

Thus it is apparent that dietary calcium deficiency as manifested by clinical rickets is being recognized in several areas of the world. It is unclear, however, how widespread the problem is, as vitamin D deficiency and dietary calcium may coexist. Furthermore, treatment of rickets often comprises both vitamin D and calcium supplements which treat both conditions effectively. The picture is complicated further by the role of low dietary calcium intakes in increasing the catabolism of vitamin D through the elevation of serum $1,25\text{-}(OH)_2D$ levels, resulting in increased requirements of vitamin D in children on low calcium intakes [36].

Here the presence of rickets due to low dietary calcium intakes has been used as a measure of dietary calcium deficiency. It is likely, however, that the clinical manifestation of rickets is the tip of the iceberg and that disturbances in the biochemical markers of mineral homeostasis are much more common findings. How common or widespread the biochemical changes of hypocalcemia, and elevated alkaline phosphatase, PTH and $1,25\text{-}(OH)_2D$ levels are, is unknown, although in one study from South Africa these findings were frequently found in a rural community [37].

The assessment of the prevalence of dietary calcium deficiency worldwide is complicated further by the lack of a clear understanding of what calcium intakes are necessary to promote optimal bone health in growing children, which in the Caucasian population in industrialized countries has been a subject of much research. Maximizing peak bone mass, which is achieved during the third decade of life, is considered to be an important objective, as bone mass at this time of life might influence the incidence of minimal trauma fractures in later life. Although a few studies have suggested an improvement in bone mass through calcium supplementation during childhood in Caucasian children, no information is available on the effect of the supplementation of the generally lower calcium intakes in children in the developing world. Further the relevance of such supplementation is unclear as the incidence of minimal trauma fractures in the elderly in the developing world is generally considered to be very much lower than that in the developed world.

It is thus apparent that much research needs to be done to clarify the indicators of dietary calcium deficiency worldwide, and to assess the role of current dietary calcium intakes on the prevalence of these indicators.

References

1 Pettifor JM, Moodley GP, Hough FS, et al: The effect of season and latitude on in vitro vitamin D formation by sunlight in South Africa. S Afr Med J 1996;86:1270–1272.
2 Webb AR, Kline L, Holick MF: Influence of season and latitude on the cutaneous synthesis of vitamin D_3: Exposure to winter sunlight in Boston and Edmonton will not promote vitamin D_3 synthesis in human skin. J Clin Endocrinol Metab 1988;67:373–378.
3 Holick MF: Environmental factors that influence the cutaneous production of vitamin D. Am J Clin Nutr 1995;61:638S–645S.
4 Norman AW: Sunlight, season, skin pigmentation, vitamin D, and 25-hydroxyvitamin D: Integral components of the vitamin D endocrine system. Am J Clin Nutr 1998;67:1108–1110.
5 Matsuoka LY, Wortsman J, Dannenberg MJ, et al: Clothing prevents ultraviolet-B radiation-dependent photosynthesis of vitamin D_3. J Clin Endocrinol Metab 1992;75:1099–1103.
6 Pettifor JM: What is the optimal 25(OH)D level for bone in children? in Norman AW, Bouillon R, Thomasset M (eds): Vitamin D Endocrine System: Structural, Biological, Genetic and Clinical Aspects. Riverside, University of California, 2000, pp 903–907.
7 Holick MF: McCollum Award Lecture, 1994: Vitamin D – New horizons for the 21st century. Am J Clin Nutr 1994;60:619–630.
8 Hollis BW, Roos BA, Draper HH, Lambert PW: Vitamin D and its metabolites in human and bovine milk. J Nutr 1981;111:1240–1248.
9 Reeve LE, Chesney RW, DeLuca HF: Vitamin D of human milk: Identification of biologically active forms. Am J Clin Nutr 1982;36:122–126.
10 Rothberg AD, Pettifor JM, Cohen DF, et al: Maternal-infant vitamin D relationships during breast-feeding. J Pediatr 1982;101:500–503.
11 Specker BL, Tsang RC: Cyclical serum 25-hydroxyvitamin D concentrations paralleling sunshine exposure in exclusively breast-fed infants. J Pediatr 1987;110:744–747.
12 Salimpour R: Rickets in Tehran. Arch Dis Child 1975;50:63–66.
13 Chick DH: Study of rickets in Vienna 1919–1922. Med Hist 1976;20:41–51.
14 Ford JA, McIntosh WB, Butterfield R, et al: Clinical and subclinical vitamin D deficiency in Bradford children. Arch Dis Child 1976;51:939–943.
15 Lulseged S, Fitwi G: Vitamin D deficiency rickets: Socio-demographic and clinical risk factors in children seen at a referral hospital in Addis Ababa. East Afr Med J 1999;76:457–461.
16 Fida NM: Assessment of nutritional rickets in Western Saudi Arabia. Saudi Med J 2003;24:337–340.
17 Bhattacharyya AK: Nutritional rickets in the tropics; in Simopoulos AP (ed): Nutritional Triggers for Health and in Disease. Basel, Karger, 1992, pp 140–197.
18 Plehwe WE: Vitamin D deficiency in the 21st century: An unnecessary pandemic? Clin Endocrinol (Oxf) 2003;59:22–24.
19 Kreiter SR, Schwartz RP, Kirkman HN Jr, et al: Nutritional rickets in African American breast-fed infants. J Pediatr 2000;137:153–157.
20 Lubani MM, Al-Shab TS, Al-Saleh QA, et al: Vitamin-D-deficiency rickets in Kuwait: The prevalence of a preventable disease. Ann Trop Paediatr 1989;3:134–139.
21 DeLucia MC, Mitnick ME, Carpenter TO: Nutritional rickets with normal circulating 25-hydroxyvitamin D: A call for reexamining the role of dietary calcium intake in North American infants. J Clin Endocrinol Metab 2003;88:3539–3545.

22 Clements MR: The problem of rickets in UK Asians. J Hum Nutr Diet 1989;2:105–116.
23 Department of Health: Nutrition and Bone Health, ed 49. London, Stationary Office, 1998.
24 Kaluski N, Basch CE, Zybert P, et al: Calcium intake in preschool children − A study of dietary patterns in a lower socioeconomic community. Public Health Rev 2001;29:71–83.
25 Murphy SP, Beaton GH, Calloway DH: Estimated mineral intakes of toddlers: Predicted prevalence of inadequacy in village populations in Egypt, Kenya, and Mexico. Am J Clin Nutr 1992; 56:565–572.
26 Thacher TD, Fischer PR, Pettifor JM, et al: Case-control study of factors associated with nutritional rickets in Nigerian children. J Pediatr 2000;137:367–373.
27 Eyberg C, Pettifor JM, Moodley G: Dietary calcium intake in rural black South African children. The relationship between calcium intake and calcium nutritional status. Hum Nutr Clin Nutr 1986;40C:69–74.
28 Dibba B, Prentice A, Ceesay M, et al: Effect of calcium supplementation on bone mineral accretion in Gambian children accustomed to a low-calcium diet. Am J Clin Nutr 2000;71:544–549.
29 Kooh SW, Fraser D, Reilly BJ, et al: Rickets due to calcium deficiency. N Engl J Med 1977; 297:1264–1266.
30 Maltz HE, Fish MB, Holliday MA: Calcium deficiency rickets and the renal response to calcium infusion. Pediatrics 1970;46:865–870.
31 Pettifor JM, Ross P, Wang J, et al: Rickets in children of rural origin in South Africa: Is low dietary calcium a factor? J Pediatr 1978;92:320–324.
32 Okonofua F, Gill DS, Alabi ZO, et al: Rickets in Nigerian children: A consequence of calcium malnutrition. Metabolism 1991;40:209–213.
33 Oginni LM, Worsfold M, Oyelami OA, et al: Etiology of rickets in Nigerian children. J Pediatr 1996;128:692–694.
34 Thacher TD, Fischer PR, Pettifor JM, et al: A comparison of calcium, vitamin D, or both for nutritional rickets in Nigerian children. N Engl J Med 1999;341:563–568.
35 Fischer PR, Rahman A, Cimma JP, et al: Nutritional rickets without vitamin D deficiency in Bangladesh. J Trop Pediatr 1999;45:291–293.
36 Clements MR, Johnson L, Fraser DR: A new mechanism for induced vitamin D deficiency in calcium deprivation. Nature 1987;325:62–65.
37 Pettifor JM, Ross FP, Moodley GP, Shuenyane E: Calcium deficiency in rural black children in South Africa − A comparison between rural and urban communities. Am J Clin Nutr 1979;32: 2477–2483.

Discussion

Dr. Guesry: I believe in the role of latitude to explain differences in synthesis in vitamin D in the derm. But with all due respect, I doubt that the difference in latitude that you mentioned between Johannesburg and Cape Town would explain more than 5–10% of the difference you showed us, and the rest is probably due to altitude, cloudiness.

Dr. Pettifor: I think that is right, we are talking about season. It is not just latitude, it is also the issue of cloud cover which makes a major difference.

Dr. Guesry: You could ask a specialist to calculate the angle and to extrapolate on the maximum effect and it is probably something like 5%.

Dr. Pettifor: I accept that seasonal weather changes are relevant.

Dr. Castillo-Durán: Infants born preterm or small-for-gestational age can be a very highly prevalent group in many developing countries, from 50 to 60%. How can this be included as a risk factor for rickets?

Dr. Pettifor: The infants that are born in many developing countries, the low birth weight group of infants, are in fact mainly small-for-gestational age rather than premature. We have looked at the problem of rickets in these children, and if they are breast-fed then the problem appears to be mainly phosphate deficiency rather than calcium deficiency, and it tends to occur in premature rather than small-for-gestational age babies. I don't have any data on what the long-term effects of perhaps mild

29

biochemical changes such as elevated alkaline phosphatase or low phosphorus levels are during this period. They certainly may be present with rickets during this period, although it is relatively uncommon. We see very little rickets due to what we think is hypophosphatemic rickets in this age group.

Dr. Endres: You showed nicely that the renal excretion of calcium increased when you gave calcium. I think most of us know as pediatricians that, when we are treating rickets, not only should vitamin D be given but also calcium because otherwise tetany might occur in these hypocalcemic infants. Did you investigate this in your studies when you gave vitamin D to these children?

Dr. Pettifor: In the calcium-deficient group the children were randomized to either receive calcium, vitamin D, or calcium and vitamin D. We didn't find any difference in calcium excretion in urine. Calcium excretion in these children is very low once they become calcium-deficient; it is 1 or 2 mg/day basically, which is very low indeed. When we talk about raising urine calcium, that calcium rise is relatively small as well. I haven't studied this problem in vitamin D-deficiency rickets, so I really can't answer the question as it relates to vitamin D deficiency. We generally do not give calcium supplements to infants who have vitamin D deficiency because we believe that their milk intake is generally adequate to meet the calcium demands of the growing child. So calcium is not supplied, except if the infants have tetany in the early stages of presentation. But if they have rickets, they should just be given a normal milk intake and vitamin D. We haven't run into tetany problems in these children. Whether it slows down the healing, I don't know.

Dr. Gebre-Medhin: I very much enjoyed your presentation and your words are well taken that to extrapolate from different populations to others leads to a lot of problems. My question is what do we know now about the body's ability to store vitamin D during periods of plenty, for instance the summer months, then use it towards the end of the year when there is less sunshine? I am asking you this question because in the early 1970s vitamin D-deficiency rickets was very prevalent in highland Ethiopia, I would say close to 80%. We have not changed the vitamin D supply program, protein energy malnutrition has not changed but rickets is now very rare, even in highland areas, and the main reason for this has been a huge program encouraging mothers to take their children outside during the sunny months. Does this mean that the body is capable of storing quite a lot for later use?

Dr. Pettifor: It appears that vitamin D is stored in fat and muscle and 25-hydroxyvitamin D may also be stored. The duration of storage is difficult to assess because it certainly depends on whether it is stored in the fat and how fat an individual is. If you take individuals who have vitamin D toxicity, the duration of vitamin D toxicity may persist for many months after cessation of giving vitamin D. So there is good evidence that vitamin D is continuously being pulled out to produce the effects of vitamin D toxicity. I am not sure if Dr. Specker has an answer to the actual half life of this in a normal individual. Certainly if you take individuals who have reasonable vitamin D sufficiency during the summer, their 25-hydroxyvitamin D levels fall during the winter, but not to the same level as in an individual who starts off relatively vitamin D insufficient during summer. These individuals tend to develop vitamin D deficiency during the winter months. So to answer your question, I am not sure I can give you an actual figure.

Dr. Specker: We found, at least in newborn infants, that the maternal and infant 25-hydroxyvitamin D levels correlate up until about 8 weeks of age in the baby [1]. So if you assume that this is placental transfer, it appears that the storage in the infant lasts about 2 months, which can also explain why you see vitamin D deficiency rickets at higher latitudes around March, the very end of winter or early spring. So as a sort of consensus, if there is one out there, it is that the half life is about 8 weeks.

Dr. Pettifor: The neonate may of course be a different issue because the major transfer across the placenta is 25-hydroxyvitamin D, and we know that the half life is about 2–3 weeks. So as we saw from the studies that we did in Johannesburg, the levels dropped significantly by 6 weeks of age, but these concentrations protect the infant from rickets in the first 3 months of life unless the mother is vitamin D-deficient.

Mr. Parvanta: In South Africa do you have a national recommendation with regard to vitamin D supplementation for breast-fed infants? In relation to the data you showed in which the controls had a better calcium intake than the children with rickets; can you give us a description of what the primary dietary sources of calcium were in that population?

Dr. Pettifor: To answer the first question about the vitamin D supplementation policy in South Africa: no, there isn't one. The pediatric community is divided as to whether we should be recommending vitamin D supplementation to breast-fed infants or whether the amount of sunlight that we have is adequate for a small daily exposure to maintain vitamin D supply. Certainly vitamin D deficiency is an uncommon problem in infants in South Africa these days. In the 1960s when breast-feeding was not as prevalent and the infant food that was given at that time was diluted cow's milk (two thirds cow's milk and a bit of sugar), rickets was very common particularly in Cape Town with 15% of children presenting with rickets, but that has almost disappeared completely now. However, we are seeing it now in the inner city areas where parents are living under poor socioeconomic conditions, where there is a lot of crime, and children and mothers are not getting outside. Thus it is a problem in the high-rise, high-density residential areas, but otherwise not. To discuss the issue of the difference in calcium intakes between the children who presented with dietary calcium deficiency, the only difference in the diet was that those who had calcium intakes of 300–400 mg/day had some sort of dairy product on a reasonably regular basis. So the parents may have kept cows; they may have had family members sending back milk powder to those families, so that they may have been drinking a little bit of milk in their tea or half a glass of milk a day, and that was the only difference. Otherwise the diet is very similar, it is mainly a corn maize-based diet with vegetables and occasional meat.

Dr. Zlotkin: I think the vitamin D issue is a wonderful example of the problematic application for the prevention of a micronutrient deficiency, and let me just give you Canada as an example. In the 1930s at the Hospital for Sick Children the most frequent diagnosis for children admitted to our hospital was actually rickets, and in the 1930s the first fortified food was developed. This is a great example of the use of fortification to solve a micronutrient problem. It was for young children but not for children of school age. 50 years ago, when I was a child, we used a supplementation to prevent rickets. As children many of my friends and I took cod liver oil because the liver of the codfish has a very high concentration of vitamin A and vitamin D. Again it is a good example of supplementation, the prevention. The next step of course was the use of foods for children, that is formula and infant cereals with calcium and vitamin D concentrations. But there was general recognition that, for infants who are exclusively breast-fed, fortification would not work because their needs are different, and possibly 10 years ago there were recommendations for vitamin D supplementation of all exclusively breast-fed infants. In Canada the prevalence of vitamin D deficiency rickets is very low and there is a strong voice among pediatricians in Canada that we no longer need supplementation because the prevalence of this entity is so low due to the successful supplementation program. So I think it is an interesting case model of how fortification and supplementation work to prevent the disease. In Canada there is a new recommendation that all infants after 6 months of age should not be exposed to sunlight in the noon hours or if they are going to be exposed to sunlight they be provided with sunscreen. So my question is: is it likely that the provision of sunscreen to infants is going to increase the prevalence of rickets? What is the effect of the sun blockers on the endogenous synthesis of vitamin D?

31

The Epidemiology of Vitamin D and Calcium Deficiency

Dr. Pettifor: I think you have actually written a paper on the issue of sunscreens as a factor in the causation of vitamin D deficiency [2]. I think there is a lot of ambivalence about what we should be recommending to mothers. Certainly I think the dermatologists would scream blue murder if one recommended any sunlight exposure to infants. The recommendation now is that as soon as a baby is put outside, it is to be covered from head to toe with sunscreen. I do believe we are going to run into problems, and we are seeing an increased prevalence of rickets in the US and Canada, although it happens particularly in the dark-skinned African-American population. Whether this is only due to vitamin D deficiency or whether there is also a role for dietary calcium deficiency in this situation is not clear. Certainly the data from DeLucia et al. [3] suggest that calcium deficiency may well be a factor here because calcium intakes drop after weaning because of the introduction of mainly nondairy low calcium-containing foods. They suggest that dietary calcium deficiency plays a significant role. If we accept this then you have a synergistic effect of dietary calcium deficiency plus vitamin D insufficiency leading to an increased prevalence of rickets, and we need to look at both of these. We should look at either increasing calcium and/or providing an adequate vitamin D intake to optimize calcium absorption during these periods.

Dr. Lozoff: Although the pediatric recommendations are for calcium and vitamin D supplementation, some advocates of exclusive breast-feeding find this recommendation problematic. I was wondering if you could comment on this.

Dr. Pettifor: That is true. There are groups that say breast milk and breast milk only, and one doesn't need to supplement with anything. In that situation there are some studies suggesting that if one supplements the mother with adequate levels of vitamin D, sufficient vitamin D will cross in the breast milk to prevent vitamin D sufficiency or insufficiency in this age group. Some researchers are recommending 4,000 units of vitamin D/day. Now I may be wrong, it may be 2,000, but I think it is about 4,000 that it is being recommended for supplementation of the mother, which is quite a high dose actually.

Dr. Guesry: I would like to come back to the data that you showed from Dibba et al. [4] who collected data on the dairy calcium intake in Africa and Asia. We have to be careful in these countries that there are other sources of calcium and that dairy calcium is not the only source of calcium intake. We also have to balance these calcium intake data by a coefficient of bioavailability, and you know better than me that when less calcium is given, it is usually better absorbed.

Dr. Pettifor: I would argue that the form in which the calcium exists in many of the developing countries is in fact relatively non-bioavailable because of high phytates and other factors, so I am not sure.

Dr. Specker: One of the things that is also important is that people forget about phosphorus in the diet, and when you get calcium from dairy products you also have phosphorus. This might also be an explanation for why we see higher rates of rickets in exclusively breast-fed infants. I think that in the 1-year-old child who is exclusively breast-fed the phosphorus content in human milk has dropped significantly since birth, whereas the calcium content stays the same. You have proposed this idea about calcium deficiency, but we should not forget phosphorus, and we should think more about the calcium phosphorus product in the etiology of rickets. Perhaps that could explain the Nigerian results with phosphorus.

Dr. Pettifor: We looked at phosphorus intake in these groups and could not find a difference. In fact the phosphorus intake is very good in these groups because their diets are all cereal-based with a high phosphorus content. I accept that some of this is phytate phosphorus which may not be absorbed. But even then there is still a significant amount of phosphorus. The serum phosphorus values are all over the place in affected children, but they are not generally severely hypophosphatemic, which I think in the issue of phosphate depletion is a factor. But having said that, Greek research done some 20 or 30 years ago suggested that there are two different types of rickets in the infant period [5]. One was a phosphate depletion rickets that was seen in the older children and the other was vitamin D deficient.

Dr. Albar: I want to ask you about the supplementation of calcium to pregnant mothers because some milk products contain calcium, and it is advised that it be given to the mothers during pregnancy and 6 months after delivery. According to the recommendations you mentioned, the mother's calcium content level does not influence the level of calcium in the baby. What is your comment about obstetric products for pregnancy and lactation including milk or vitamin-mineral supplementation, especially calcium and vitamin D, that advertise that during pregnancy and lactation mothers should consume these products to prevent their babies from developing rickets? An example of an advertisement for obstetric products goes as follows: Best assurance for a healthy baby is a healthy mother – special milk or vitamin-mineral supplement for pregnancy and lactation.

Dr. Pettifor: I think the data suggesting that calcium supplementation is beneficial in either pregnancy or lactation is negligible. In fact, the British recommendations have not increased the calcium intake during lactation [6]. They suggest that there is no need for that. Prentice et al. [7] studied calcium supplementation in the Gambia where calcium intakes were very low, and were unable to show any effect of calcium supplementation during that period on the mothers, on breast milk calcium levels or on the well-being of the babies. The issue though is whether long-term calcium supplementation may influence breast milk calcium levels, and there are no data on that. But the issue of vitamin D supplementation might be more relevant in those communities where vitamin D insufficiency is a relatively common problem. Most of Europe and the Middle East need to make sure that the mother's vitamin D status is adequate during pregnancy and lactation.

Dr. Albar: Do you agree on giving calcium supplementation to malnourished pregnant mothers?

Dr. Pettifor: If we talk about malnourished pregnant mothers, I am not sure that calcium supplementation is the answer. What the mother needs is a general improvement in the diet, and if that actually happens to include increasing the calcium intake that is well and good, but calcium supplementation is not the major factor in improving the nutritional status one hopes to achieve for the baby at birth.

Dr. Albar: There are a lot of milk products fortified with calcium and vitamin D whose advertising is directed toward pregnant and lactating mothers, but calcium supplementation to the mothers has no effect on their babies. So it is useless for the mothers to consume these products to prevent their babies from calcium deficiency.

Dr. Pettifor: I think the issue of protein or nutrient supplementation during pregnancy, except in the very severely malnourished mother, makes very little difference on the birth weight of the infant.

Dr. Hurrell: I would like to come back to the phytic acid question and the absorption of calcium. In adults phytic acid has been shown to reduce calcium absorption slightly, not as much as iron, and I don't know of any studies in infants which have shown that phytic acid reduces calcium absorption. It reminds me of a study we did several years ago with a high phytate infant cereal in which we measured calcium absorption in infants. We compared Cerelac with a very high phytate cereal, and there was no difference in calcium absorption between the high and the low phytate cereals, and the absorption was about 80% in these infants who were 5–8 months old. So I would say that there is no evidence that phytic acid reduces calcium absorption other than in adults, and there the reduction is not so high.

Dr. Pettifor: Perhaps Dr. Abrams might want to comment on that as well. We are busy planning a study in Nigeria to look exactly at this, using stable isotopes in the children that we see there. For instance whether the children who develop rickets are less able to adapt to the low calcium intakes is a question, and if a child already has a low calcium intake, whether the addition of phytate or oxalate for that matter may just drop calcium absorption enough to produce rickets on the long-term basis, I don't think we know.

Dr. Hurrell: Obviously oxalate has a big impact on calcium absorption, it is not very well absorbed, but phytate I am not so sure.

Dr. Abrams: In Nigeria we measured calcium absorption because we thought that perhaps these children with rickets can't absorb calcium very well, and we found that their calcium absorption is completely normal. So we were wondering if there is a critical value by which certain children get rickets, it is not very obvious at all. In general in developing weaning foods, calcium has been consider to be kind of a bad guy and it hasn't been used for the most part, except in some commercial foods, because of larger concerns about iron, zinc and vitamin A. Given the considerable prevalence of calcium-deficiency rickets, do you think this should be reconsidered as a public policy matter?

Dr. Pettifor: I would take issue with your statement about the considerable prevalence of dietary calcium deficiency. I don't think that dietary calcium deficiency, certainly clinical rickets, is that prevalent. The issue of whether there is a subclinical situation is another question: we have certainly suggested that children on low calcium intakes in some communities have biochemical perturbations with elevated alkaline phosphatase and low serum calcium, but did not have any radiological evidence of rickets [8]. Whether these children are disadvantaged long-term, we don't know. So to make recommendations on a policy of calcium supplementation or fortification of foods, particularly in developing countries where it is very difficult or very expensive for the families to buy ready-prepared, ready-made food, I am not sure. I think it may well be appropriate to supplement with micronutrients at the moment. I am not sure that we should be recommending a broad spread of calcium supplementation at this stage. If one looks at osteoporosis in adults, the issue of long-term consequences may be relatively unimportant as osteoporosis is lowest in those countries that have the lowest calcium intake. Why is this, why don't we see osteoporosis in Africa for instance where calcium intakes have always been around 200–400 mg/day. Is it a genetic factor or are they able to adapt their calcium homeostasis to maintain bone mass, I don't know.

Dr. Mannar: A few years ago in Bangladesh there was a sudden increase in the prevalence of rickets, probably calcium deficiency induced, and I was wondering whether there are any underlying factors that increase the prevalence of rickets in children?

Dr. Pettifor: In fact, a study was reported recently at the NIH Conference on Vitamin D Requirements, and I am afraid there is no conclusive evidence that it is dietary calcium deficiency. There is evidence that it might be that supplementation improves the condition. There are data suggesting that it is of recent onset. There may be many factors: one that has been put forward is related to the increased irrigation of rice fields and therefore being able to get more rotations of rice in any given year, and thus the diet has become very much more monotonous than it used to be 20 or 30 years ago. Whether this is a factor, we don't know.

References

1   Specker BL, Valanis B, Hertzberg V, et al: Sunshine exposure and serum 25-hydroxyvitamin D concentrations in exclusively breast-fed infants. J Pediatr 1985;107:372–376.
2   Zlotkin S: Vitamin D concentrations in Asian children living in England. Limited vitamin D intake and use of sunscreens may lead to rickets. BMJ 1999;318:1417.

3 DeLucia MC, Mitnick ME, Carpenter TO: Nutritional rickets with normal circulating 25-hydroxyvitamin D: A call for reexamining the role of dietary calcium intake in North American infants. J Clin Endocrinol Metab 2003;88:3539–3545.

4 Dibba B, Prentice A, Ceesay M, et al: Effect of calcium supplementation on bone mineral accretion in Gambian children accustomed to a low-calcium diet. Am J Clin Nutr 2000;71: 544–549.

5 Lapatsanis P, Makaronis G, Vretos C, Doxiadis S: Two types of nutritional rickets in infants. Am J Clin Nutr 1976;29:1222–1226.

6 Department of Health: Nutrition and Bone Health: With Particular Reference to Calcium and Vitamin D. London, Her Majesty's Stationary Office, 1998.

7 Prentice A, Jarjou LM, Cole TJ, et al: Calcium requirements of Gambian mothers: Effects of a calcium supplement on breast-milk calcium concentration, maternal bone mineral content, and urinary calcium excretion. Am J Clin Nutr 1995;62:58–67.

8 Pettifor JM, Ross FP, Moodley GP, Shueyane E. Calcium deficiency in rural black children in South Africa – A comparison between rural and urban communities. Am J Clin Nutr 1979;32: 2477–2483.

Pettifor JM, Zlotkin S (eds): Micronutrient Deficiencies during the Weaning Period and the
First Years of Life. Nestlé Nutrition Workshop Series Pediatric Program, vol 54, pp 37–52,
Nestec Ltd., Vevey/S. Karger AG, Basel, © 2004.

Epidemiology of Micronutrient Deficiencies in Developing and Developed Countries, Specifically Zinc, Copper, Selenium and Iodine

Carlos Castillo-Duran[a] *and Manuel Ruz*[b]

[a]Institute of Nutrition and Food Technology, and
[b]Department of Nutrition, Faculty of Medicine, University of Chile, Santiago, Chile

Micronutrient Deficiencies around the World

Trace mineral deficiencies in humans were first studied in relation to iodine deficiency and thyroid function, and iron deficiency and anemia. Zinc, copper and selenium deficiencies have become a matter of concern only over the last 40 years. Micronutrient deficiencies are frequently found to be combined in the same communities, especially in those less privileged. The effects of micronutrient deficiencies on population health have received great attention in the last years in studies dealing with the burden of disease [1, 2]. The World Health Organization has proposed epidemiological screening for populations at risk of disease based on suspected micronutrient deficiencies and on indices linked to long-term ill health [1]. An approach to defining the level of population risk based on subclinical signs of micronutrient deficiencies has been proposed taking into account: seasonal weight loss; women's low body mass index; low birth weight; rate of stunted children, and iodine, vitamin A and iron deficiencies (table 1). Recent studies on the burden of disease have also included zinc deficiency [2, 3].

Zinc Deficiency

One of the main constraints to determining the prevalence of zinc deficiency in population groups around the world is the lack of reliable biomarkers. Despite the large number of zinc status indices proposed, none of them present high

Table 1. An approach to defining the level of population risk based on subclinical signs of micronutrient deficiencies

	IV (severe prevalence)	III (moderate to severe)	II (mild and widespread)	I (mild and clustered)
Seasonal weight loss	>3	≥2 to <3	≥1 to <2	<0.5
Women's low body mass index	≥40	≥30 to <40	≥20 to <30	≥10 to <20
Low birth weight	≥25	≥10 to <25	≥5 to <10	<5
Stunted children	≥40	≥20 to <40	≥10 to <20	<10
Iodine deficiency	>99	≥50 to <99	≥20 to <50	<20
Vitamin A deficiency	≥20	≥10 to <20	≥2 to <10	<2
Iron deficiency	≥80	≥50 to <80	≥30 to <50	<12

From the Commission on the Nutritional Challenges of the 21st Century [1].

sensitivity and specificity to detect subnormal degrees of zinc status, especially mild and moderate. Instead, severe zinc deficiency shows markedly decreased zinc tissue concentrations. Thus, the diagnosis of zinc deficiency has frequently been based on clinical signs suggestive of zinc deficiency and a positive response to zinc supplementation in some biological functions. Currently, a suitable, although still imperfect, approach to screening for zinc deficiency is the assessment of the adequacy of zinc intake, which can be complemented by plasma zinc levels [4]. In addition, a post-intervention positive effect on some zinc-related clinical variables provides supportive evidence to characterize the community studied in terms of its zinc levels.

Dietary zinc adequacy is related to the total zinc content of food and zinc bioavailability. One of the most important dietary factors that reduce intestinal zinc absorption is phytic acid. It has been estimated that a phytate:zinc ratio of >15 significantly decreases zinc absorption, thus increasing the zinc needed to be provided by the diet. Most of the developing world presents phytate:zinc ratios above this cutoff point (e.g., Sub-Saharan Africa 26.9, South Asia 26.9, Latin America 21.1). Instead, the developed world has ratios well below that cutoff point [4].

With the exception of women of childbearing age, in which menstrual losses are the main determinant of iron status, the prevalence of zinc deficiency is probably similar to that of nutritional iron deficiency in all other age groups. In these, the characteristics of the diet are the key factors. Dietary patterns high in unrefined grains and fiber and low in animal protein, especially meat, induce a high risk of both iron and zinc deficiencies. Iron deficiency anemia has been estimated to have a low prevalence in Europe, medium prevalence in the Americas (14% as a whole), and high prevalence in the South-East Asian, African, East Mediterranean and West Pacific areas (29–39%) [5].

Probability estimates for the risk of zinc deficiency can be calculated from dietary data alone. Diets with a proportion of animal protein between 10 and 25% are adequate to support zinc nutrition [6]. However, to determine the severity of zinc inadequacies, dietary information must be analyzed along with biochemical and functional indices. Since zinc-rich foods are mainly animal products, it is possible to estimate a higher risk of zinc deficiency in regions where the consumption of livestock products is low. Estimates based on the production, import and export of these foods by countries and regions show a very low consumption in South Asia and Sub-Saharan Africa [7].

Zinc deficiency has been included as a related exposure variable for risk of disease in populations (defined as less than the US recommended dietary allowances for zinc, and with a theoretical minimum intake established as the entire population consuming sufficient dietary zinc to meet the physiological needs, taking into account routine and illness-related losses and bioavailability). The outcomes associated with zinc deficiency are diarrhea, pneumonia and malaria in children aged <5 years. In the 2002 report by the WHO [3], analysis of the disabilities-adjusted life years (DALYs) associated with zinc deficiency estimated 11–18% DALYs for diarrheal disease, 19% for lower respiratory disease and 18–19% for malaria in developing countries with high mortality; 3–5% for the same diseases in developing countries with low mortality, and 1–3% in developed countries [2, 3] (table 2). In total 800,000 deaths worldwide were attributable to zinc deficiency, 1.4% in males and 1.5% in females.

Zinc Deficiency in Developing Countries

The main conditions accompanying zinc deficiency in developing countries are: low consumption of meat or fish along with increased phytate and fiber consumption; protein-energy malnutrition; infectious diseases, particularly acute diarrhea and malaria, and fetal growth retardation [4].

Protein-Energy Malnutrition

Protein-energy malnutrition is a condition associated with multiple macro- and micronutrient deficiencies, including zinc. Thus, in communities where this condition is prevalent, zinc deficiency is also present. Analysis of DALYs shows childhood and maternal undernutrition as the main isolated condition associated with burden of disease (140 million years). Over 16% DALYs have been estimated in Africa and South-East Asia [3]. According to the WHO, approximately 27% (168 million) of children under 5 years are underweight [8].

Zinc and Growth

There is consistent evidence on the relationship between zinc deficiency and postnatal growth retardation, including a recent refined meta-analysis [9] (fig. 1). The effect of zinc supplementation was greater in stunted children (height/age < −2 z score). Countries or communities with a stunting prevalence

Table 2. Selected population attributable risk factors (% DALYs for each cause)

	World	High mortality developing	Low mortality developing	Developed countries
Underweight				
Diarrheal disease	45	49	21	12
Low birth weight	10	12	3	3
Lower respiratory infection	40	46	25	8
Malaria	45	45	14	0
Measles	33	34	23	10
Protein-energy malnutrition	88	88	92	78
Iron deficiency				
Anemia	100	100	100	100
Maternal mortality	11	13	6	1
Perinatal mortality	19	22	13	2
Vitamin A deficiency				
Diarrheal disease	18	19	9	0
Malaria	16	17	7	0
Maternal mortality	10	12	5	0
Measles	15	15	13	0
Zinc deficiency				
Diarrheal disease	10	11	3	2
Lower respiratory infection	16	19	5	2
Malaria	18	18	3	1

From the WHO [3].

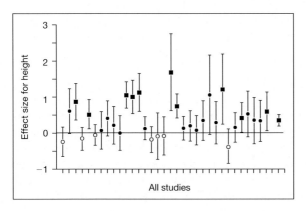

Fig. 1. Mean effect size and 95% CI for the effect of zinc supplementation on children's linear growth. Results of individual studies and a meta-analysis. Adapted from Brown et al. [9].

Table 3. Studies analyzing the effect of zinc supplementation during pregnancy on fetal growth (birth weight and prematurity) in humans

Citation	Country	Zinc mg	Controls	n	Birth weight	Prematurity
Hunt, 1984	USA	20	MVM	213	–	–
Hunt, 1985	USA	20	MVM	138	–	–
Ross, 1985	South Africa	30	Placebo	127	–	–
Kynast, 1986	Germany	20	No placebo	524	↑	–
Mahomed, 1989	UK	20	Placebo	494	–	–
Cherry	USA	30	Placebo	556	–	↓(multip.)
Simmer, 1991	UK	22.5	Placebo	56	↑	–
Garg, 1993	India	45	No placebo	168	↑	↓
Goldenberg, 1995	USA	25	MVM	580	↑	↓
Jonsson, 1996	Denmark	44	Placebo	1,206	–	–
Caulfield, 1999	Peru	15	Placebo	1,100	–	–
Osendarp, 2000	Bangladesh	30	Placebo	559	–	–
Castillo-Durán, 2001	Chile	20	Placebo	507	–	↓
Wieringa, 2001	Indonesia	30	β-carot.	228	± boys, Zn carotene	–

MVM =Multivitamin mineral supplement. From Castillo-Durán and Weisstaub [10].

of >20% are at high risk of associated micronutrient deficiencies, including zinc [1].

Low birth weight, as an index of fetal growth retardation, may also be associated with zinc deficiency. Nevertheless, evidence gathered to date [10–12] on the effect of zinc supplementation during pregnancy on birth weight has not confirmed this expectation (table 3). This issue is still being studied.

Zinc and Infections

There are several studies analyzing the magnitude of zinc intakes, but not many on zinc losses during infectious diseases. Zinc losses of >100 µg/kg/day as found in acute or protracted diarrhea may induce zinc deficiency, especially when associated with a decreased zinc intake [13]. Ruz and Solomons [14] showed that for each day of acute diarrhea, the increased loss of zinc duplicates the need for zinc. Studies on zinc supplementation in poor communities in India, Bangladesh and other countries have found decreased risks of acquiring infectious diarrhea, respiratory infections (pneumonia) or impetigo and sepsis [15–18] (table 4). Others have shown a decrease in the duration of diarrheal processes [16, 17]. Zinc supplementation, added to other micronutrients from 1 to 9 months of age, also decreased the mortality of small-for-gestational age infants (RR = 0.32; CI = 0.12−0.89) mainly by decreasing diarrhea and sepsis [17, 18]. Breast-feeding was also independently associated with lower mortality.

41

Table 4. Trials evaluating the preventive effects of zinc supplementation on prevention of diarrhea and pneumonia

Country	Author	Number of subjects	Age months	Other criteria	Diarrhea incidence	Pneumonia incidence
Vietnam	Ninh, 1996	146	4–36	W/A or W/L <-2 z score	44% lower	44% lower
India	Sazawal, 1997 Sazawal, 1998	579	6–35	Recovery from diarrhea	8% lower	43% lower
Mexico	Rosado, 1997	194	18–36	–	37% lower	–
Guatemala	Ruel, 1997	89	6–9	–	18% lower	–
Jamaica	Meeks-Gardner, 1998	61	6–24	W/A <-2 z score	8% lower	88% lower
Brazil	Lira, 1998	205	0–6	Low BW	28% lower	–
Peru	Penny, 1999	159	6–35	Recovered persistent diarrhea	12% lower	15% lower
Papua New Guinea	Shankar, 1999	274	6–60	–	12% lower	–
Burkina Faso	Muller, 2001	709	6–31	–	16% lower	–
India	Bhandari, 2002	2,482	6–30	–	–	26% lower

W/A = Weight-for-age; W/L = weight-for-length; BW = body weight. Adapted from Black [18].

In spite of some initial evidence suggesting a positive effect of zinc supplementation on the incidence of malaria in children, recent studies have failed to find such an effect [19, 20].

Zinc Deficiency in Developed Countries

These countries present, as a whole, a low risk of zinc deficiency. Nevertheless, there have been some reports suggesting zinc deficiency in some specific groups.

The classic studies by Walravens and Hambidge [21] in Denver, USA, showed a subnormal zinc status in a pediatric population from poor districts of Denver in the 1970s. Similar evidence was added later in other American and Canadian cities [22, 23]. In 1989 in pregnant African-American adolescents, Cherry et al. [24] found a decrease in the rate of low birth weight when zinc supplementation started before the 25th week of gestation in normal and overweight pregnant women. In the early 1990s in Paris, France, Walravens et al. [25] found an increased risk of zinc deficiency in infants of migrant African families who exclusively breast-fed their babies beyond 6 months of age. Zinc supplementation (5 mg/day) increased the length and weight of male infants, but not females. This practice of prolonged breast-feeding along with delayed introduction of complementary foods may be a risk factor for zinc deficiency in the second semester of life. Preliminary results of zinc supplementation in Mexican-American children, 6–8 years old, from Brownsville, Tex., suggest that zinc deficiency may be prevalent in that community [26].

In summary, zinc deficiency is highly prevalent in developing countries, probably similar to iron deficiency. It is associated with low zinc diets, diets high in phytates and fiber, protein-energy malnutrition, diarrheal disease, and low birth weight. This condition affects most of the poor countries in South-East Asia and Africa, and also countries in the Middle East and Latin America. Zinc deficiency can also be found in specific groups in developed countries, especially among those migrating from less affluent communities.

Copper Deficiency

Copper deficiency was described in the 1960s in infants recovering from malnutrition and fed unfortified cow's milk. The effects of copper deficiency have been described: hematological signs such as neutropenia, leucopenia and anemia; immune compromise, and increased risk of infections. Growth delay and bone disease may also be other clinical signs. Protein-energy malnutrition and low birth weight appear as risk factors of copper deficiency, along with early weaning and feeding with unfortified cow's milk. A history of acute diarrheal episodes and the increased fecal loss of copper associated with it increase the risk of copper deficiency. The magnitude of copper deficiency has not been studied in large community settings. Because copper is widely distributed in foods and absorption is larger than other trace elements, it is not likely that apparently healthy individuals consuming mixed foods present with copper deficiency. Copper deficiency becomes an issue, particularly in children, under certain conditions in which some of the following factors interact: malnutrition; low copper recovery diets; prematurity, and diarrhea. The prevalence of copper deficiency here is unknown. Limited data in malnourished children indicate that up to 50–80% may have low plasma copper [27, 28].

Selenium Deficiency

Among the main determining factors of selenium status is selenium intake, rather than selenium absorption. Both organic and inorganic forms of selenium are absorbed at high rates, i.e. >70%. Likewise, selenite and selenate forms are absorbed at a similar rate (Van Dael, personal commun.). The selenium content of foods is strongly affected by soil characteristics. As a consequence, the selenium content of foods, especially those of vegetable origin, may vary over such a wide range that the use of food composition tables becomes meaningless. In general terms, the best sources of dietary selenium are seafood and meats; grains are highly variable depending on soil conditions; fruits and vegetables do not contribute significantly to the total intake. Variations in selenium in soils and foods are important. They determinate that certain geographic locations around the world have been classified as areas of 'low' and 'high' selenium [29].

Current recommended selenium intakes are $20\,\mu g/day$ for children 1–3 years old, $30\,\mu g/day$ for those 4–8 years old, $40\,\mu g/day$ for 9–13 years, and $55\,\mu g/day$ 14 years old and beyond [30]. No differences have been established by gender. Excess selenium is toxic. Clinical symptoms of its toxicity include severe irritations of the respiratory system, metallic taste in mouth, signs of rhinitis, lung edema, and bronchopneumonia.

Studies Conducted in Developing Countries

Iyengar et al. [31] studied the dietary intake of essential minor and trace elements from Asian diets by analyzing about 700 diet samples. The average dietary selenium supply ranged from 52 to $141\,\mu g/day$. In Latin America, Venezuela has been the focus of attention due to the existence of areas with naturally high selenium in soils. Bratter et al. [32] measured a selected set of parameters of selenium, red blood cells, serum and hair of children, and breast milk from seleniferous areas of Venezuela. In these areas, selenium intakes can be ten times or more than that observed in areas considered as 'low selenium' such as Finland or New Zealand. Ruz et al. [33] studied the selenium distribution in Chile by using free-range hen's eggs as a selenium monitor. This was followed by direct dietary analysis and biochemical determinations (red blood cell count and serum glutathione peroxidase, serum selenium and toenail selenium) in adults living in three distinct cities. The mean selenium intake ranged from 52 to $99\,\mu g/day$. The first city was a cold and rainy midland location, whereas the third was a coastal town by the Atacama Desert [34]. A further study was conducted in schoolchildren in the city with the lowest selenium intake to investigate the potential association between iodine supplementation, selenium status and goiter prevalence. The children in this city, despite having a relatively greater iodine intake, tended to have a higher goiter prevalence and, concomitantly, a lower selenium status [35].

The relationships between selenium and iodine metabolism have been a matter of concern in a number of studies in animals and humans. Vanderpas et al. [36] suggested that the high frequency of myxedematous cretins observed in certain areas of Zaire may result from a combined severe deficiency of both iodine and selenium. In 7- to 12-year-old Turkish children, Aydin et al. [37] attributed the high goiter prevalence to iodine and selenium deficiency. Untoro et al. [38] suggested that low environmental selenium availability may be an additional determinant for goiter in East Java, Indonesia. Zimmermann et al. [39], studying children from rural villages in the western Ivory Coast, concluded that although more severe selenium deficiency partially blunts the thyroid response to iodine supplementation, oral iodized oil is an effective method for iodine repletion in goitrous children who are selenium-deficient. Correction of selenium status without a previous restoration of iodine status can worsen the altered thyroid metabolism [40].

Ahmed et al. [41] found indications of low selenium status in Sudanese children with marasmic-kwashiorkor. Subotzky et al. [42] studied children with kwashiorkor during the first 30 days of recovery. After this period a full clinical recovery was reached, with normalization of the plasma levels of selected trace elements, with the exception of zinc and selenium, indicating that this period of time may not be sufficient to allow a full recovery with respect to these two micronutrients.

Studies in Developed Countries

A number of studies have been carried out in Eastern Europe. A common feature has been the finding of rather low selenium intakes. Zachara and Pilecki [43] studied the daily selenium intake of breast-fed infants and the selenium concentration in the milk of lactating women in western Poland. The calculated mean daily selenium intake by breast-fed infants was 7.71 (range 3.67–17.17)µg/day. The selenium concentration in human milk in the region studied was uniform, but the daily selenium intake of breast-fed infants was lower than the recommended daily requirement. The authors attributed this to the low selenium content of the soil and consequently of the foodstuffs from this region [43]. Wasowicz et al. [44], also in Poland, reported average selenium intakes in children and adults of 30–40 µg/day. In Slovakia, Kadrabova et al. [45] found that the daily dietary selenium intake was 43.3 µg/day for men and 32.6 µg/day for women. In 1992 in the former Yugoslavia, Beker et al. [46] studied the selenium status of 8- to 15-year-old individuals of both sexes and from four distinct geographic locations by analyzing serum samples. The authors reported significant differences regarding age and sex but not by location; the mean serum selenium was 57 µg/l [46].

In Nordic Europe, Samuelson [47] studied the dietary intakes of vitamins and minerals in adolescents from Denmark, Finland, Norway and Sweden. Dietary calcium intake was high, whereas the intake of fiber, vitamin D, zinc and selenium and, in girls, iron were below the Nordic recommendations.

As a consequence of the naturally low selenium in Finnish soil, the addition of selenium to fertilizers began in the early 1980s. Kantola et al. [48] determined the impact of soil selenium supplementation over a 10-year period. selenium intake rose from 30–40 to 85 µg/day.

Recently, data on the dramatic decline of selenium intakes in the UK over the past 20–25 years have become available. In 1974 the reported selenium intake was 60 µg/day, whereas the current figure is as low as 30–40 µg/day. Although no functional consequences have been recognized, the significance of the biochemical changes observed in UK individuals supplemented with selenium is under study [49].

Table 5. Current magnitude of iodine deficiency disorders by goiter by WHO Region (1999)

	Population in millions	Population affected by goiter	
		in millions	% of the region
Africa	612	124	20
The Americas	788	39	5
South-East Asia	1,477	172	12
Europe	869	130	15
East Mediterranean	473	152	32
Western Pacific	1,639	124	8
Total	5,858	741	13

From WHO-UNU and the International Council for Control of Iodine Deficiency Disorders [50].

Iodine Deficiency

The most common indicators used to assess iodine status are urinary iodine, as determined in a casual urine sample, and thyroid volume, as measured by ultrasonography. Evaluations of iodine deficiency throughout the world by the WHO show differences in the various regions, with the highest prevalence of iodine deficiency in East Mediterranean countries and Africa. The iodine deficiency disorders (IDDs) prey upon poor, pregnant women and preschool children, posing serious public health problems in 130 developing countries. IDDs affect over 740 million people, 13% of the world's population, and 30% of the remainder are at risk. It has been estimated that nearly 50 million people suffer from some degree of IDD-related brain damage [50]. Associated with salt iodinization, the prevalence of goiter has decreased in the Americas to <5% (table 5).

References

1   Commission on the Nutrition Challenges of the 21st Century: Ending malnutrition by 2020: An agenda for change in the millennium. Issues to be considered by regional and national meetings. Food Nutr Bull 2000;21(suppl):74–81.
2   Ezzati M, Lopez AD, Rodgers A, et al, and the Comparative Assessment Collaborative Group: Selected major risk factors and global and regional burden of disease. Lancet 2002;360: 1347–1360.
3   WHO Report: Reducing Risks, Promoting Healthy Life. Geneva, World Health Organization, 2002.
4   Brown KH, Wuehler SE, Peerson JM: The importance of zinc in human nutrition and estimation of the global prevalence of zinc deficiency. Food Nutr Bull 2001;22:113–125.
5   UNICEF/UNU/WHO/MI: Preventing Iron Deficiency in Women and Children. Technical Consensus on Key Issues. Boston, International Nutrition Foundation, 1999.

6 WHO/FAO Report: Preparation and Use of Food-Based Dietary Guidelines. Nutrition Programme. Geneva, WHO, 1996.
7 Bruinsma J (ed): World Agriculture: Towards 2015/2030. An FAO Perspective. Rome, Food and Agriculture Organization of the United Nations/London, Earthscan, 2003.
8 WHO Global Database on Child Growth and Malnutrition. Geneva, World Health Organization, 2002. Available from: http://www.who.int/nutgrowthdb/
9 Brown KH, Peerson JM, Rivera J, Allen LH: Effect of supplemental zinc on the growth and serum zinc concentrations of prepubertal children: A meta-analysis of randomized controlled trials. Am J Clin Nutr 2002;75:1062–1071.
10 Castillo-Durán C, Weissstaub G: Zinc supplementation and growth of the fetus and low birth weight infant. J Nutr 2003;133(suppl):1S–4S.
11 Osendarp SJ, West CE, Black RE, and Maternal Zinc Supplementation Study Group: The need for maternal zinc supplementation in developing countries: An unresolved issue. J Nutr 2003;133:817S–827S.
12 Goldenberg RL, Tamura T, Neggers Y, et al: The effect of zinc supplementation on pregnancy outcome. JAMA 1995;274:463–468.
13 Castillo-Duran C, Vial P, Uauy R: Trace mineral balance during acute diarrhea in infants. J Pediatr 1988;113:452–457.
14 Ruz M, Solomons NW: Mineral excretion during acute, dehydrating diarrhea treated with oral rehydration therapy. Pediatr Res 1990;27:170–175.
15 Bhutta ZA, Bird SM, Black RE, et al: Therapeutic effects of oral zinc in acute and persistent diarrhea in children in developing countries: Pooled analysis of randomized controlled trials. Am J Clin Nutr 2000;72:1516–1522.
16 Black RE, Sazawal S: Zinc and childhood disease morbidity and mortality. Br J Nutr 2001; 85(suppl 2):S125–S129.
17 Sazawal S, Black RE, Menon VP, et al: Zinc supplementation in infants born small for gestational age reduces mortality: A prospective, randomized, controlled trial. Pediatrics 2001;108: 1280–1286.
18 Black RE: Zinc deficiency, infectious disease and mortality in the developing world. J Nutr 2003;133(suppl):1485S–1489S.
19 Zinc Against Plasmodium Study Group: Effect of zinc on the treatment of *Plasmodium falciparum* malaria in children: A randomized controlled trial. Am J Clin Nutr 2002;76: 805–812.
20 Muller O, Becher H, van Zweeden AB, et al: Effect of zinc supplementation on malaria and other causes of morbidity in west African children: Randomized double blind placebo controlled trial. BMJ 2001;322:1567–1570.
21 Walravens PA, Hambidge KM: Growth of infants fed a zinc supplemented formula. Am J Clin Nutr 1976;29:1114–1121.
22 Gibson RS, Vanderkooy PDS, MacDonald AC, et al: A growth-limiting, mild zinc-deficiency syndrome in some southern Ontario boys with low height percentiles. Am J Clin Nutr 1989;49:1266–1273.
23 Goldenberg RL, Tamura T, Neggers Y, et al: The effect of zinc supplementation on pregnancy outcome. JAMA 1995;274:463–468.
24 Cherry FF, Sandstead HH, Rojas P, et al: Adolescent pregnancy: Associations among body weight, zinc nutriture and pregnancy outcome. Am J Clin Nutr 1989;50:945–954.
25 Walravens PA, Chakar A, Mokni R, et al: Zinc supplements in breastfed infants. Lancet 1992; 340:683–685.
26 Egger N, Sandstead H, Penland J, et al: Zinc supplementation improves growth in Mexican-American children (abstract). FASEB J 1999;13:A246.
27 Castillo-Duran C, Uauy R: Copper deficiency impairs growth of infants recovering from malnutrition. Am J Clin Nutr 1988;47:710–714.
28 Fisberg M, Castillo-Duran C, Egaña JI, Uauy R: Zinc y cobre plasmáticos en lactantes con desnutrición proteínico-energética. Arch Latinoam Nutr 1984;34:568–577.
29 Levander OA: A global view of selenium nutrition. Annu Rev Nutr 1987;7:227–250.
30 Food and Nutrition Board, Institute of Medicine: Dietary Reference Intakes for Vitamin C, Vitamin E, Selenium, and Carotenoids. Washington, National Academy Press, 2000.
31 Iyengar GV, Kawamura H, Parr RM, et al: Dietary intake of essential minor and trace elements from Asian diets. Food Nutr Bull 2002;23(suppl):124–128.

32 Bratter P, Negretti de Bratter VE, Jaffe WG, Castellano MH: Selenium status of children living in seleniferous areas of Venezuela. J Trace Elem Electrolytes Health Dis 1991;5: 269–270.
33 Ruz M, Codoceo J, Hurtado S, et al: Characterization of the regional distribution of selenium in Chile by using selenium in hens' eggs as a monitor. J Trace Elem Med Biol 1995;9:156–159.
34 Ruz M, Codoceo J, Rebolledo A, et al: Selenium intake and selenium status of Chilean adults from three distinct geographical locations. J Trace Elem Exp Med 1995;8:112A.
35 Ruz M, Codoceo J, Galgani J, et al: Zinc-selenium Iodine interactions and thyroid function in school-children. J Trace Elem Exp Med 1998;11:461A.
36 Vanderpas JB, Contempré B, Duale NL, et al: Iodine and selenium deficiency associated with cretinism in northern Zaire. Am J Clin Nutr 1990;52:1087–1093
37 Aydin K, Kendirci M, Kurtoglu S, et al: Iodine and selenium deficiency in school-children in an endemic goiter area in Turkey. J Pediatr Endocrinol Metab 2002;15:1027–1031.
38 Untoro J, Ruz M, Gross R: Low environmental selenium availability as an additional determinant for goiter in East Java, Indonesia? Biol Trace Elem Res 1999;70:127–136.
39 Zimmermann MB, Adou P, Torresani T, et al: Effect of oral iodized oil on thyroid size and thyroid hormone metabolism in children with concurrent selenium and iodine deficiency. Eur J Clin Nutr 2000;54:209–213.
40 Contempré B, Dumont JE, Bebe N, et al: Effect of selenium supplementation in hypothyroid subjects of an iodine and selenium deficient area: The possible danger of indiscriminate supplementation of iodine-deficient subjects with selenium. J Clin Endocrinol Metabol 1991;73: 213–215.
41 Ahmed HM, Lombeck I, el-Karib AO, et al: Selenium status in Sudanese children with protein-calorie malnutrition. J Trace Elem Electrolytes Health Dis 1989;3:171–174.
42 Subotzky EF, Heese HD, Sive AA, et al: Plasma zinc, copper, selenium, ferritin and whole blood manganese concentration in children with kwashiorkor in the acute stage and during refeeding. Ann Trop Paediatr 1992;12:13–22.
43 Zachara BA, Pilecki A: Daily selenium intake by breast-fed infants and the selenium concentration in the milk of lactating women in western Poland. Med Sci Monit 2001;7:1002–1004.
44 Wasowicz W, Gromadzinska J, Rydzynski K, Tomczak J: Selenium status of low-selenium area residents: Polish experience. Toxicol Lett 2003;137:95–101.
45 Kadrabova J, Mad'aric A, Ginter E: Determination of the daily selenium intake in Slovakia. Biol Trace Elem Res 1998;61:277–286.
46 Beker D, Romic Z, Krsnjavi H, Zima Z: A contribution to the world selenium map. Biol Trace Elem Res 1992;33:43–49.
47 Samuelson G: Dietary habits and nutritional status in adolescents over Europe. An overview of current studies in the Nordic countries. Eur J Clin Nutr 2000;54(suppl):S21–S28.
48 Kantola M, Mand E, Viitak J, et al: Selenium contents of serum and human milk from Finland and neighbouring countries. J Trace Elem Exp Med 1997;10:225–232.
49 Jackson MJ, Broome CS, McArdle F: Marginal dietary selenium intakes in the UK: Are there functional consequences? J Nutr 2003;133(suppl):1557S–1559S.
50 WHO-UNU, and International Council for Control of Iodine Deficiency Disorders: Assessment of Iodine Deficiency Disorders and Monitoring Their Elimination. A Guide for Programme Managers, ed 2. Geneva, WHO, 2001.

Discussion

Dr. Vasquez-Garibay: Do you think that pneumonia is a good indicator of infections in zinc deficiency because only a few studies have found some results?

Dr. Castillo-Durán: At this time all the studies on the association between zinc deficiency and pneumonia are related to very severe zinc deficiency in countries like India, Bangladesh, and Indonesia where severe deficiency is prevalent. Some studies have well demonstrated an effect of zinc deficiency on immunity, mainly cellular immunity, and there are some studies showing an association with IgA deficiency. There are several studies at this time that also demonstrate the effect well.

I don't know if this effect is also prevalent in countries where marginal zinc deficiency is prevalent.

Dr. Guesry: What type of criteria would you recommend to define zinc deficiency? We know that plasma zinc is not a good indicator, particularly during infection when there is sequestration of zinc in other pools.

Dr. Castillo-Durán: There is a lot of discussion at this time. Several studies propose that plasma zinc with a cutoff close to 80 μg/dl or 12.3 μmol/l may be one of the markers for analyzing the prevalence. Brown et al. [1] have used another approach which is to add the prevalence of low absorbable zinc associated with phytate intake to this factor; the molar ratio of >15:1 between phytate and zinc could possibly be associated with a high prevalence of zinc deficiency or high/low zinc absorption. At this time we need more information but we must use the information available. Plasma zinc is useful. Another measurement which is very difficult to use is white blood cell content. If red cells are used, then another measurement is needed because red cells are very difficult to use in community populations. At this time, the clinical effects, growth and infections are good markers for the suspicion of zinc deficiency, but we cannot say what the prevalence is because we have no reliable markers. For iron deficiency, it is 40–50%, but for zinc we suspect that it is similar to iron, but we cannot say if it is the same rate as iron or another nutrient.

Mr. Parvanta: Following up on this discussion of the indicator. For example, you mentioned that in some countries foodstuffs are being fortified with zinc. Do you think it is possible to use a marker like serum zinc as a way to track the potential impact of that fortification program rather than being concerned about what the deficiency is? Basically, in a way, it is more like looking at whether the intervention has actually been effective.

Dr. Castillo-Durán: Perhaps I can give you an example of fortification in my country. We have a cow's milk powder which is fortified with iron 10 mg/l, zinc 5 mg/l, copper 0.5 mg/l. Two years after it was introduced in Chile iron deficiency decreased from 30 to 10 or 8%. We analyzed the rate of low plasma zinc. At that time, when the program was beginning, we had about 40%, and presently we have 30% in 18-month-old children. What is the explanation? Can we say that 5 mgZn/l is not enough to produce a favorable response in low plasma zinc, or is there a negative interaction between the 10 mgFe/l and the 5 mgZn/l for this result in plasma zinc? In spite of this effect, growth increased during the last years and these children have improved from −1 to −0.3 length-for age z-score. This is only an example, I cannot give you the exact answer and we need more studies.

The erythrocyte zinc content has been analyzed in many studies. With experimental zinc deficiency it was demonstrated that the zinc content in the membrane could be a useful marker for zinc deficiency. But we did a study in our community and after some months could not find any effect of zinc supplementation on the content of red blood cell membranes. I think it is very difficult to use this marker for communities.

Dr. Gia-Khanh: I would like to ask about the interaction between iron and zinc. In a community of children we had 3 groups: 1 receiving iron only, 1 receiving zinc only, and 1 receiving iron and zinc, and the results were very clearly different between the 3 groups. In the group receiving iron, anemia is clearly decreased. In the group receiving zinc, diarrhea and pneumonia clearly increased. But in the group receiving iron and zinc supplementation, the results are not as clearly different. Is there an interaction between zinc and iron when they are given to children from 6 to 12 months?

Dr. Castillo-Durán: I think Dr. Lozoff will analyze the interaction between zinc and iron, or Dr. Lönnerdal in the next presentation.

Dr. Zlotkin: Just sort of focusing on epidemiology. It has been my observation that most of us talk in terms of prevalence in developed countries and prevalence in developing countries, as your slides demonstrated. Yet it is quite clear to me, in Canada for example, that there are pockets of individuals within our developed country where micronutrient deficiency is in fact a significant problem. In Canada among our aboriginal populations, the prevalence of a micronutrient deficiency, like iron deficiency, may be as high as 40%. Yet if you look at national prevalence the number might be as low as 5–7%. In the developing world, and Mexico may be a good example where there is a burgeoning middle class, is it still fair for us to lump our prevalence data on the entire developing country, or in fact, as we sit here, is there a change going on where the 15 or 20% of the population who are becoming middle class are no longer at risk of micronutrient deficiencies. In fact if our national prevalence is 40% it means that in certain pockets it may be as high as 60 or 70%, whereas in other pockets it is as low as 5 or 10%. Should we be splitting rather than mounting at this point?

Dr. Castillo-Durán: We need more information from developing countries because, as you said, there are many pockets. In some countries these pockets are increasing because migration is increasing, and zinc deficiency is suspected in this kind of community. It would be an advantage if we could study these groups which may present with isolated deficiencies. This would allow us to analyze zinc deficiency or to control for a few other deficiencies. The problem in underprivileged communities in developing countries is that there are many deficiencies such as protein energy, many micronutrient deficiencies such as iron, copper, vitamin A, iodine, and many diseases. Fortification or supplementation can be tried but, in Guatemala or other countries, if the children present with acute diarrhea and environmental enteropathy, it is sometimes difficult to demonstrate very positive effects. In the future we may be able to compare these isolated deficiencies in developed countries with those mild deficiencies in developing countries.

Dr. Hurrell: I would like to question the assumption that zinc deficiency or the prevalence of zinc deficiency is as high as iron deficiency. My thoughts would be that phytic acid, which is often given as the reason, is much less inhibitory to zinc that it is to iron, and that most of the zinc studies have been in adults and not in children. Those that have been made in children, at least one of those studies, showed no effect of phytic acid on zinc absorption [2], and studies in infants are also nonexistent. The other reason would be that one of the main risk factors for iron deficiency is blood loss, which is not really a risk factor for zinc deficiency. Would you like to make some comments?

Dr. Castillo-Durán: I agree with you that we cannot use iron deficiency to define the suspicion of zinc deficiency, but there are some common effects. If we say that a low zinc intake is one of the risk factors, the same products in complementary foods contain iron and zinc. Another common factor is low birth weight related to low zinc and iron stores, which has been found to be common. As you said, it is not common that phytic acid is more related or more demonstrated for zinc status, but we need more information about the amount of phytate intake in children during complementary feeding after 6 months or between 6 months to 2 years old. It is different with the information related to blood loss, intestinal loss, which is more related to iron deficiency than to zinc deficiency. In the future we will be able to control for these confounding factors and analyze them. If we control these factors we can demonstrate some common effect of low zinc intake related to high zinc intake.

Dr. Gebre-Medhin: This is more a comment rather than a question, and I would like to reinforce what Dr. Guesry and Mr. Parvanta as well as Dr. Zlotkin have mentioned, and that is that these individual nutrients rarely occur without being associated with two fundamental things, protein energy malnutrition and infection. As long as this issue of criteria markers and indicators for pure authentic individual iron deficiency is not rushed, we will be in great trouble. Dr. Lönnerdal will go into basic issues on interrelations and interactions using experimental situations, but in humans it is getting more and more frustrating. The other comment I have is that if you give an individual any nutrient you are likely to increase the serum level, and this has been known for perhaps 100 years. Anything that is given to anybody will usually increase the serum level. The other thing is that it will be compromised by protein energy status and infection. Now as long as these issues are not rushed, we will continue to be in trouble.

Dr. Neufeld: I just want to come back to Dr. Zlotkin's comment about the distribution of deficiencies in a country. We have recently conducted a nationally representative nutrition survey and found quite large differences for some micronutrients and for some nutritional problems within Mexico and less for other problems. For example iron deficiency anemia occurs all over Mexico, whereas with zinc deficiency there were differences, vitamin A, etc. I think it is very important to make sure that we look out for those differences in terms of monitoring progress and also in defining programs, something we need to focus on more.

Mr. Parvanta: I wonder whether you have some comments on indicators for diagnosing individuals versus diagnosing or assessing populations? I also wonder whether an indicator may be more applicable to a population assessment rather than in individually diagnosed subclinical cases or individual patients? I wonder whether there might be some way to assess populations using certain indicators that may not be as regressive to monitoring or assessing or diagnosing an individual, and specifically with zinc? Do you have any comment on that?

Dr. Castillo-Durán: For a good analysis it is sometimes difficult to find children without infection, in good condition and fasting. At this time, for individuals, when we get a good sample for zinc with no infection, we can say that it is a reliable marker if there is some information on plasma zinc under 80 µg/dl. Also if the history of these children presents other suspicious risk factors, for instance in the first years of life or repeated infections, then we can only suspect zinc deficiency. The purpose is to supplement and to demonstrate an effect. Similar to vitamin A, there are some studies that are trying to find out if there is some effect after zinc supplementation on plasma zinc, but there is no indication that the change is a good indicator for zinc deficiency. If we have 80 µg and we supplement this and increase to 90, the change is an indicator of zinc deficiency. At present we can only use the information available. For individuals plasma zinc is the only measurement associated with history. For communities we must analyze the problem. At this time there is a very high risk for very underprivileged communities. The problem at this time is to demonstrate whether marginal zinc deficiency is associated with some clinical effects, growth and infection. If an association is found, even at a marginal level, we can advance in this definition.

Dr. Gibson: New Zealand has just completed a national survey examining plasma zinc levels in children between 5 and 14 years of age. We are actually analyzing these data and I certainly believe, at the population level, that serum zinc can tell you very useful things about the distribution of zinc status in a population. It appears, with our New Zealand data, that the low zinc status is restricted to certain ethnic groups [3].

Dr. Cozzolino: We have been working with zinc and selenium in Brazil for a long time. I think at the moment the major problem is to discover a biomarker that will be useful to say that a patient is deficient or not, because plasma is always alright, the level is normal, but sometimes the patient has a deficiency. Do you think we need another biomarker to really tell us whether there is a deficiency or not, also with selenium? In Brazil we have found different levels of selenium, and we are trying to discover more about this mineral in Brazil. I think it is also important to know what biomarker is useful in this case. What do you think about the biomarkers?

Dr. Castillo-Durán: I agree with you. New information is appearing all the time proposing new biomarkers for selenium, for zinc and trying to demonstrate efficiency. Biomarkers are needed which are easy to perform and analyze in a population. There are some reliable markers but they are too difficult or too expensive to use. They are not useful for us. If we can perhaps demonstrate that the changing zinc pool is useful to measure marginal zinc deficiency that would be very nice, but it is not available for individuals because it is too expensive. For selenium we might analyze glutathione peroxidase for zinc and selenium content in some tissues. But at this time we must also demonstrate what the selenium outcome is. Is the outcome perhaps an iron deficiency disorder because we have no other clinical outcome at this time? In the case of selenium we need much more metabolic information to advance to the communities, and we also need new information for zinc.

Dr. Yin: I would like to make some comments about selenium. As you know, China was probably a good example for selenium deficiency in the past. About 30 years ago, we had a long belt area from north-eastern to south-western China with a population of 200 million, in which there was a high incidence of Keshan disease and also Kaschin-Beck's disease. After selenium supplementation, the prevalence of the two diseases was significantly decreased. In the last 20 years, the prevalence and the great extent of these diseases have been alleviated along with improvements in the socioeconomic and living standards and nutritional status. In recent years in some low-selenium areas, although there was no selenium supplementation, the incidence of Keshan disease and Kaschin-Beck's disease has decreased. From this I think the general nutritional status should be considered, and if we improve the general nutritional status we can also decrease some micronutrient deficiencies.

Dr. Gibson: I would like to comment on the collection of blood samples for plasma serum zinc. When we were setting up the protocol for the national children's nutrition survey in New Zealand, we actually did a lot of work trying to establish standardized methods. One of the things I would like to just emphasize is that if you don't refrigerate the blood samples or store them on ice immediately after collection [4], and also separate the serum/plasma within a certain short space of time (i.e. within 2 h), you will find that your plasma or serum zinc levels do go up; during clotting, zinc may be released from platelets [5]. I think this is one of the reasons why we have such difficulty in interpreting so much of the data in the literature: the standardization procedures have not necessarily been rigorous enough. So sometimes you might find that actually if you use the proper procedures you will end up with a lower plasma zinc than you would otherwise have.

References

1   Brown KH, Peerson JM, Rivera J, Allen LH: Effect of supplemental zinc on the growth and serum zinc concentrations of prepubertal children: A meta-analysis of randomized controlled trials. Am J Clin Nutr 2002;75:1062–1071.
2   Manary MJ, Hotz C, Krebs NF, et al: Dietary phytate reduction improves zinc absorption in Malawian children recovering from tuberculosis but not in well children. J Nutr 2000;130: 2959–2964.
3   Parnell W, Scragg R, Wilson N, et al: NZ Food NZ Children. Key Results of the 2002 National Children's Nutrition Survey. Wellington, Ministry of Health, 2003.
4   Tamura T, Johnston KE, Freeburg LE, et al: Refrigeration of blood samples prior to separation is essential for the accurate determination of plasma or serum zinc concentrations. Biol Trace Elem Res 1994;41:165–173.
5   English JL, Hambridge KM: Plasma and zinc concentrations: Effects of time between collection and separation. Clin Chim Acta 1988;175:211–216.

Pettifor JM, Zlotkin S (eds): Micronutrient Deficiencies during the Weaning Period and the
First Years of Life. Nestlé Nutrition Workshop Series Pediatric Program, vol 54, pp 53–65,
Nestec Ltd., Vevey/S. Karger AG, Basel, © 2004.

Stable Isotope Methods in Micronutrient Research

S.A. Abrams

USDA/ARS Children's Nutrition Research Center, and Section of Neonatology,
Department of Pediatrics, Baylor College of Medicine, Houston, Tex., USA

Introduction

We will consider specific examples of three areas in which mineral stable
isotopes are used, and then discuss the issues regarding increasing the use of
stable isotope-based research.

Evaluation of Food Fortification in Indonesia

We assessed iron and zinc absorption in fortified wheat flour in
collaboration with the Nutrition Research and Development Center in Bogor,
Indonesia. One of the important questions weighed in this study was whether
the bioavailability of zinc sulfate added as a fortificant to wheat flour would
be the same as that of zinc oxide [1, 2].

Zinc fortification is increasingly frequent in developed countries, where the
most common forms of zinc used are zinc oxide and zinc sulfate. In Indonesia,
consideration is being given to co-fortifying iron-fortified flour with zinc.
Identifying the optimal form of zinc to add (best bioavailability and lowest
cost) is crucial to implementing such a program. Ninety healthy children (45
male and 45 female) were recruited from a rural clinic south of Jakarta,

This work is a publication of the US Department of Agriculture (USDA)/Agricultural Research
Service (ARS), Children's Nutrition Research Center, Department of Pediatrics, Baylor College
of Medicine and Texas Children's Hospital, Houston, Tex. This project has been funded in part
with federal funds from the USDA/ARS under Cooperative Agreement number 58–6250–6-001.
Contents of this publication do not necessarily reflect the views or policies of the USDA, nor does
mention of trade names, commercial products, or organizations imply endorsement by the US
Government.

Indonesia. Healthy subjects, 4–8 years old, were enrolled after informed written consent was obtained.

We prepared ^{67}Zn as both the oxide and the sulfate. Doses were mixed with steamed dough balls of the food product to be fortified. The iron and zinc isotopes were added to water, which in turn was added to the dough. After an overnight fast, subjects received an intravenous infusion of ^{70}Zn. Shortly thereafter, the subjects received a meal consisting of the dough balls. Subjects collected urine samples for zinc isotope ratio analysis at 48 and 72 h. Urinary zinc isotope ratios were measured following acid digestion and anion exchange. Isotope enrichments were measured by magnetic sector thermal ionization mass spectrometry. Isotope ratios were expressed with respect to the non-administered isotope, ^{66}Zn, and corrected for differences in fractionation using the ^{64}Zn/^{66}Zn ratio.

We found no difference in zinc absorption between the children who received the zinc oxide (24.1 ± 8.2%) and those who received the zinc sulfate (23.7 ± 11.2%; p = 0.87). This result was somewhat unexpected. Because zinc oxide is less soluble than zinc sulfate, it has been generally expected that zinc absorption would be greater from zinc sulfate than from zinc oxide. However, there is little objective evidence to support a bioavailability difference. As zinc absorption was similar from zinc sulfate and zinc oxide, we suggest that zinc oxide might be a preferable choice, especially as it is cheaper than zinc sulfate (a significant consideration) [1]. Whether these findings would hold true for smaller children including those in the first 2 years of life, however, is uncertain and should be further tested before choosing a zinc fortificant for foods intended for this age group.

Children with Chronic Illnesses

The use of stable isotopes may be especially relevant in studies involving children and adolescents with chronic illnesses [3, 4]. Such patients are unlikely to tolerate the dietary regulation and long-term collections associated with metabolic balance studies. One recent study used stable isotopes to assess calcium absorption in children in cystic fibrosis (CF). Earlier radio-isotope studies suggested that adults with CF had decreased calcium absorption but data using a dual tracer system and data in children were lacking [5].

Schulze et al. [3] studied children with CF who were pre-, early-, or late-pubertal. Data were compared with results from similarly studied healthy children (table 1) [6, 7]. They found no evidence of decreased calcium absorption in the children with CF. This might be related to the relatively high calcium intakes and normal vitamin D levels in their study subjects. These findings suggest that it may not be simple to enhance calcium status in children with chronic illnesses by increasing their calcium or vitamin D

Table 1. Total calcium absorption (mmol/day) in children and adolescents with CF

	Healthy girls	Girls with CF
Pre-pubertal	6.1 ± 1.9 (n = 6)	6.9 ± 1.6 (n = 4)
Early pubertal	10.7 ± 3.4 (n = 7)	12.8 ± 0.9 (n = 4)
Late pubertal	5.9 ± 1.9 (n = 6)	8.2 ± 3.5 (n = 4)

intake. This area of research also points out another potential use of stable isotopes. That is, evaluating the effects of medical interventions on mineral homeostasis in adults with CF. Brown et al. [8] administered calcitriol and demonstrated an increase in radioisotope calcium absorption. Ultimately, it is reasonable to assume that this type of therapy or therapy with direct bone-acting agents, such as bisphosphonates, may be evaluated by their effects on calcium absorption and bone kinetics (see below) as determined using stable isotopes. This would obviate the need for radiation exposure and allow the studies to be more readily performed in children.

It is important that future studies also address the secretory losses of minerals in children with conditions that might affect gut losses of nutrients such as inflammatory bowel disease or CF. Although measuring dietary absorption is useful in assessing the bioavailability of fortificants and supplements, ultimately it is the net mineral retention which matters. In the case of healthy subjects, especially for calcium, and magnesium, it is likely that relatively little regulation is via endogenous excretion and oftentimes this can be omitted [9–10]. However, this assumption may not be valid in cases of chronic bowel-related illnesses.

Kinetic Studies of Mineral Metabolism

Although the majority of published radioisotope or stable isotope mineral kinetic studies have involved calcium and more recently zinc, we will use magnesium as our example in this report (fig. 1) [9, 11–14]. This is because, until recently, analytical difficulties and dosing issues made the use of magnesium stable isotopes extremely limited and therefore many are not aware of the potential involving magnesium stable isotopes. Even radioisotope studies of magnesium metabolism were severely limited by the limited availability and safety concerns with using ^{28}Mg [11]. Recently, the use of high-resolution mass spectrometric analytical techniques has led to the opportunity to expand our knowledge on the physiology of this crucial, but under-researched, mineral.

Stable isotope techniques permit a unique approach to the assessment of magnesium metabolism, including absorption, excretion, pool sizes, and turnover [10, 11, 15]. We evaluated the relationship between magnesium

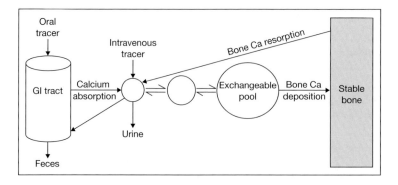

Fig. 1. Typical kinetic model showing use of multiple tracers to track the course of a mineral over time in the body. Model shown is for calcium, although a very similar model may also be used for magnesium.

Table 2. Correlation coefficients for body composition/ anthropometric values and mineral kinetics (n = 22) [14]

	Mg pool mass	Mg turnover[1]
Age	0.39	0.50*
Weight	0.76**	0.55**
Height	0.62**	0.68**
Body mass index	0.72**	0.45*
Fat-free mass	0.77**	0.67**

*p < 0.05; **p < 0.01.
[1]Mg turnover refers to the forward flow of magnesium from the largest identifiable pool to long-term storage, primarily in bone.

kinetic values and other measures of body composition. We found that fat-free mass represents the single body composition parameter that most closely correlates with magnesium kinetic data [14] (table 2). Of note is that body composition has a stronger relationship with magnesium kinetics than with calcium kinetics. These relationships provide justification for basing dietary magnesium requirements in children on body composition measures such as body weight or, where available, fat-free mass. Further studies to evaluate these relationships are indicated in situations where either magnesium status or body composition is abnormal.

Based on available human data, it is not currently possible to directly relate magnesium deficiency conditions to changes in the exchangeable pool or pool turnover rates. As with calcium and zinc, whole-body deficiency conditions may lead to an increase in both the mass and turnover of magnesium

Table 3. Recommended guidelines for purchasing mineral stable isotopes [2, 9]

It is recommended that purchasers obtain, or be able to readily obtain from any distributors the following documents:
1 Original manufacturer's assay (translated)
2 A certificate of origin from the country of isotope production
3 Independent assay of composition
Accompanying letter from the manufacturer that provides the date of manufacture, the company to which the material was sold, when it was sold, and how it was transported from the source country to the distributor.

from some of these pools [10, 11]. However, unlike calcium, there is no readily available method (e.g., dual energy X-ray absorptiometry) for determining whole-body magnesium content during growth. Therefore, development and enhancement of stable-isotope based methods of evaluating magnesium kinetics offers a unique opportunity to study this mineral and the effects of nutritional and medical conditions on it.

Methodological Issues

An important aspect of mineral stable isotope studies is that they can be used in any subject population [9]. This includes children of all ages, as well as pregnant and lactating women. However, special considerations are involved when performing pediatric studies. First, it is frequently difficult to obtain the same volume or sampling frequency in children relative to adults. Secondly, isotope doses must be tailored based on the body pool distribution and turnover rates which are affected by growth and puberty [15]. Finally, analgesia during painful procedures, as well as ethical issues, must be carefully considered in performing pediatric studies.

Mineral stable isotopes have been used in thousands of clinical studies with no reported complications related to their use. Complications would only be expected related to inappropriate isotope preparation or administration, especially of intravenous doses. That these have not been reported provides testimony to the exceptional safety profile of the isotopes and the care used in their clinical administration.

Our foremost concern is that the isotopes be obtained from sources which have thoroughly tested and demonstrated their purity, and which provide evidence, in the form of formal certification, documenting the origin of the isotopes, the isotopic content (enrichment), and the lack of excessive trace mineral contamination (table 3). Isotopes prepared for intravenous dosing must always be prepared in a sterile environment and rigorously tested before human dosing, which must also be done in a sterile fashion by trained medical personnel who monitor patient status during and after the infusion.

An important consideration is that infusion procedures be made as painless as possible. Children have a limited ability to tolerate uncomfortable procedures, a concern which should be kept in mind when interacting with those who volunteer to participate in research studies. It should be noted that often, pediatric subjects receive no direct benefit from the study. Clearly, on principle, any potential risks and discomforts that may be associated with a child's participation in an individual study should be very carefully scrutinized and minimized. To minimize discomfort from venipuncture, we utilize an analgesic agent for all phlebotomies. The universal use of numbing creams has made such studies better tolerated by children.

Ongoing Issues Related to Mineral Stable Isotope Studies

There is little doubt that the central issue remaining currently for mineral stable isotope studies, especially those involving iron, is identification of the optimal form and method for dosing. This issue extends to a long-standing controversy regarding the benefits, risks and interpretation related to the use of an intravenous iron stable isotope dose. A detailed description of these issues is beyond the scope of this review, but it remains to be determined whether the relatively smaller particle size and greater purity of centrifuge-produced isotopes leads to levels of absorption, especially for iron, that substantially exceed those obtained in food-fortification programs. This issue does not seem to be a concern for calcium where stable isotope absorption values have been shown over many years to be comparable to those obtained from both mass balance studies and radioisotope studies.

An important issue is developing the supply line and enhancing the connection between the various contributors to research regarding stable isotopes (table 4). This line begins with the scientist or physician, frequently in a developing country who has a question he or she wishes to ask. They must then find collaborators, suppliers, funding sources, research subjects and ultimately a 'market', such as government agencies, for the research. This is an extremely daunting task whether in the United States or other countries.

It is crucial to organize these efforts both to enhance the quality of the science, by standardizing approaches and methods, and more importantly, to make it feasible for these studies to be conducted. This requires organizing the analytical laboratories and suppliers so that scientists know who and how these may be accessed. Organization would involve providing consistent availability, purity and source information for the isotopes and analytical speed, precision and cost by the analytical laboratory. There are, in reality, many geology and other non-biological science laboratories that have the equipment to perform very high precision analysis of mineral stable isotopes.

Table 4. Critical components of enhancing mineral stable isotope-based research

---

Researchers:
- Identify clinical and scientific questions
- Contact collaborators to assist with:
  Analyzing samples
  Clinical administration of isotopes
  Data interpretation
- Identify sources of funding
- Identify study population and obtain needed ethical permission from participants and ethical review boards

Collaborating laboratories:
- Provide readily available information regarding
  Cost
  Accuracy
  Time to perform analyses
- Assist in teaching methods of isotope administration
- Collaborate with data interpretation
- Interact with other laboratories to harmonize methods and limit duplication of studies.

Funding agencies:
- Harmonize sources and cost of isotope
- Encourage multi-component nutritional research studies
- Support global training in isotope methods and interpretation

---

Organization of these efforts might induce some of them to more readily consider participating in this research thereby providing more opportunities for nutritional scientists searching for analytical collaborators.

Funding agencies that have supported this type of research include, notably, the International Atomic Energy Agency, other United Nations-based organizations, the National Institutes of Health, the National Research Council (UK), and many other such government and non-governmental organization. Important research has been funded via private corporations, either directly or via foundations such as the Nestlé Foundation [16, 17].

Of note is that our group has found that virtually everyone who initially contacted us about conducting such research has overestimated the costs involved in doing these studies. We believe that many more potential scientists do not even get that far in proposing mineral stable isotope studies because they believe that these studies are impossibly expensive or even that the isotopes cannot be obtained.

This thinking is no doubt a legacy issue generated from the fact that before 1990, virtually all of the mineral stable isotopes were obtained from the US Department of Energy Calutron Program in Oak Ridge, Tenn. This program was based on full-cost recovery and thus prices for isotopes increased substantially over a short period of time, especially between 1980 and 1990. Moreover, since the Oak Ridge calutrons were placed in a shut-down mode at

Stable Isotope Methods in Micronutrient Research

various times in the 1990s (they are now completely out of service), it was thought that isotopes were in either short supply or very expensive [18].

Technological advances in isotope separation, namely gas centrifugation, have allowed large quantities of isotopes to be isolated at a relatively low cost. While not applicable to all elements the isotopes of zinc, iron and selenium are now available at higher enrichments at lower prices using the gas centrifugation approach. With respect to the isotopes of calcium and magnesium, which cannot be produced by gas centrifugation, there is an abundant supply produced on an ongoing basis from the calutrons located in Russia. There are reputable distributors who validate, assay, and alter the chemical form of the isotope when this is required for the nutrition market (table 3). Russia has been thought of as an 'unstable source' of isotopes but in fact they have been the key supplier to the industry for over 10 years, and reliability has not been an issue when dealing with reputable agents.

Advocacy for this type of research is also important. Often both public policy administrators as well as those trained in other nutrition disciplines may not appreciate the value or the way such data may be used. The rapidly expanding publication list of mineral stable isotope studies may alleviate much of this problem, but it remains important to emphasize the inter-relationship of epidemiological and physiological research as represented by mineral stable isotope studies.

References

1 Herman S, Griffin IJ, Suwarti S, et al: Co-fortification of iron fortified flour with zinc sulfate, but not zinc oxide, decreases iron absorption in Indonesian children. Am J Clin Nutr 2002;76: 813–817.
2 Abrams SA, Griffin IJ, Herman S: Using stable isotopes to assess the bioavailability of minerals in food-fortification programs. Food Nutr Bull 2002;23:158–165.
3 Schulze KJ, O'Brien KO, Germain-Lee EL, et al: Efficiency of calcium absorption is not compromised in clinically stable prepubertal and pubertal girls with cystic fibrosis. Am J Clin Nutr 2003;78:110–116.
4 Perez MD, Abrams SA, Loddeke L, et al: Effects of rheumatic disease and corticosteroid treatment on calcium metabolism and bone density in children assessed 1 year after diagnosis, using stable isotopes and dual-energy X-ray absorptiometry. J Rheumatol 2000;27(suppl 58): 38–43.
5 Aris RM, Lester GE, Dignman S, Ontjes DA: Altered calcium homeostasis in adults with cystic fibrosis. Osteoporos Int 1999;10:102–108.
6 Abrams SA, Stuff JE: Calcium metabolism in girls: Current dietary intakes lead to low rates of calcium absorption and retention during puberty. Am J Clin Nutr 1994;60:739–743.
7 Abrams SA, Griffin IJ, Davila PM, Hawthorne KM: Calcium absorption is similar from milk and two types of fortified orange juice. J Bone Miner Res 2003, in press.
8 Brown SA, Ontjes DA, Lester GE, et al: Short-term calcitriol administration improves calcium homeostasis in adults with cystic fibrosis. Osteoporos Int 2003;14:442–449.
9 Abrams SA: Using stable isotopes to assess mineral absorption and utilization by children. Am J Clin Nutr 1999;70:955–964.
10 Griffin IJ, King JC, Abrams SA: Body weight specific zinc compartmental masses in girls significantly exceed those reported in adults: A stable isotope study using a kinetic model. J Nutr 2000;130:2607–2612.

11 Avioli LV, Berman M: 28 Mg kinetics in man. J Appl Sci 1996;21:1688–1694.
12 Sojka J, Wastney M, Abrams S, et al: Magnesium kinetics in adolescent girls determined using stable isotopes: Effects of high and low calcium intake. Am J Physiol 1997;273:R710–R715.
13 Abrams SA: Stable isotope studies of mineral metabolism: Calcium, magnesium, and iron; in Abrams SA, Wong WW (eds): Stable Isotopes in Nutrition. Oxon, CABI, 2003, pp 35–60.
14 Abrams SA, Ellis KJ: Multicompartmental analysis of magnesium and calcium kinetics during growth: Relationships with body composition. Magnes Res 1998;11:307–313.
15 O'Brien KO, Abrams SA: Effects of development on techniques for calcium stable isotope studies in children. Biol Mass Spectromet 1994;23:357–361.
16 O'Brien KO, Zavaleta N, Caulfield LE, et al: Influence of prenatal iron and zinc supplements on iron absorption, red blood cell incorporation and iron status in pregnant Peruvian women. Am J Clin Nutr 1999;69:509–515.
17 Zavaleta N, O'Brien KO, Abrams SA, Caulfield LE: Maternal iron status influences iron transfer to the fetus during the third trimester of pregnancy. Am J Clin Nutr 2003;77:924–930.
18 Abrams SA, Klein PD, Young VR, Bier DM: Letter of concern regarding a possible shortage of separated isotopes. J Nutr 1992;122:2053.

Discussion

Dr. Guesry: I know the cost is very different for bioavailability studies, but do you think that extrinsic tags give as reliable data as intrinsic labeling?

Dr. Abrams: I think that one cannot assume that this is the case. For every mineral and every circumstance one has to look at the data out there. The good thing is that, for the last 50 or so years, people have been looking into this issue and there is a lot of information about where the extrinsic tag is working and where it doesn't work, so one is entirely in the dark. In general, for example, cow's milk extrinsically tagged with calcium is a very good marker, whereas more complex markers, for instance soy milk with calcium, are very bad, it is overestimated. So it is not simple, but it is also not true that it can't be done. For iron one virtually has to use the same source at least as what you are measuring, but it depends on the circumstances.

Dr. Castillo-Durán: For infants, what is the amount of the fluid, urine, saliva, that you need for this kind of analysis?

Dr. Abrams: For blood analysis of iron we routinely use 0.5 ml of whole blood, so that is not really problematic. Usually between 5 and 10 ml of urine is plenty for calcium and zinc. We had a problem in Nigeria because the children had such low calcium in their urine that in fact we could not find it, so occasionally one runs into special problems. But in general it is extreme volumes for what we are doing.

Dr. Castillo-Durán: And for saliva?

Dr. Abrams: Saliva is widely used by NASA for astronauts. I have to check to see how much they got, but it was not very much, the astronauts routinely did that. The question is just how accurate saliva analyses are? They have been used especially for calcium, but not very much.

Dr. Castillo-Durán: Concerning the selection of stable isotopes or radioisotopes. I understand that radioisotopes are still a lot cheaper, and I wonder whether stable isotopes are good mainly in terms of safety or accuracy?

Dr. Abrams: The shift of stable isotopes is certainly not a cause of accuracy. Stable isotope is more accurate in terms of the measurement of absorption for different things you do. It has primarily been safe, and also the overall cost of isotope studies has come down quite a bit. We can talk about details of cost, but it is a typical subject in terms of iron and zinc study. It might cost between USD 500 and 1,000 for the isotope after analysis for single subjects. If studies involve 20–50 people we might be talking about USD 10–15,000 for a study, which is not very large relative to a USD 1 million supplementation trial. I think the real issue has been safety and the maintenance of global levels of safety.

Dr. Hurrell: I think that radioisotopes are much less expensive. In Kansas City we have done a lot of radioisotope studies and we calculate on maybe USD 3,000/study. With stable isotopes it is somewhat more expensive. With radioisotopes we investigate many more variables; we could look at many more levels of phytate for example. However, one of the main differences between the radioisotope and the stable isotope studies is that with radioisotope studies no additional mineral is added, but with the stable isotope studies there is. So with stable isotope studies we are always investigating a food which has milligrams of iron added to it. You can never investigate meals which are not iron fortified, which you can do with the extrinsic tag radio iron studies.

Dr. Abrams: In terms of the cost, I fully agree in terms of the total amount. There are issues of disposal, transport of isotopes and things like that in different areas that may affect the cost, but I would not deny that radioisotope studies are cheaper than stable isotope studies, only that the safety margin prefers the use of stable isotope in my opinion, that is why I said not everybody agrees with me. The issue of adding the mineral too is a very real one. I think for the most part, for most of the clinically relevant issues that we must ask about whether this food is a good source of iron, is this iron supplement useful, can we give doses of the isotopes so that we are not exceeding what would otherwise be given in a food that we are testing as supplement? There are some special issues certainly involved in breast milk that may be problematic, but for most issues I think that we can make use of the stable isotopes for practical questions.

Dr. Pettifor: Just one issue related to what Dr. Hurrell said about the use of non-labeled iron or calcium. If we talk about the calcium issue, there is going to be a difference if one adds non-isotope calcium to the meal compared to when you are using a purely tracer amount of calcium. When you are looking at absorption, just a very small amount of absorption, then you may well be looking at the effects of diffusion of calcium across the gut as opposed to the active transport of calcium.

Dr. Abrams: We can do studies using the stable isotope ^{46}Ca, giving a dose of less than 1 mg of calcium total in an adult.

Dr. Pettifor: But the issue is which is the most relevant? I think the issue of just using a tracer amount is not particularly helpful in assessing what is happening in real life.

Dr. Abrams: I guess it doesn't mix in again with the query of calcium and that again depends on the circumstances. There are certainly some questions one might ask.

Dr. Vasquez-Garibay: Could you explain a little bit about the use of iron incorporation and iron absorption in babies with iron deficiency anemia because that can influence the results and also the rate of erythrocyte incorporation of iron in this particular case.

Dr. Abrams: I will pass on the clinical aspects of segmentation rate because that is not my field, but I will say that red blood cell incorporation of iron well reflects the iron absorption of small babies, and this an area of considerable controversy right now. There is some evidence that the 14-day incorporation method does not really represent true incorporation. Comparing the studies, I am not entirely sure that it is a big effect, but there is some effect. The bigger concern is that small babies don't actually incorporate most of the iron that they absorb. So I think that at least for now we have to recognize that for small babies there are some limitations in the red blood cell method, but it does give you at least some basis for comparison. The only way to correct that would be to do fecal collections at the same time and therefore do simultaneous mass balance, which has extreme limitations, or to give an intravenous dose which is what we did in premature infants and some others have also done, which also has extreme limitation, so I think there are still some unknown issues here.

Dr. Barclay: Coming back to the question raised earlier, could you comment on whether to use short-term or longer-term bioavailability studies depending on the question being asked?

Dr. Abrams: The iron/calcium interaction is one of my favorites and we took 12-month-old babies and gave them calcium supplement and iron, actually gave milk and iron, and found a marked decrease in iron absorption with calcium. We adapted them for anywhere from 2 to 6 weeks in different studies and we found complete adaptation just as in adults. So one of the big questions in the studies is, let's suppose you have a weaning food and you want to know how much iron is absorbed from it. You have two basic choices: tomorrow you can bring in 30 children from the community, give them the food, label with the isotope and measure the absorption, or you can put them on it for 2, 4 or 6 weeks, 1 year, and then measure the absorption. You are going to get different numbers, so you have to decide what the question is that you are asking, and I think they answer very different questions. My personal bias is to go ahead and adapt them for a brief period of time beforehand, but that gives you a different answer than just bringing them in tomorrow.

Dr. Gebre-Medhin: Would you comment on the issue of steady-state. Do the individuals have to be in a steady-state? How do you measure that? Does it have any importance if they are not?

Dr. Abrams: Other than what I just said, upon the change in isotope absorption or any mineral absorption over time as the iron status improved, the biggest problem we have for steady-state is when we look at body pool masses and turnover rates, especially in small children. So they are ways mathematically within the SAMM program that actually counts and models growth into those. So it is not an impossible thing to model within the SAMM program but it is certainly true that there are some limitations there. The reality is when you are looking at absorption, there isn't any real steady-state. As long as you continue to give somebody a supplement the status is going to change and the absorption may change. So you simply have to identify some points on which you are going to make your measurement.

Dr. Zlotkin: In your institution there are some people who have been using stable isotopes to intrinsically label growing plants. I wonder if you could just talk about that for a moment because I think that the use of plant breeding is important for understanding the bioavailability of minerals from new plant sources. It might be important in the future.

Dr. Abrams: There is no question that the extrinsic tag is not the way to go if you are working with broccoli, it has to be labelled intrinsically. The use of hydropomax allows that to be done. The really big problem is that of cost because a considerable amount of isotope is going to be lost in the growing process. So one of the things that plant physiologists have to do is to recycle the water and keep the losses to a minimum. In fact, depending on the plant and the situation, they have become pretty good at that. As we see all sorts of new types of crops develop a stable isotope, with higher levels of iron or whatever, there is no question that, if scientifically the technique currently exists to intrinsically label them and to test those in people, it could be done today.

Dr. Hurrell: You mentioned pools, and I am a little unclear what you mean by the fast pool and the slow pool. Could you explain what parts of our physiology they are? The second question is about trying to use the size of the pools to measure micronutrient status. Can you explain this?

Dr. Abrams: One of the things noticed about calcium a long time ago is when a patient became deficient in calcium some of the body pools increased. The same thing is probably true for zinc as well. When a kinetic study is made it is critical what the model is and how it is divided up, what type of equations are used, and a multi-equation model or a multi-component exponential model are the same model to determine what period of time you are looking at. These are purely theoretical constructs until animal studies are done. This has been done somewhat with zinc to try to figure out where they are and what tissues they are in. For example, for calcium we know that even the fastest turnover pool is mostly serum plasma versus a small amount of bone. With zinc we have all sorts of tissues that are mixed into these, including liver and so on. But the bottom line is that the pool is a theoretical construct, and there is no question that being deficient may make some of your pools increase because when there is a deficiency the turn over increases to protect the initial serum pool.

Dr. Barclay: Could you comment on the doses of stable isotopes or the amounts of calcium administered in calcium absorption studies? If you look at absorption values for different calcium fortification compounds, there are large differences between studies and a lot of this could be due to methodological differences. What are the most important factors to take into consideration in this context?

Dr. Abrams: Calcium absorption intensely depends upon the role of total calcium given and what the meal components of that are. Heaney et al. [1] have spent many years documenting that beautifully. They have a perfect curve relating the dose of total calcium and absorption, and this was published about 12 years ago. So there is no question that when these things are used, they must be standardized. The high dose of the isotope itself isn't much of an issue, it is only a tiny amount. When giving the meal, typically a glass of milk in a calcium study, it depends on whether the isotope is given at the beginning or at the end of the meal or half an hour after a meal. So any given group certainly has to standardize what it is doing and recognize those supplementations. We have done a lot of studies trying to relate what we get with isotopes to other methods including mass balances, so we have a reasonable idea of what the best way is to do them, but it is very critically time dependent. That is one of the reasons why the numbers vary all over the place and why there is so much controversy about things like whether or not calcium citrate or calcium carbonate is better absorbed.

Dr. Villalpando-Carrión: I was wondering if you are aware of this pool model? Does the iron pool model stimulate, correlate or to some point move from one pool to the zinc model?

Dr. Abrams: Theoretical kinetics, that is working with iron pools, is a method that pretty well died with radioisotope studies about 30 years ago. Very few people have done them in humans since then. We are doing them because until very recently it was hard technically to do iron isotope ratios and anything other than red blood cells.

Dr. Barclay: One calcium isotope that has not been discussed today is ^{41}Ca.

Dr. Abrams: I removed that slide. For those of you who are not familiar with it, ^{41}Ca is an extreme along isotope with a half life of millions of years. It is somewhat radioactive and somewhat stable and it has a multi-million year half life with a radiation exposure that is essentially negligible. The nice thing is that it exists naturally in every one's tissues so you could have a tiny dose in the permanent lifetime turnover rates. The drawbacks are first of all that special isotope analysis techniques are not widely available, and the second is that you have to be looking over a very long period of time. It is the cutting edge of calcium isotope work. The reason I am not too involved in it is that I decided a long time ago that I would not give a radioisotope to a child no matter what, and I stand by that. Other people might have another ethical perspective because the doses are extremely small in practical terms, the problem is really safety. In adults I think it is a tremendous opportunity to look at long-term turnover rates. It is something that will be seen in the future. A Swiss group and some others are actively involved in this work.

Dr. Barclay: Would you also give a rough estimate of the cost per subject of an iron or a calcium bioavailability study?

Dr. Abrams: Just to give you an idea, right now a ^{58}Fe study runs at more than USD 50 or 60/mg. A study in a typical child might use 1–2 mg ^{58}Fe. So if you are going to give that, it again depends upon what you are doing, you may be talking about USD 100. If you are going to give a reference dose of 2–5 mg ^{57}Fe, it is running at about USD 10–15/mg. So we are roughly talking about USD 200 to study a small child. That can be roughly doubled or tripled if you are talking about a pregnant woman. As you go up, it depends on what you are looking at. So from USD 200 to 500 is the current price for the isotope analysis. We would generally charge anywhere between USD 50 and 150/sample, and iron study is one sample so we are not talking that much in general. A zinc study is 1 or 2 samples, a calcium is 1 or 2 samples. So I think we are talking about isotope dosing in the range of USD 300–500, 600/mineral tested.

I only want to comment that in terms of safety it is not causing any harm. There is nothing different to what we do than draw blood. I think every single one of you would not hesitate to do a research study in which you draw blood from the subject. There is not one bit of difference between that and the stable isotope study in terms of what the child must go through. We use numbing cream for every single child, for every single blood sample draw, any single site, we have a very large team of medical college students in the laboratory to provide amusements and distractions, etc. But it does involve a velocity of research, and we have done this in many of the countries that are represented here, virtually all of them are represented here.

Dr. Zlotkin: I think that understanding physiology in the year 2003 really does involve using stable isotopes in children to understand both the normal child and a pathological condition. This really does demonstrate that it can be done. It can be done safely; it can be done within a reasonable price range. We have an obligation to understand the metabolism of micronutrients as we go forward with programs, and I think this exemplifies that very well.

Reference

1   Heaney RP, Weaver CM, Fitzsimmons ML, Recker RR: Calcium absorptive consistency. J Bone Miner Res 1990;5:1139–1142.

Pettifor JM, Zlotkin S (eds): Micronutrient Deficiencies during the Weaning Period and the
First Years of Life. Nestlé Nutrition Workshop Series Pediatric Program, vol 54, pp 67–81,
Nestec Ltd., Vevey/S. Karger AG, Basel, © 2004.

Interactions between Micronutrients: Synergies and Antagonisms

Bo Lönnerdal

Department of Nutrition and Program of International Nutrition,
University of California, Davis, Calif., USA

Introduction

There is growing awareness that the micronutrient status of large segments of populations is inadequate and causing adverse effects on infants and
children. Iron, vitamin A and iodine deficiencies are common and the long-
term consequences are well known. Many programs have been and are being
launched to prevent and treat such micronutrient deficiencies. However,
whereas some micronutrients have mutually beneficial or synergistic effects,
i.e. providing more of one micronutrient will improve the status/metabolism
of another, other micronutrients interact negatively with each other, such that
providing too much of one micronutrient will impair the status of another
micronutrient. It is therefore important that there is a thorough knowledge of
micronutrient interactions when designing and interpreting programs to
combat micronutrient deficiencies. Without such knowledge, unexpected and
unfortunate outcomes may be experienced and, perhaps less serious, the
evaluations of interventions in different settings/populations may become
difficult or impossible. Meta-analysis of studies performed by different
researchers in various settings/populations is a powerful tool to evaluate outcomes of interventions; however, if the underlying micronutrient status is
highly variable and the outcome is dependent upon this, a 'true' picture of the
global situation may be difficult to obtain.

Iron and Zinc

When it was recognized that suboptimal zinc nutrition may be common in
large segments of the population, various strategies to prevent zinc deficiency
were considered. Since zinc is stable in water solution and non-toxic, oral

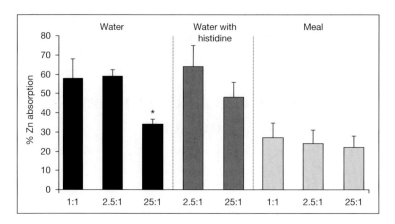

Fig. 1. The effect of iron:zinc ratio on the absorption of zinc in human healthy adults as measured when the elements were given in water, water with histidine (dietary zinc chelator) or in a standardized meal. Adapted from Sandström et al. [2].

supplements would be one possible avenue. However, in areas where zinc deficiency may be expected, iron deficiency is frequently common, and iron supplements may be used. Therefore, Solomons and Jacob [1] evaluated the effect of oral iron on zinc absorption by giving zinc and ferrous sulfate to human subjects in different molar ratios. They found that iron lowered zinc uptake as measured by the increase in plasma zinc at a molar ratio of 2:1. This obviously could be a concern if iron and zinc were to be given together. However, very large amounts of iron and zinc were given because of the method used (plasma area-under-the-curve) and it is conceivable that these two elements would only compete with each other when given in water solution and possibly not when food is present. This was investigated by Sandström et al. [2] who studied zinc absorption at physiological intakes using radioisotopes. When excess iron was added (25:1 ratio), zinc absorption from a water solution was inhibited significantly, whereas no effect was observed when they were given in a meal (fig. 1). As the inhibitory effect was abolished when histidine (chelator of zinc) was added, it was believed that when iron and zinc are chelated to their 'normal' ligands, resulting from digestion of foods, they will be absorbed via different pathways and no interaction would occur. A study by Rossander-Hulthén et al. [3] showed that similar results were obtained for iron absorption in humans when excess zinc was added, i.e. an inhibitory effect of zinc on iron absorption was found when they were given in water solution, whereas no effect was seen if they were given with a meal (fig. 2). These studies strongly suggested that iron and zinc may interact when given as supplements, but that this would not occur when they are given as food fortificants.

Two recent studies on iron and zinc supplementation of Indonesian infants [4, 5] show that antagonistic interactions between iron and zinc in fact do

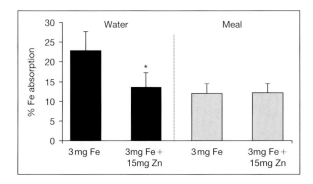

Fig. 2. The effect of added zinc on iron absorption in healthy human adults as measured when the elements were given in water solution or in a standardized meal. Adapted from Rossander-Hulthén et al. [3].

occur when they are given as supplements (drops). In a study by Dijkhuizen et al. [4] infants were given iron alone (10 mg/day), zinc alone (10 mg/day), both elements together (10 + 10 mg/day) or placebo from 4 to 10 months of age. Supplementation significantly reduced the prevalence of anemia, iron deficiency anemia and zinc deficiency. Iron supplementation did not negatively affect plasma zinc concentrations, and zinc supplementation did not increase the prevalence of anemia. However, iron supplementation combined with zinc was less effective than iron supplementation alone in reducing the prevalence of anemia (20 vs. 38% reduction) and in increasing hemoglobin and plasma ferritin concentrations. There were no differences in growth among the groups, and the growth of all groups was insufficient to maintain their z scores for height-for-age and weight-for-height, showing that overcoming these micronutrient deficiencies is not sufficient to improve growth performance in these infants.

In the study by Lindh et al. [5], the infants received the same treatments, but from 6 to 12 months of age. After supplementation, the iron group had higher hemoglobin and serum ferritin than did the iron+zinc group, indicating an effect of zinc on iron absorption (table 1). The zinc group had higher serum zinc than did the placebo group, whereas this was not the case for the iron and iron+zinc groups, suggesting an effect of iron on zinc absorption. Thus, supplementation with iron+zinc was less efficacious than single supplements in improving iron and zinc status, with evidence of a negative interaction between iron and zinc when the combined supplement was given. In this study, significant effects on growth were observed.

The reason why different results for growth were obtained in these two studies, which were performed in similar populations, is not known, but the different ages for the introduction of the supplements is one possibility. A stable isotope study by Domellöf et al. [6] showed that at 6 months (and

Table 1. Effect of iron (10 mg/day), zinc (10 mg/day), iron+zinc (10 + 10 mg/day) or placebo on iron status and plasma zinc in Indonesian infants supplemented from 6 to 12 months of age[1]

	Fe group	Zn group	Fe+Zn group	Placebo group	p value
Hemoglobin, g/l	119 ± 15[2,3]	116 ± 15	115 ± 14	113 ± 16	0.012
Serum ferritin, µg/l	46 ± 2[2,3]	13 ± 4	32 ± 32[2]	13 ± 4	<0.001
Serum zinc, µmol/l	8.8 ± 1.2	11.6 ± 1.4[2]	10.8 ± 1.3[2]	9.1 ± 1.3	<0.001

[1]Adapted from Lindh et al. [5].
[2]Significantly different from placebo.
[3]Significantly different from Fe+Zn group.

presumably at lower age), iron absorption was immature and that there was no downregulation of iron absorption with increased iron status. At 9 months, however, regulation of iron absorption appeared to be similar to that in adults, i.e. iron-replete infants absorbed much less iron than iron-depleted infants. Experiments in experimental animals show that regulation of iron transport mechanisms is immature at young age, but matures in late infancy [7]. Thus, competition for absorptive pathways may be more pronounced during late infancy. Further studies using stable isotopes are needed to elucidate the interaction between iron and zinc at different ages.

A crucial question is whether the interaction between iron and zinc has any functional consequences. In the study by Lindh et al. [5], weight-for-age was significantly higher in the zinc-supplemented group than in the other groups, and psychomotor development (Bayley Scales of Infant Development) was significantly higher in the iron-supplemented group than in the placebo group. Thus, the combination of iron and zinc supplements did not improve growth or development as compared to placebo. Iron supplementation has recently been shown to adversely affect the growth and morbidity of Honduran and Swedish infants [8] and to cause a redistribution of vitamin A (lower plasma retinol, higher liver retinol) in Indonesian infants [9]. Whether these consequences are a direct effect of iron or an indirect effect on zinc metabolism is not yet known. However, these observations may have considerable implications when designing programs for micronutrient interventions. It should be emphasized that, similar to adults, there does not appear to be an interaction when formulas or weaning foods are fortified with iron or zinc [10, 11].

Iron and Copper

Iron and copper are known to compete for absorptive pathways, although the mechanism behind this negative interaction has not been delineated.

Although most studies on this interaction have been done in experimental animals, there are some human studies suggesting that this may be an underestimated nutritional problem. Haschke et al. [12] showed that copper absorption in infants was significantly lower from infant formula fortified with a high level of iron (10.2 mg/l) than from formula with a low level of iron (1.1 mg/l). In another study, feeding infants a formula with a higher level of iron (7 mg/l) resulted in a significantly lower concentration of ceruloplasmin, or ferroxidase I, the major copper-binding protein in serum [10]. In a recent study of breast-fed infants given iron supplements (1 mg/kg/day), the activity of erythrocyte Cu,Zn-superoxide dismutase (SOD), which has been suggested as a long-term marker of copper status, was significantly lower than in unsupplemented infants [13]. Thus, copper status may be compromised by excessive iron supplementation. Impaired copper status has been shown to compromise immune function [14] and the decreases in ceruloplasmin and Cu,Zn-SOD may affect iron metabolism and the defense against free radicals negatively. Whether these observations had any functional consequences in the infants is not known, but should be studied further.

Iron and Ascorbic Acid

It is well known from a multitude of studies that ascorbic acid has an enhancing effect on iron absorption. This may be due in part to the reducing effect of ascorbic acid, keeping iron in the absorbable ferrous (+II) form, and in part to a weak chelating effect of ascorbic acid, also helping to keep iron soluble. Although it is known that the iron intake of several populations is adequate but inhibitory compounds limit the bioavailability of iron, there have been relatively few studies exploring this synergistic effect in fortification programs. Derman et al. [15] showed that fortifying infant formula with ascorbic acid significantly enhanced iron absorption in human adults, but studies on infants fed formulas with various levels of ascorbic acid were not done. Davidsson et al. [16] evaluated the addition of ascorbic acid to a Peruvian school breakfast meal and found that iron absorption was significantly enhanced in a dose-dependent manner. It is likely that the addition of ascorbic acid can overcome the inhibitory effect of phytic acid in the meal as has been shown previously [17]. Whether this enhancing effect of ascorbic acid on iron absorption is sustainable in populations with diets high in phytate was explored by Garcia et al. [18]. In a food-based community trial in Mexico they found that ascorbic acid from lime juice twice daily (50 mg/day) for 8 months did not improve the iron status of iron-deficient women, although a stable iron study showed an enhancing effect on iron absorption [19]. Although further long-term studies are needed on ascorbic acid fortification, it is possible that the initial enhancing

Table 2. Supplementation of anemic pregnant women in Indonesia with vitamin A and iron[1]

	Women without anemia	
	n	95% CI
Placebo (n = 62)	10 (16%)	7–29
Vitamin A (n = 63)	22 (35%)	22–48
Iron (n = 63)	43 (68%)	54–79
Vitamin A + Iron (n = 63)	61 (97%)	88–99

[1]Adapted from Suharo et al. [24].

effect of ascorbic acid on iron absorption is downregulated by homeostatic mechanisms.

Iron and Vitamin A

Studies on children in Central America showed that low plasma retinol concentrations were correlated to low hemoglobin, serum iron and transferrin saturation values [20]. These observations were made when iron intake was adequate; no correlation was found when dietary iron was low. In a study on experimental vitamin A deficiency in human adult volunteers, Hodges et al. [21] found that hemoglobin values decreased in a pattern similar to that of plasma vitamin A and that during repletion with vitamin A, hemoglobin values increased with plasma vitamin A. Studies in experimental animals have shown that liver and spleen iron increase concomitantly with the decrease in serum iron and hemoglobin [22]. When following the absorption of iron (with the radioisotope ^{59}Fe) in vitamin A-deficient rats [23], no difference in iron absorption or iron turnover was observed between vitamin A-deficient and control animals. The incorporation of ^{59}Fe into red blood cells, however, was significantly lower in the vitamin A-deficient animals than in controls. Consistent with this observation was the increased accumulation of ^{59}Fe in the liver of vitamin A-deficient animals. Thus, it appears that the mechanism of interaction between vitamin A and iron is an impairment in the mobilization of iron from the liver and/or incorporation of iron into the erythrocyte. Consequently, in order to optimize the outcome, it appears important to normalize vitamin A status in populations being given additional iron. Studies in some populations [24] have shown that supplementation with both iron and vitamin A increases hemoglobin concentrations to a greater extent in anemic pregnant women than does iron supplementation alone (table 2), although the magnitude of this effect varies considerably.

A synergistic effect between vitamin A and iron on iron absorption has been suggested by one group of investigators [25]. Both preformed retinol and β-carotene were shown to have a positive effect on the absorption of radio-iron from single meals in adult human volunteers. The mechanism between such an interaction remains elusive, but it was suggested that a physico-chemical interaction between iron and vitamin A occurs, which results in a complex being formed, enhancing iron absorption. However, a recent thorough study in human subjects did not find an enhancing effect of vitamin A on iron absorption [26]. These authors suggested that it may only occur in populations with low vitamin A status and that the effect in that case may be more related to the repletion in vitamin A status than a direct effect on iron absorption. Whether the enhancing effect of vitamin A on iron absorption in itself is biologically relevant in human populations or a consequence of the experimental method used also remains to be elucidated.

Zinc and Vitamin A

Zinc deficiency is known to impair vitamin A metabolism; thus, interventions intended to prevent or treat vitamin A deficiency may vary in efficacy depending on the subject's zinc status. It was found early that experimental animals fed low zinc diets had low levels of serum retinol and that these levels could not be increased by large supplements of retinyl acetate. Smith et al. [27] showed that rats fed a low zinc diet had markedly reduced levels of plasma retinol as compared to zinc-adequate animals, in spite of similar and adequate levels of vitamin A in the diet. They suggested that the mobilization of vitamin A from the liver was impaired by zinc deficiency. In a subsequent study [28], they showed that whereas plasma protein concentrations were lower in zinc-deficient animals, concentrations of retinol-binding protein (RBP) was dramatically reduced. Thus, the lower levels of circulating vitamin A may be due to a decrease in liver RBP synthesis. Studies in non-human primates fed a diet marginally low in zinc showed that plasma retinol was positively correlated to plasma zinc concentrations, and plasma RBP concentrations were also positively correlated to plasma zinc [29].

There have been few studies on the interaction between zinc and vitamin A in humans. In several conditions manifested by low zinc status in humans, such as alcoholic cirrhosis and protein-energy malnutrition, zinc supplementation sometimes but not always resulted in improved vitamin A status [30]. Similarly, some studies on preterm infants [31] and children [32] have shown positive effects on serum retinol, RBP and conjunctival epithelium, but not all studies show such effects. Christian et al. [33] showed that zinc potentiated the effect of vitamin A in restoring night vision among night-blind pregnant women, but this only occurred in women with low initial serum zinc concentrations. Thus, careful assessment of both initial zinc status, which is notoriously difficult, and vitamin A status before evaluating the effect of zinc on vitamin A status may be required.

Iron and Riboflavin

Riboflavin deficiency in human adults is known to result in low hemoglobin levels. When riboflavin deficiency was induced in human volunteers, the subjects got anemia, which was restored when riboflavin status was restored [34]. Studies in the Gambia have also shown that iron given with riboflavin supplements was more efficient in restoring hematologic parameters than iron given alone [35, 36]. Studies in experimental animals showed that the activity of NADH-FMN oxidoreductase was low in riboflavin-deficient animals and that this may be the underlying mechanism for the abnormal iron metabolism observed [37]. A study by Powers [38] showed that ariboflavinosis was more rapidly induced in young animals than in adult ones and that NADH-FMN oxidoreductase activity was dramatically reduced in riboflavin-deficient animals as compared to controls (2.9% of controls). Since iron stores, as measured by ferritin, were low in the riboflavin-deficient animals, it was possible that iron absorption was impaired. Adelakan and Thurnham [39] demonstrated such an impairment by showing that ^{59}Fe appearance was slower and lower in riboflavin-deficient animals than in controls. More unabsorbed ^{59}Fe remained in the gastrointestinal tract of riboflavin-deficient animals, supporting the idea of impairment in the uptake phase of iron. Taken together, these studies show that NADH-FMN oxidoreductase activity is low in riboflavin-deficient animals and that iron absorption is impaired, possibly because NADH-FMN oxidoreductase is involved in the mobilization of iron from ferritin. Thus, in riboflavin-deficient animals the release of iron (temporarily stored in mucosal ferritin) may be reduced significantly and more iron than normal would be lost by mucosal sloughing.

Further, assimilated iron may be diverted to the erythroid marrow at the expense of repleting iron stores. This is supported by a study in pregnant and lactating women in the Gambia [36] in which riboflavin given in addition to iron resulted in a significant increase in circulating plasma iron and in iron stores, relative to placebo. Additional studies in experimental animals [40] showed that riboflavin deficiency is associated with an increase in small intestine crypt depth and a twofold increase in the rate of crypt cell production. Thus, although there may be a contribution from turnover of enterocytes with an increased iron content, enhanced iron loss associated with riboflavin deficiency is likely due to an accelerated rate of small intestine epithelial turnover.

Iron and Iodine

A synergism between iron status and the efficacy of iodine fortification and supplementation in human populations was recently discovered. Zimmermann et al. [41] reported that in children with goiter, the therapeutic

Table 3. Change in goiter prevalence and thyroid volume in goitrous children in Cote d'Ivoire given iodized salt[1]

Time and group	Thyroid volume, ml	Subjects with goiter, %
Baseline		
Fe-treated	5.6 (3.5–16.4)	100
Placebo	5.8 (3.4–24.7)	100
6 weeks		
Fe-treated	5.6 (2.9–15.4)	68
Placebo	5.8 (2.9–22.5)	78
12 weeks		
Fe-treated	4.9 (2.5–16.0)	54
Placebo	5.2 (2.4–22.7)	63
20 weeks		
Fe-treated	4.3 (2.1–12.9)	43
Placebo	5.1 (2.1–21.4)[2]	62[2]

[1] Adapted from Hess et al. [42].
[2] Significantly different from placebo at 20 weeks.

response to orally given iodized oil was lower in children with iron deficiency anemia than in iron-replete children. Further, iron treatment of goitrous children with iron deficiency [42, 43] improved their response to iodized salt (table 3) or oil. It is known from studies in experimental animals that iron deficiency impairs central nervous system control of thyroid metabolism [44] and modifies nuclear triiodothyronine binding [45]. In human subjects with iron deficiency anemia, plasma concentrations of thyroxine and triiodothyronine are decreased, the conversion of thyroxine to triiodothyronine is lower and concentrations of thyrotropin are elevated [46, 47]. Thus, it appears likely that key steps in iodine metabolism are iron-dependent and that adequate iron status is a prerequisite for effective iodine treatment of goiter. Further studies in cells and experimental animals are needed to better define the molecular mechanisms behind the effect of iron deficiency on thyroid hormone metabolism.

Conclusions

Supplementation and fortification with single micronutrients has led to highly variable outcomes, making evaluations of the relative efficacy of each type of intervention difficult. It is likely that the results have been confounded by underlying deficiencies of other micronutrients. Thus, synergistic effects of providing two or more micronutrients may be expected. On the other hand, several studies have shown that supplementation and fortification with multiple micronutrients also have had mixed success, and in some cases adverse

effects of multinutrient supplementation as compared to single-nutrient supplementation [48]. In this case, interactions between micronutrients are likely,
i.e., one or more of the added micronutrients is already adequate and further
amounts may interfere with the absorption or metabolism of another one. Far
better knowledge and awareness of micronutrient interactions and their
underlying mechanisms are needed to institute improved interventions without negative side effects.

References

1 Solomons NW, Jacob RA: Studies on the bioavailability of zinc in humans: Effects of heme and
  nonheme iron on the absorption of zinc. Am J Clin Nutr 1981;34:475–482.
2 Sandström B, Davidsson L, Cederblad Å, Lönnerdal B: Oral iron, dietary ligands and zinc
  absorption. J Nutr 1985;115:411–414.
3 Rossander-Hulthén L, Brune M, Sandström B, et al: Competitive inhibition of iron absorption
  by manganese and zinc in humans. Am J Clin Nutr 1991;54:152–156.
4 Dijkhuizen MA, Wieringa FT, West CE, et al: Effects of iron and zinc supplementation in
  Indonesian infants on micronutrient status and growth. J Nutr 2001;131:2860–2865.
5 Lind T, Lönnerdal B, Stenlund H, et al: A community-based randomized controlled trial of iron
  and zinc supplementation in Indonesian infants: Interactions between iron and zinc. Am J Clin
  Nutr 2003;77:883–890.
6 Domellöf M, Lönnerdal B, Abrams SA, Hernell O: Iron absorption in breast-fed infants:
  Effects of age, iron status, iron supplements and complementary foods. Am J Clin Nutr 2002;
  76:198–204.
7 Leong W-I, Bowlus CL, Tallkvist J, Lönnerdal B: Iron supplementation during infancy –
  Effects on expression of iron transporters, iron absorption and iron utilization in rat pups. Am
  J Clin Nutr 2003;78:1203–1211.
8 Dewey KG, Domellöf M, Cohen RJ, et al: Iron supplementation affects growth and morbidity
  of breast-fed infants: Results of a randomized trial in Sweden and Honduras. J Nutr 2002;
  132:3249–3255.
9 Wieringa FT, Dijkhuizen MA, West CE, et al: Redistribution of vitamin A after iron supplementation in Indonesian infants. Am J Clin Nutr 2003;77:651–657.
10 Lönnerdal B, Hernell O: Iron, zinc, copper and selenium status of breast-fed infants and
   infants fed trace element fortified milk-based infant formula. Acta Paediatr 1994;83:367–373.
11 Fairweather-Tait SJ, Wharf SG, Fox TE: Zinc absorption in infants fed iron-fortified weaning
   food. Am J Clin Nutr 1995;62:785–789.
12 Haschke F, Ziegler EE, Edwards BB, Fomon SJ: Effect of iron fortification of infant formula
   on trace mineral absorption. J Pediatr Gastroenterol Nutr 1986;5:768–773.
13 Domellöf M, Dewey KG, Cohen RJ, et al: Iron supplements reduce erythrocyte superoxide
   dismutase activity in term, breast-fed infants. FASEB J 2003;17:A697.
14 Percival SS: Copper and immunity. Am J Clin Nutr 1998;67:1064S–1068S.
15 Derman DP, Bothwell TH, MacPhail AP, et al: Importance of ascorbic acid in the absorption
   of iron from infant foods. Scand J Haematol 1980;25:193–201.
16 Davidsson L, Walczyk T, Zavaleta N, Hurrell RF: Improving iron absorption from a Peruvian
   school breakfast meal by adding ascorbic acid or Na₂EDTA. Am J Clin Nutr 2001;73:283–287.
17 Hallberg L, Brune M, Rossander L: Iron absorption in man: Ascorbic acid and dose-dependent
   inhibition by phytate. Am J Clin Nutr 1989;49:140–144.
18 Garcia OP, Diaz M, Rosado JL, Allen LH: Ascorbic acid from lime juice does not improve the
   iron status of iron-deficient women in rural Mexico. Am J Clin Nutr 2003;78:267–273.
19 Diaz M, Rosado JL, Allen LH, et al: The efficacy of a local-ascorbic acid-rich food in improving iron absorption from Mexican diets: A field study using stable isotopes. Am J Clin Nutr
   2003;78:436–440.
20 Mejia LA, Hodges RE, Arroyave G, et al: Vitamin A deficiency and anemia in Central American
   children. Am J Clin Nutr 1977;30:1175–1184.

21 Hodges RE, Sauberlich HE, Canham JE, et al: Hematopoietic studies in vitamin A deficiency. Am J Clin Nutr 1978;31:876–885.
22 Mejia LA, Hodges RE, Rucker RB: Clinical signs of anemia in vitamin A-deficient rats. Am J Clin Nutr 1979;32:1439–1444.
23 Mejia LA, Hodges RE, Rucker RB: Role of vitamin A in the absorption, retention and distribution of iron in the rat. J Nutr 1979;109:129–137.
24 Suharno D, West CE, Muhilal, et al: Supplementation with vitamin A and iron for nutritional anaemias in pregnant women in West Java, Indonesia. Lancet 1993;342:1325–1328.
25 Garcia-Casal MN, Layrisse M, Solano L, et al: Vitamin A and β-carotene can improve nonheme iron absorption from rice, wheat and corn by humans. J Nutr 1997;128:646–650.
26 Walczyk T, Davidsson L, Rossander-Hulthen L, et al: No enhancing effect of vitamin A on iron absorption in humans. Am J Clin Nutr 2003;77:144–149.
27 Smith JC Jr, McDaniel EG, Fan FF, Halsted JA: Zinc: A trace element in vitamin A metabolism. Science 1973;181:954–955.
28 Smith JE, Brown ED, Smith JC Jr: The effect of zinc deficiency on the metabolism of retinol binding protein in the rat. J Lab Clin Med 1974;84:692–697.
29 Baly DL, Golub MS, Gershwin ME, Hurley LS: Studies on marginal zinc deprivation in rhesus monkeys. III. Effects on vitamin A metabolism. Am J Clin Nutr 1984;40:199–207.
30 Smith JC Jr: Interrelationship of zinc and vitamin A metabolism in animals and human nutrition: A review; in Prasad AS (ed): Clinical, Biochemical and Nutritional Aspects of Trace Elements. Current Topics in Nutrition and Disease. New York, Liss, 1982, vol 6, pp 239–247.
31 Hustead VA, Greger JL, Gutcher GR: Zinc supplementation and plasma concentration of vitamin A in preterm infants. Am J Clin Nutr 1988;47:1017–1021.
32 Udomkesmalee E, Dhanamitta S, Sirisinha S, et al: Effect of vitamin A and zinc supplementation on the nutriture of children in Northeast Thailand. Am J Clin Nutr 1992;56:50–57.
33 Christian P, Khatry SK, Yamini S, et al: Zinc supplementation might potentiate the effect of vitamin A in restoring night vision in pregnant Nepalese women. Am J Clin Nutr 2001:73: 1045–1051.
34 Lane M, Alfrey CP Jr, Mengel DE, et al: The rapid induction of human riboflavin deficiency with galactoflavin. J Clin Invest 1964;43:357.
35 Powers H, Bates CJ, Prentice AM, et al: The relative effectiveness of iron and iron with riboflavin in correcting a microcytic anemia in men and children in rural Gambia. Hum Nutr Clin Nutr 1983;37C:413–425.
36 Powers HJ, Bates CJ, Lamb WH: Haematological response to supplements of iron and riboflavin to pregnant and lactating women in rural Gambia. Hum Nutr Clin Nutr 1985;39:117–129.
37 Sirivech S, Driskell J, Frieden E: NADH-FMN oxidoreductase activity and iron content of organs from riboflavin-deficient and iron-deficient rats. J Nutr 1977;107:739–745.
38 Powers HJ: Investigation into the relative effects of riboflavin deprivation on iron economy in the weanling rat and the adult. Ann Nutr Metab 1986;30:308–315.
39 Adelakan DA, Thurnham DI: The influence of riboflavin deficiency on absorption and liver storage of iron in the growing rat. Br J Nutr 1986;56:171–179.
40 Powers HJ, Weaver LT, Austin S, Beresford JK: A proposed intestinal mechanism for the effect of riboflavin deficiency on iron loss in the rat. Br J Nutr 1993;69:553–561.
41 Zimmermann MB, Adou P, Torresani T, et al: Persistence of goiter despite oral iodine supplementation in goitrous children with iron deficiency anemia in the Côte d'Ivoire. Am J Clin Nutr 2000;71:88–93.
42 Hess SY, Zimmermann MB, Adou P, et al: Treatment of iron deficiency in goitrous children improves the efficacy of iodized salt in Côte d'Ivoire. Am J Clin Nutr 2002;75:743–748.
43 Zimmermann MB, Adou P, Torresani T, et al: Iron supplementation in goitrous, iron-deficient children improves their response to oral iodized oil. Eur J Endocrinol 2000;142:217–223.
44 Beard JL, Brigham DE, Kelley SK, Green MH: Plasma thyroid hormone kinetics are altered in iron-deficient rats. J Nutr 1998;128:1401–1408.
45 Smith SM, Finley J, Johnson LK, Lukaski HC: Indices of in vivo and in vitro thyroid hormone metabolism in iron-deficient rats. Nutr Res 1994;14:729–739.
46 Beard JL, Borel MJ, Derr J: Impaired thermoregulation and thyroid function in iron-deficiency anemia. Am J Clin Nutr 1990;52:813–819.
47 Dillman E, Gale C, Green W, et al: Hypothermia in iron deficiency due to altered triiodothyronine metabolism. Am J Physiol 1980;239:R377–R381.

48 Penny ME, Peerson JM, Marin RM, et al: Randomized, community-based trials of the effect of zinc supplementation, with and without other micronutrients, on the duration of persistent childhood diarrhea in Lima, Peru. J Pediatr 1999;135:208–217.

Discussion

Dr. Specker: I am curious, you talk about iron fortification or supplementation and its relationship to copper deficiency, but I guess I was not playing close enough attention. Do you think that it is a short- or a long-term effect?

Dr. Lönnerdal: I think it is a long-term effect. The copper absorption study was conducted during a short period of time but the study in which we saw the effects was a long-term fortification study [1]. So I think it is a long-term effect rather than an acute one. There may also be an acute effect, but I think here the concern should be about the long-term outcome because again when we give iron we tend to do it for the long-term. We want to have a program in place where we give iron as a supplement or as a fortificant, but very few studies have looked at copper status.

Dr. Barclay: In Indonesia, was that a supplementation study or a fortification study?

Dr. Lönnerdal: That was a supplementation study, iron drops or zinc drops or a combination.

Dr. Pettifor: Your study on iron supplementation and the reduction in growth, do you have any idea of the cause for this reduction of growth? Was it an anorexia issue, or was it an intake problem?

Dr. Lönnerdal: No, it was not an intake problem, we did not see an effect on that. I can only speculate. We are doing some secondary data analysis right now looking in particular at the Honduran cohort. We were surprised that we saw it in Honduras actually because we didn't think that we had the statistical power to detect this but we did. My guess right now is that we are impairing zinc status, and we know that zinc, certainly zinc deficiency or even marginal zinc deficiency, reduces IGF-I, and there is a potential link to linear growth. So possibly it could be an indirect effect via zinc. There is the possibility that other micronutrients could be affected but zinc and growth are ultimately connected, and again we know that iron certainly does have an effect on zinc as we saw in these studies. It will also be interesting to complete the iron absorption study we published [2], and that is what I referred to earlier together with Dr. Abrams; we saw no downregulation at a young age but we saw it in older infants. In the same cohort we actually have stable zinc and stable copper absorption results, but we have not completed the data calculation yet. Hopefully, these results will aid in our interpretations.

Dr. Abrams: Has anyone thought to give iron in the morning and zinc in the evening, or some approach like that?

Dr. Lönnerdal: That was my conclusion from these studies but I have not pursued it yet. I think that is what we need to try because supplementation can be very effective, and in many settings it may be the only practical way to prevent or treat deficiencies. I believe it will be necessary to take the supplements on separate occasions, like morning/evening (red pill, blue pill or whatever to try to distinguish them), but my feeling is that gastric emptying needs to be complete before the next one is given. It may also be possible to give them on alternate days. The problem may be that for zinc you cannot skip too many days because we don't have any stores for zinc. For iron there has been discussion about whether we can give weekly instead of daily supplements; would it be possible to give it every other day? We need to have some new approaches: either on the same day but spread apart or alternate days or something like that.

Dr. Delgado: What is your opinion on the delivery interactions of micronutrients in the special condition of catch-up growth in premature babies? A better evolution of catch-up growth in premature babies supplemented with zinc has recently been shown.

Dr. Lönnerdal: I haven't really worked on that myself. There are many studies that show a very positive effect of zinc on catch-up growth [3]. I think we need to go back and look a little bit at interactions because the hematologists really like to give a lot of iron to these premature babies to make them catch up when it comes to hematology. Many pediatricians caring about the growth of the infants like to give zinc. So there are all kinds of possibilities for interactions. In reference to what Dr. Abrams eluded to, we really don't know how effective infants are when it comes to turning iron into hemoglobin at a young age. We have done radioisotope studies on infant rhesus monkeys showing similar results as stable isotope studies in human infants [4]. When infants are young they are not very good at incorporating iron into hemoglobin. The question is what do they do with the iron in the case that they are not putting it into hemoglobin? It would be nice if they put iron into ferritin because that is a fairly innocuous form of iron, but I am not quite sure they are doing that judging from our human data. So the question is: if you have iron floating around in the system and not making ferritin or hemoglobin, what is it doing? I think we need to go back and look critically at those studies because zinc researchers have usually looked at the zinc effect, the iron researchers have looked at the iron effect, and very few studies have looked at them together, which is a bit surprising to me.

Dr. Zlotkin: We recently completed a study with Sprinkles which I call a fortification methodology because it is a supplement added to food. This was a double-labeled stable isotope study in which we actually gave the ^{50}Fe intravenously and the ^{57}Fe orally. There were 3 groups and each group received 30 mg iron and 50 mg ascorbic acid: 1 group had no zinc; the 2nd group had 5 mg, and the 3rd group had 10 mg zinc. The question we asked was: does the provision of zinc as a fortificant impact on iron absorption? What we saw was a significant impact of 10 mg but not of either 0 or 5 mg. This has not been published yet but for the sake of this discussion, again as a fortificant.

Dr. Lönnerdal: I think that the ratio between iron and zinc is very critical. I prefer fortification because I think it is a much more biologically safe way of providing minerals like iron and zinc. We have done a fortification study and we know how much iron can be added and how absorbable is it. It may be safer but it is not as effective as one would like.

Dr. Zlotkin: The dietary reference intake (DRI) process has recently come up with upper limits or upper levels, and for zinc the level recommended is in fact lower than the 10 mg that you used in your studies in Indonesia. There has been a lot of discussion and controversy around the relatively low upper limit that was defined for infants under the age of 2 years, and I believe the upper limit was something like 6 mg/day, between 5 and 6 mg/day. Any comments on whether or not the potentially adverse effects you might be seeing have anything to do with going above the upper limit?

Dr. Lönnerdal: Not really, I think that actually the safe level is quite a bit higher, and we know that from our Swedish studies, for example. The formula zinc level has been 10 mg/l for quite some time, but when it was increased, there was more iron so the iron problem was taken care of first. Then the zinc content was balanced in order to not interfere with iron, but at the same time making sure that there was enough zinc. This example was a formula with a very high phytate content. It is not that I don't believe in the DRI but I think that we can overcome the problems by carefully considering the dietary matrix and the ratio between iron and zinc.

Dr. Lozoff: We just completed a large trial on preventing iron deficiency anemia in Chile and found no effect of iron supplementation on growth in that study [5]. There were over 1,600 babies between 6 and 12 months old who were supplemented. In this situation there was a lot of iron deficiency in the first place. But in Honduras there may be a different effect.

Dr. Lönnerdal: We saw no overall effect on growth in Honduras, but when we split them up by initial iron status, it was found.

Dr. Lozoff: This is one of the things that we haven't done yet. These babies were all breast-fed, but should we look at those who are exclusively breast-fed separately? There is another thing I wanted to ask you about. A new study, recently published in the *Journal of Pediatrics* [6], reports iron supplementation to totally breast-fed babies in Canada beginning at 1 month of age. In this small study, an increase in hemoglobin was found in those given iron both at 6 and 12 months, but no differences in growth. A very low dose of iron was given (7.5 mg/day). If prevention with such a low dose of iron is used, would there still be concern about interactions or growth?

Dr. Lönnerdal: In the Swedish and Honduras studies we also used 1 mg/kg/day, definitely a very modest level. We have also seen some studies that used designs similar to ours with the iron/zinc combination, but at different sites [7], and when the amount was adequately small no effect was found. To find an effect on growth of course a large sample size is needed, and we found an effect at that level when the groups were larger. More studies need to be done on that. In a population like the Canadian one I would be hesitant to give iron starting at 1 month of age. Even though I believe that iron is good for us, it is a very toxic element and I think we have underestimated the negative effects of iron. A balanced approach should be used.

Dr. Mannar: In your studies on the use of ascorbic acid in fortified foods in which you found no effect of ascorbic acid, I was wondering whether one of the possible reasons could be that ascorbic acid is lost during food processing?

Dr. Lönnerdal: It was not my study, it was a study by Garcia et al. [8]. It was prepared with freshly made lime juice and consumed as a drink, so it was not part of the food preparation. They also analyzed the vitamin C content.

Dr. Hurrell: I was quite surprised by the efficacy study of Garcia et al. [8] showing no effect of ascorbic acid on iron status. I suppose the drinks were fed with the meal. Perhaps one of the explanations could be that the phytic acid content of the diet was higher than the meal which was tested as a single meal absorption study. If we consider the various studies which have been made on the molar ratios of ascorbic acid to iron needed to overcome the inhibitory effect of phytate, when the phytic acid content is high, what is now recommended is a 4:1 molar ratio of ascorbic acid to iron, that is 12:1 by weight. So if the diet contains 10 mg iron you would need to have something like 120 mg ascorbic acid in order to expect an increase in iron absorption. I think in the study by Garcia et al. 2 × 25 mg of ascorbic acid was fed. I would imagine that this is not a high enough level. I don't know how high the phytic acid was in their meals, but perhaps this is an explanation for why they failed to show an effect of ascorbic acid on iron status.

Dr. Lönnerdal: It could be and I can check with Dr. Allen. In the 8-month study they used meals of similar composition to the one used in the stable isotope study. Of course in the stable isotope study the meals were very well defined, but in the free-living setting they were typical Mexican meals. Just as there are no really typical American or Swedish meals, I don't think there is a typical Mexican meal, the diet varies. It could be that there was regularly more phytate than in the defined meal; this is quite possible. It is also potentially possible that when vitamin C faces the intestinal mucosa, the iron-regulatory mechanism adapts to this situation just as it does for calcium. However, more studies are needed.

Dr. Zlotkin: I just want to get back to your point of iron supplementation versus fortification. Again the American/Canadian DRI of iron for infants at about 1 year of age is 11 mg/day. That is the current recommended dose. The assumption is that that would be not as a supplement but as the iron found in food, and in fact when you look at the intake of iron from any data from America the intake of iron is around this range or even higher for the 1-year-old in America today. Again, although I can't recall that anyone has specifically done placebo-controlled trials looking at growth, we really do define our growth expectations internationally based on that population. So I just want to make sure and be clear on what you are saying. You are not suggesting that an intake of 10 or 11 mg/day from food as recommended in the DRI would have specifically negative effects on growth, you are specifically talking about when it is given as a supplement at a young age, and that is perhaps under 6 months of age.

Dr. Lönnerdal: Exactly, I think it is only as a supplement. There are many studies showing that when iron is in the diet these effects are not seen at all.

Dr. Castillo-Durán: One of my concerns is whether this interaction also remains in the condition of disease. For instance in the studies from India or other countries, all the children have diseases, parasitic infections and so on. Does this interaction remain on the same level or is it higher? Do you have any information about this confounding variable which is important for many countries?

Dr. Lönnerdal: I think you are hitting on something very sensitive here and I think you are right, and Dr. Semba will talk more about this. For example, if this is a zinc-mediated effect certainly growth is affected and I would certainly expect immune function to be affected, and then again these effects could be expected for a variety of diseases. We were very close to seeing a significant effect on infection, both upper respiratory disease and diarrheal disease, but statistical significance was not reached for that. In a larger cohort it would perhaps have been seen. But in studies like those in Honduras and Sweden, all infants with acute infection were omitted from the studies by analyzing C-reactive protein. There were not many; in neither Honduras nor Sweden did we find many with elevated C-reactive protein.

References

1 Lönnerdal B, Hernell O: Iron, zinc, copper and selenium status of breast-fed infants and infants fed trace element fortified milk-based infant formula. Acta Paediatr 1994;83:367–373.
2 Domellöf M, Lönnerdal B, Abrams SA, Hernall O: Iron absorption in breast-fed infants: Effects of age, iron status, iron supplements and complimentary foods. Am J Clin Nutr 2002;76: 198–204.
3 Brown KH, Peerson JM, Rivera J, Allen LH: Effect of supplemental zinc on the growth and serum zinc concentrations of prepubertal children: A meta-analysis of randomized controlled trials. Am J Clin Nutr 2002;75:1062–1071.
4 Fomon SJ, Ziegler EE, Serfass RE, et al: Less than 80% of absorbed iron is promptly incorporated into erythrocytes of infants. J Nutr 2000;130:45–52.
5 Lozoff B, De Andraca I, Castillo M, et al: Behavioral and developmental effects of preventing iron-deficiency anemia in healthy full-term infants. Pediatrics 2003;112:846–854.
6 Friel JK, Aziz K, Andrews WL, et al: A double-masked, randomized control trial of iron supplementation in early infancy in healthy term breast-fed infants. J Pediatr 2003;143:582–586.
7 Dijkhuisen MA, Wieringa FT, West CE, et al: Effects of iron and zinc supplementation in Indonesian infants on micronutrient status and growth. J Nutr 2001;131:2860–2865.
8 Garcia OP, Diaz M, Rosado JL, Allen LH: Ascorbic acid from lime juice does not improve the iron status of iron-deficient women in rural Mexico. Am J Clin Nutr 2003;78:267–273.

Pettifor JM, Zlotkin S (eds): Micronutrient Deficiencies during the Weaning Period and the
First Years of Life. Nestlé Nutrition Workshop Series Pediatric Program, vol 54, pp 83–103,
Nestec Ltd., Vevey/S. Karger AG, Basel, © 2004.

Influence of Food Intake, Composition and Bioavailability on Micronutrient Deficiencies of Infants during the Weaning Period and the First Year of Life

R.S. Gibson[a], *C. Hotz*[1] *and L.A. Perlas*[2]

[a]Department of Human Nutrition, University of Otago, Dunedin, New Zealand

Introduction

In recent years, the promotion of breast-feeding has received much attention. This emphasis, however, has overshadowed efforts in many developing countries to provide safe and nutritionally adequate complementary foods for infants and young children, and this critical aspect of young child feeding has been severely neglected. This is unfortunate in view of the overwhelming importance of complementary feeding practices and behaviors on the growth, development, health and wellbeing of young children. Indeed, the World Health Organization has urged that programs to improve complementary feeding practices and behaviors are given the highest priority [1].

It is now well established that at about 6 months of age, the supply of energy and certain nutrients from breast milk is no longer adequate to meet an infant's needs [2]. Consequently, complementary foods, preferably with a relatively high energy and nutrient density, must be provided after 6 months of age until the child is ready to consume the same foods as those consumed by the rest of the family members. Increasingly, research has shown that in developing countries and in some more affluent countries, the nutritional adequacy of these complementary foods is compromised in terms of their quantity and/or dietary quality [2]. Such inadequacies are especially serious

---

[1]Currently at the Centro de Investigacion en Nutricion y Salud, Instituto Nacional de Salud Publica, Cuernavaca, Mexico.
[2]Currently at Food and Nutrition Research Institute, Metro Manila, Philippines.

for children less than 2 years of age, whose nutritional requirements at this time are higher per kilogram body weight than at any other time during the life cycle. The challenge of meeting these high requirements is exacerbated by the limited gastric capacity of infants ($\sim$30–40 g/kg body weight) [2], and the frequency with which meals can be provided, coupled in developing countries with high rates of infection.

Effect of Total Food Intake on Micronutrient Intakes

Several factors are known to affect the total amount of complementary foods consumed during the weaning period, and thus in turn the adequacy of micronutrient intakes. These factors have been reviewed in detail elsewhere [2–4], and are classified into three groups: caregiver behaviors; child-related factors, and dietary factors. Only the latter two will be considered here.

Child-Related Factors

Of the child-related factors, those related to appetite have received the most attention in part because of the repeated reports of poor appetite in young children in developing countries [4]. Studies have shown that appetite and, hence, food intake is often reduced during illness. Moreover, the incidence of illness, especially diarrhea, peaks during the second half of infancy, coinciding with the period when the contribution of complementary foods to total dietary requirements increases markedly [2].

Nonetheless, among Peruvian infants, $\sim$30% of days with reported anorexia occurred regardless of the presence of other illnesses, suggesting that other important causes of anorexia exist [3, 4]. In these same infants, the energy intake from complementary foods was reduced by $\sim$25–35% on those days when mothers reported poor appetite. Such a reduction in energy intake was probably accompanied by a concomitant decrease in micronutrient intakes, although the latter were not reported in this Peruvian study. In a community-based study in rural Malawi, a 30% reduction in energy intake from complementary foods for those infants whose mothers reported poor appetites [5] was accompanied by nearly a 33% reduction in iron, zinc, and vitamin A intakes.

Additional factors that may induce alterations in appetite and thus food intake are micronutrient deficiencies per se, specifically deficiencies of iron and zinc [2, 3]. Whether these effects are mediated by changes in physical activity, rates of infection, or direct changes in neuropeptides that control appetite is unknown. Some iron and zinc supplementation studies have reported increases in appetite or weight gain in response to additional iron or zinc [6].

Diet-Related Factors

The main dietary factors known to influence total complementary food intake are the frequency of feeding and the energy density, as well as the physicochemical, and organoleptic characteristics of the food [3, 4].

Feeding Frequency. In many developing countries infants may receive only 2–3 complementary feedings per day on average because they eat together with adult family members [2]. Experimental studies on fully weaned, recovering malnourished children have shown that a marked increase in energy intake can be achieved by increasing feeding frequency, when the level of energy density has been controlled [2–4].

Energy/Nutrient Density. Some studies have shown that children consume less food or formula (g/kg/day) as the energy densities of the complementary foods increase, thus apparently compensating in part, for the differing energy densities of their diets [2, 3]. Despite this apparent adjustment, however, the resultant total daily intakes of energy and micronutrients are increased when more energy-dense diets are consumed [3], provided micronutrient-containing sources of energy and not oil or sugar are used. Experimental studies have confirmed similar increases in total energy and thus micronutrient intakes after reducing the viscosity of stiff high-energy porridges by the addition of amylase-rich flours [3, 5, 8].

Food Variety. Increasing the variety of complementary foods may also enhance food intake, and thus in turn energy and micronutrient intakes. Underwood [9] and later Brown et al. [10] in an experimentally controlled study reported that, when children received a varied dietary regimen, they consumed ~10% more than when consuming monotonous diets.

Combined Strategies. A combination of these strategies discussed above can be used to increase food intake, and hence energy and micronutrient intakes during complementary feeding in developing countries. These may include increasing feeding frequency, probably to a maximum of 4 meals/day, increasing the energy/nutrient density of the complementary diets, and increasing the variety and tastefulness of nutritious foods in the diet. The choice of the most effective combination to implement will depend on the limitations of current feeding practices within the population group, as discussed by the WHO [2].

In a study in rural Malawi, a nutrition education intervention employed a combination of strategies to increase the amount of complementary foods consumed, and their energy and nutrient densities [5]. Results are shown in figure 1. Significant increases in the amount of complementary food consumed and the energy density of the diets in the intervention compared to the control group led, in turn, to higher intakes of energy, iron and zinc, as shown in figure 1.

Effect of Dietary Quality on Micronutrient Intakes from Complementary Foods

Poor dietary quality is often inherent in complementary foods in developing countries where the poor socioeconomic and environmental factors

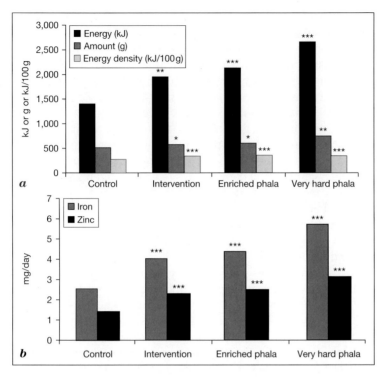

Fig. 1. Dietary intakes from complementary foods by Malawian children (9–24 months of age) compared between the control (n = 40) and intervention groups (n = 71) and users of enriched porridge (phala; n = 34) or very hard phala (16% dry matter; n = 21) on the day of dietary recall. **a** The energy intake, amount, and energy density of the complementary diet are shown. **b** The corresponding intakes of iron and zinc are shown. Data represent adjusted means with the number given above each column. Significant differences between control group and other groups: *p < 0.05; **p < 0.01; ***p < 0.001 (linear regression model controlling for age, sex, and whether intakes were considered by the mother to be usual or unusually poor).

limit the types of foods available [11]. Typically the complementary foods are based on starch-based staple foods (i.e. cereals, roots/tubers); very few sources of animal foods, rich sources of several key micronutrients, are included [12]. This pattern poses two important barriers to adequate micronutrient nutriture for weanlings. First, a low diversity of food sources, especially few animal-source foods, limits dietary quality as it decreases the chance of acquiring good food sources of all nutrients [13]. Secondly, the antinutrient content of plant-based staples such as unrefined cereals and legumes, pose further limitations to dietary quality through their negative impact on bioavailability [12].

Dietary Diversity

The relationship between the dietary diversity and dietary quality of complementary diets has been studied by several investigators [2, 5, 13, 14]. Results have confirmed that when complementary diets with a higher dietary diversity are consumed, micronutrient intakes (per day) and micronutrient densities (per 100 kcal) increase [13, 14]. Moreover, in Mexican preschoolers [15], lower rates of stunting were linked with more diverse diets, attributed to enhanced bioavailability of calcium, iron and zinc, compared to that from diets based on high phytate, maize-based tortillas. Promoting dietary diversity also provides infants with an important opportunity to appreciate different tastes and textures of food, both critical attributes for developing good eating habits in the future [2].

Micronutrient Bioavailability

It is noteworthy that the nutrients consistently reported to be most limiting in the complementary diets of infants in developing countries during the first years of life, calcium, iron, and zinc, and in some cases, vitamin A, are also those for which the reported inadequacies are often exacerbated by poor bioavailability. The latter arises because the complementary diets are predominantly based on cereals and legumes, especially in developing countries where consumption of animal source foods is low [2, 5, 12, 14]. Moreover, these plant-based complementary foods are often provided during the first 3 months, when they displace breast milk [2, 3, 5, 14]. Even in the more affluent countries, consumption of meat and fish during infancy is low [16, 17].

To date there have been very few in vivo isotope studies in humans that have measured the bioavailability of micronutrients in complementary foods; some exist for iron and zinc in complementary foods used in developed countries [18, 19]. Several dietary components modify the bioavailability of these limiting micronutrients: some enhance and others inhibit absorption. Of the dietary inhibitors, phytate is of particular concern for complementary foods based on cereals and legumes, depending on the preparation or processing methods used [2, 5, 12, 14, 19]. Phytate chelates certain minerals, and inhibits their absorption across the intestinal mucosa. The inhibition of zinc absorption by phytate is well established, and follows a dose-response effect. Phytate in unprocessed food is composed primarily of the hexa- and penta-inositol phosphate forms that inhibit zinc absorption [5, 12, 14]. Some processing methods (e.g. fermentation) can cause the dephosphorylation of the inositol phosphates to lower inositol forms (i.e., mono- to tetra-inositol phosphates) via microbial phytase enzymes, which do not have an inhibiting effect on zinc absorption. Soaking can also reduce the total content of phytate in cereal flours (e.g. maize and rice) and most legume flours because it is stored in a relatively water-soluble form, and hence can be removed by diffusion [5, 12, 14]. Phytate also inhibits non-heme iron absorption in cereal-based

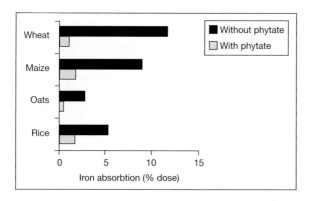

Fig. 2. Influence of phytic acid degradation on iron absorption from wheat, maize, oats, and rice porridges. Adapted from Hurrell et al. [19].

complementary foods [18, 19]. Even small amounts produce an inhibitory effect and, unlike zinc, the myo-inositol phosphates must contain less than 3 phosphate groups before iron absorption is no longer inhibited [20].

Any reduction in the total phytate content of complementary porridges based on cereals and legumes has the potential to enhance absorption of iron and zinc. This has been confirmed by two in vivo human stable isotope studies in which adults consumed tortillas or polenta prepared with a low phytic acid maize strain and wild-type unmodified maize [20, 21], and by a recent study by Hurrell et al. [19]. They demonstrated increases in iron absorption from porridges prepared from a variety of dephytinized cereals compared to those with their native phytate content. Dephytinization of rice, oat, maize and wheat porridges prepared with water resulted in 3- to 12-fold increases in iron absorption as shown in figure 2. In this study, the phytic acid was degraded by the addition of exogenous phytase, and iron absorption was measured in adult humans with an extrinsic-label radioiron technique.

The inhibitory effect of phytate on zinc absorption may be further exacerbated by high levels of calcium, which reduce the solubility of the phytate-mineral complex [12]. Some single meal isotopic studies suggest that high levels of calcium (both supplemental and dairy products) inhibit non-heme iron absorption, although whole diet studies have produced conflicting results [2]. The conflict may be due in part to differences in the iron status of the individuals being studied. However, the calcium content of most plant-based complementary foods is too low to have any detrimental effect [12].

Polyphenols and tannins are also important inhibitors of non-heme iron absorption; they form insoluble iron-phenolic compounds [19]. Complementary foods based on certain cereals (e.g. red sorghum and finger millet) and legumes (e.g. red kidney beans, black beans and black grams) may contain high levels of polyphenols. As well, beverages such as tea or coffee that contain

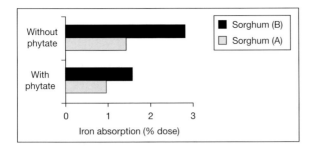

Fig. 3. Iron absorption from low (B) and high (A) tannin sorghum porridges with and without native phytate. Modified from Hurrell et al. [19].

polyphenols are sometimes introduced into an infant's diet, and have been associated with suboptimal iron status during infancy [22, 23]. The inhibitory effect of polyphenols on iron absorption was also demonstrated in the in vivo isotope study of Hurrell et al. [19] by comparing iron absorption after dephytinization of high-tannin and tannin-free varieties of sorghum. Results are shown in figure 3. A nearly 2-fold increase in iron absorption was observed in a tannin-free variety of dephytinized sorghum (B), whereas no significant increase in iron absorption occurred in the high-tannin dephytinized variety (A) [19].

Animal source foods play an important role in optimizing iron and zinc nutriture of weanlings. Apart from their high content of bioavailable heme iron and zinc, animal protein also has an enhancing effect on non-heme iron and zinc absorption [2, 12]. This has been confirmed by stable isotope studies comparing iron and zinc absorption in infants consuming vegetable or cereal-based complementary foods with those based on meat [24, 25].

Cellular animal protein also partially counteracts the inhibition by phytate on non-heme iron and zinc absorption [2, 12]. Hence, even the addition of a small amount of animal source foods can play an important role in improving the bioavailability of both non-heme iron and zinc in complementary foods, and thus in turn iron and zinc nutriture during infancy. Nevertheless, intervention studies to examine the effect of the greater intake of meat as a complementary food on the iron and zinc status of infants have yielded inconsistent results [18]. Postulated reasons for the absence of any benefit may include that the iron and zinc nutriture of the infants was already adequate, and/or the study had insufficient power to detect any differences in the rate of iron or zinc deficiency between the 2 groups.

In view of the limited amount of in vivo absorption data from complementary foods based on human studies, the bioavailability of iron and zinc in complementary foods is often estimated from bioavailability algorithms. We have applied the bioavailability algorithms compiled by Murphy et al. [26] to estimate the intakes of available iron and zinc in the complementary

Table 1. Intakes of total iron and zinc, estimated available iron and zinc, phytate and phytate:zinc molar ratios (25th, 75th percentile) from complementary foods for Malawian infants

	Harvest season		Hungry season	
	6–8 months	9–11 months	6–8 months	9–11 months
Number	26[a]	32	20	34
Iron, mg	1.2	2.8	1.5	2.3
	(0.5, 2.5)	(1.8, 3.4)	(1.1, 2.4)	(1.5, 3.0)
Available iron, μg[a]	0.07	0.20	0.11	0.15
	(0.03, 0.19)	(0.13, 0.31)	(0.06, 0.16)	(0.12, 0.22)
Available iron, %	5.5	7.4	5.7	7.1
	(4.8, 6.6)	(5.7, 9.8)	(5.3, 8.2)	(5.9, 8.6)
Zinc, mg	0.7	1.7	1.0	1.4
	(0.4, 1.7)	(1.0, 2.2)	(0.5, 1.5)	(0.9, 1.9)
Available zinc (basal), μg[a]	0.11	0.34	0.12	0.18
	(0.05, 0.40)	(0.18, 0.43)	(0.07, 0.23)	(0.12, 0.27)
Available zinc, %	14.9	19.9	13.9	12.5
	(12.1, 20.9)	(14.4, 24.5)	(10.6, 16.2)	(10.3, 15.4)
Available zinc (normative), μg[a]	0.11	0.33	0.12	0.18
	(0.05, 0.38)	(0.18, 0.40)	(0.07, 0.21)	(0.12, 0.27)
Available zinc, %[a]	14.9	18.5	13.9	12.5
	(12.1, 20.5)	(14.4, 22.2)	(10.6, 16.0)	(10.3, 15.4)
Phytate, mg, IP5+IP6	198	332	276	432
	(112, 318)	(197, 474)	(175, 397)	(277, 605)
Phytate:zinc molar ratio	26	20	31	32
	(14, 37)	(11, 31)	(25, 39)	(25, 39)

[a]Determined from total daily intakes. Modified from Hotz and Gibson [27].

maize-based diets of infants in rural Malawi at two seasons of the year: harvest and hungry season [27]. Table 1 summarizes the data on intakes of total and available iron and zinc for infants 6–8 and 9–11 months old. Details on their phytate:zinc molar ratios are also given; ratios over 15 are associated with a half-maximal absorption of zinc [12]. Note that the median estimated bioavailabilities of both iron (5.5–7.4%) and zinc (12.5–18.5%) for all age groups were low, attributed to the low intakes of both meat/fish/poultry protein (only 0–4% of iron from meat, poultry and fish) and ascorbic acid for iron, and the high phytate:zinc molar ratios for zinc. Indeed, nearly 60% of all meals consumed had a phytate:zinc ratio of >15. Note that most complementary foods based on unrefined cereals and legumes (per 100 g as eaten) have phytate:zinc molar ratios of >15 [12].

To our knowledge, there are no in vivo studies on the bioavailability of copper, manganese, selenium, or iodine in complementary foods in developed or developing countries. Lower copper absorption from infant cereals compared to milk has been reported using a weanling rat model, but the copper content of plant-based complementary foods is usually higher than the milk-based diets. Hence, it is unlikely that copper nutriture is of concern during infancy, unless infants are fed diets based on cow's milk alone [2].

For plant-based complementary foods with a low fat content, the bioavailability of fat-soluble vitamins A, D, E, and K and carotenoids may be compromised when breast-feeding ceases. Use of mild heat treatment (i.e. preparation of porridges) may release bound carotenoids from the food matrix and binding proteins, but if severe heat treatment is used, it can be detrimental. Fiber, especially the water-soluble fiber pectin, impairs β-carotene absorption by interfering with gastric emptying and with mixed-micelle formation [2]. Recent research has emphasized that the bioavailability of provitamin A β-carotene from plant sources is only half that of previous estimates [28]. Hence, if complementary diets do not include sources of preformed vitamin A from animal or dairy products, and concentrations of breast milk vitamin A content are low, deficits in vitamin A are likely to occur which cannot be overcome by the consumption of green leafy vegetables and orange-yellow fruits [28].

Evaluating the Nutritional Adequacy of Complementary Foods by Comparison with WHO Recommendations

The WHO [2] report on the estimated energy and nutrients needed from complementary foods for infants of various ages in developing countries has provided an opportunity to evaluate the nutritional adequacy of complementary foods. WHO has computed the theoretical energy and nutrient needs based on the difference between the age-specific energy and nutrient requirements and the energy and nutrients provided by breast milk, taking into account the volume and composition of breast milk consumed. The estimated needs have been compiled for low, average and high intakes of breast milk corresponding to mean -2 SD, mean, and mean $+2$ SD, respectively. Both estimated needs per day and per 100 kcal have been published; details are given in WHO [2]. Expressing the nutrient needs per 100 kcal (i.e. nutrient density) allows the identification of those nutrients most limiting in the diet because of inadequacies in total intake of complementary foods per se, or in the composition or quality of the complementary diet. As well, the adequacy of individual complementary foods to meet the estimated needs can be assessed by this method. An update of these calculations incorporating new energy and micronutrient requirements for infants is given by Dewey and Brown [3].

Comparison of micronutrient intakes (per day and per 100 kcal) from complementary foods based on assumed intakes [12] derived from data on gastric capacity [2] including actual intake data from a range of developing countries,

Table 2. Nutrient densities of complementary diets consumed by infants aged 6–8 months in seven countries compared to WHO desired densities

	WHO 1998	WHO 2002	Philippines	Bangladesh	Ghana	Malawi	Guatemala	Peru	USA
Age, months			6	6–8	6–8	6–8	6–8	6–8	6–8
Protein, g	0.7	1.0	1.7	1.9	3.3	2.3	2.2	2.6	2.6
Ca, mg	125	105	**18**	**16**	**35**	**5**	**27**	**19**	67
Fe, mg	4.0[b]	4.5[b]	**0.5**	**0.4**	**1.2**	**0.8**	**0.5**	**0.4**	3.6
Zn, mg	0.8	1.6	0.9	**0.2**	**0.6**	**0.5**	**0.4**	**0.4**	**0.4**
Vitamin A, μg RE	5	31	**0.5**	**0**	7	**2**	87	35	95
Thiamin, mg	0.04	0.08	**0.02**	0.04	0.07	0.06	0.04	0.04	0.14
Riboflavin, mg	0.07	0.08	**0.02**	**0.04**	**0.03**	**0.04**	**0.06**	0.07	0.18
Niacin, mg	1.1[a]	1.5[a]	**0.30**[a]	**0.9**[a]	**0.8**[a]	**0.7**[a]	**0.4**[a]	**0.5**[a]	1.5[a]

Values in bold print indicate that the observed density is below the reference values for the average desired density for WHO [2, 30]. Modified from Dewey and Brown [3], Perlas [14] and Hotz and Gibson [27].
[a]Excludes the contribution of dietary tryptophan to niacin synthesis.
[b]Medium bioavailability of iron assumed.

as well as the USA [2, 3], has emphasized that for certain micronutrients the amount and density from complementary foods are consistently and substantially less than the corresponding WHO [2, 3, 29] recommendations. These nutrients have been defined as 'problem nutrients'. Based on recommendations by the WHO in 1998 [2] or in 2002 [30] for the desired nutrient density levels, tables 2 and 3 clearly show that calcium, iron, and zinc are problematic for infants aged 6–8 months, and calcium and iron for those aged 9–11 months, even when moderate bioavailability is assumed. Comparable deficits exist when micronutrient intakes per day are compared with the estimated needs defined by the WHO in 1998 [2] and 2002 [30] (data not shown).

Vitamin A, riboflavin, and niacin may also be a problem nutrients for some age groups and settings, as shown in tables 2 and 3. Note that for many developing countries, the bioavailability of iron and zinc in the complementary diets may be low rather than moderate, as assumed in tables 2 and 3, because such a large proportion of energy is provided by cereals, and intake of cellular animal protein is low [2, 14, 18, 27, 29].

Deficits may also occur in the complementary diets of infants living in more affluent countries, although methodological differences limit the comparisons that can be made. Again, the micronutrient deficits most frequently reported in the diets of breast-fed and weaned infants are those for zinc and iron [2, 3, 16–18, 27], attributed to low intakes of animal source foods. Inadequacies in intakes of vitamin D, vitamin E, and vitamin B_6 have also been reported in some studies of US, Swedish, or Finnish infants [2, 18, 31, 32]. Few other studies have reported intakes of vitamin D, E, and vitamin B_6 during infancy for comparison.

Table 3. Nutrient densities of complementary diets consumed by infants aged 9–11 months in seven countries compared to WHO desired densities

	WHO 1998	WHO 2002	Philippines	Bangladesh	Ghana	Malawi	Guatemala	Peru	USA
Age, months			10	9–11	9–11	9–11	9–11	9–11	9–11
Protein, g	0.7	1	1.7	2.5	3.1	2.7	2.7	2.6	3.4
Ca, mg	78	74	**17**	**20**	**40**	**18**	**37**	**27**	**53**
Fe, mg	2.4[b]	3[b]	**0.5**	**0.4**	**1.3**	**0.8**	**0.6**	**0.4**	**1.2**
Zn, mg	0.5	1.1	1.0	**0.3**	0.6	0.5	**0.4**	**0.4**	**0.4**
Vitamin A, µg RE	9	30	**5**	**1**	9	28	62	29	88
Thiamin, mg	0.04	0.06	**0.02**	0.05	0.06	0.07	0.05	0.04	0.1
Riboflavin, mg	0.04	0.06	**0.02**	0.05	0.02	0.04	0.06	0.07	0.08
Niacin, mg	0.9[a]	1[a]	**0.35[a]**	**1.0[a]**	**0.7[a]**	**0.8[a]**	**0.5[a]**	**0.5[a]**	1.1[a]

Values in bold print indicate that the observed density is below the reference values for the average desired density [2, 33]. Modified from Dewey and Brown [3], Perlas [14] and Hotz and Gibson [27].

[a]Excludes the contribution of dietary tryptophan to niacin synthesis.

[b]Medium bioavailability of iron.

Deficits may also occur in manganese, iodine, and selenium, but accurate food composition data for these micronutrients are sparse, especially in developing countries [2]. Moreover, levels for iodine and selenium (as well as zinc) depend on soil trace element levels, so that unless region-specific food composition data are used to calculate intakes for these trace elements, or laboratory analysis is undertaken, an accurate assessment of their adequacy is difficult.

Caution must be used when extrapolating deficiencies based on dietary data alone, because the requirement estimates for some nutrients during infancy are uncertain, leading to large discrepancies among published requirement estimates [2, 3]. There is still considerable uncertainty regarding the nutrient composition values in the food-composition databases used to calculate nutrient intakes, and in the concentrations of certain nutrients in breast milk. Nevertheless, these comparisons do suggest that complementary diets for infants aged between 6 and 12 months of age from both developing and more affluent countries are limiting at least in iron, zinc, and probably calcium [2, 3].

Are These Dietary Inadequacies Associated with Micronutrient Deficiencies during the Complementary Feeding Period?

It is evident from the discussion above that deficits in both the quantity and quality of complementary foods contribute to the coexistence of several micronutrient deficits. Nevertheless, studies examining interrelationships

Table 4. Prevalence of multiple biochemical micronutrient deficiencies

Biochemical index	Vietnam [35] (n = 160) 6–24 months	Indonesia [34] (n = 478) 4 months	Ghana [33] (n = 152) 6 months	New Zealand [16, 37] (n = 22) 6–12 months
Hemoglobin <110 g/l	46	57	30	52
Plasma ferritin <12 μg/l	–	20	17	13
Plasma Zn <10.7 μmol/l	36	17	4	52
Plasma retinol <0.7 μmol/l	46	54	26	–
RBC B-2 <200 μmol/l packed RBC	–	–	14	–
Urinary iodine <50 μg/l[a]	–	–	–	51

[a]Moderate iodine deficiency.

between dietary inadequacies and biochemical micronutrient deficits among weanlings, and adverse functional health outcomes are limited. Indeed, only a few studies have quantified the prevalence of multiple biochemical micronutrient deficiencies in weanlings, notably iron, zinc, vitamin A, and riboflavin; available results are summarized in table 2 [33–38]. Note that at least a third of the infants in each developing country represented have low hemoglobin concentrations indicative of anemia, compared to <4% in New Zealand [16]. In contrast, the prevalence of low serum/plasma retinol and serum/plasma zinc values varies markedly across countries. Biochemical data confirming deficiencies of iodine, selenium, riboflavin, niacin, and vitamin B_6 among weanlings are more limited [31, 33, 34; in the New Zealand study, 51% of the breast-fed infants had low urinary iodine concentrations, 37]. Note that some of these prevalence data are based on observational studies in which it is difficult to control for the adverse environmental factors (e.g. parasitic infections), or hereditary diseases (e.g. hemoglobinopathies) that may also have a detrimental effect on micronutrient status.

Very few of the studies in table 4 have examined relationships between micronutrient intakes from complementary foods and biochemical status, with the exception of Ghana [33] and New Zealand [16]. In Ghana [33], the intakes of iron, vitamin A, and energy from complementary foods were positively associated with plasma ferritin, plasma retinol, and zinc status, respectively, in infants at 12 months, whereas the intake of calcium from foods was negatively associated with zinc status. In New Zealand infants aged

Table 5. Multi-micronutrient efficacy trials of infants and their impact on biochemical status and growth

Country	n	Initial age months	Duration months	Study design	Effects on growth	Effects on micronutrient status
China [41]	164	6–13	3	V/M fortified vs. unfortified rusk	NS	↑ Hb; ↓ Vit E; NS Vit A, riboflavin, Fe indices
Ghana [40]	208	6	6	Weanimix, ±V/M; Weanimix with fish powder; Fermented maize with fish powder vs. cross-sectional comparison group	NS among groups ↑ Wt and ht in intervention vs. comparison group	↑ Vit A, ferritin (in V/M group only); NS Hb, riboflavin, Zn
Vietnam [35]	163	6–24	3	Fe, Zn, Vit A, Vit C weekly, daily or placebo	↑ Ht only in stunted children	↑ Hb, vit A, Zn
Guatemala [42]	259	6	8	BSC+V/M, V/M, BSC or placebo	NS	NS vitamins A and E
Mexico [36]	319	8–14	12	V/M vs. placebo	↑ Ht in those <12 months at baseline	Not yet reported
Indonesia [43]	478	4	6	Fe+Zn; Fe; Zn; placebo	NS	↑ Hb in Fe; Fe+Zn; ↑ ferritin in Fe; Fe+Zn ↑ Zn in Zn; Fe+Zn

V/M = Vitamin/mineral; BSC = bovine serum concentrate; Hb = hemoglobin; NS = not significant; Wt = weight; Ht = height. Modified from Dewey [44].

6–12 months, serum ferritin was positively associated with intakes of iron and vitamin C, but negatively with calcium and dietary fiber [16], while hair zinc was significantly associated with the proportion and absolute amount of energy provided by meat (Ferguson EL, personal commun.); iodine intakes could not be calculated because of the paucity of data on the iodine content of complementary foods in New Zealand.

Some randomized trials with micronutrient supplements or fortificants, notably iron, zinc, and/or vitamin A, provided singly or in combination, have demonstrated significant reductions in the prevalence of biochemical micronutrient deficiencies, based on hemoglobin, ferritin, serum retinol, and plasma zinc; reductions in the prevalence of low riboflavin biochemical indices have not been reported [33]. In some but not all of these studies, improvements in functional outcomes, mainly growth, have also been reported after supplementation or fortification with single [6, 38, 39] or multiple micronutrients [35, 40, 41], depending on the micronutrients, study group, and the setting; these studies have been summarized elsewhere [6, 44]. Table 5 summarizes the available efficacy trials of multiple micronutrients as supplements or fortificants that have measured both biochemical indices and growth [44].

The results in tables 4 and 5 confirm that biochemical micronutrient deficiencies, notably iron, zinc, and vitamin A, do exist among weanlings, sometimes concurrently in some settings, induced at least in part by micronutrient inadequacies during the complementary feeding period. Nevertheless, the results have not been consistent. In the single micronutrient supplement or fortificant studies, some of the discordant results may be due in part to the coexistence of multiple micronutrient deficiencies, which may suppress the effect of the micronutrient under study if it is not the first limiting micronutrient [36]. Additional factors that may also play a role in both the single and multiple micronutrient supplement or fortificant trials include differences in initial age and nutritional status of infants, duration of intervention, form and level of supplements or fortificants, study design, inadequate sample size, and constraints on growth due to infection, prenatal factors, and parenteral size [45].

Conclusions and Recommendations

It is apparent that inadequacies in iron, calcium, and zinc consistently arise in complementary diets used in both developing and affluent countries. In some countries, deficits in certain vitamins (e.g. vitamin A, riboflavin, niacin, vitamin B_6) and iodine and selenium may also occur, depending on the dietary staple used and the soil iodine and selenium levels.

Nevertheless, studies examining interrelationships between dietary and biochemical micronutrient deficits among weanlings, and adverse functional health outcomes are limited.

Several non-nutritional factors, notably infection, are known to exacerbate certain micronutrient deficiency states in weanlings, and confound such relationships. Hence, ensuring adequate intakes of readily available micronutrients in complementary foods alone may not necessarily ensure optimal growth, health and development during infancy and early childhood.

To accomplish the latter, a comprehensive and integrated approach is needed. Such an approach should emphasize nutrition prior to and during pregnancy, promote exclusive breast-feeding for about 6 months, followed by the use of micronutrient-dense complementary foods, and incorporate effective nutrition and health education messages. Only when a combination of such strategies is used can optimal growth, health, motor and cognitive development during infancy and early childhood in developing countries be expected.

References

1 World Health Organization: Global Consultation on Complementary Feeding. Department of Child and Adolescent Health and Development: Department of Nutrition for Health and Development. Geneva, WHO, 2001.
2 World Health Organization: Complementary feeding of young children in developing countries: A review of current scientific knowledge Geneva, WHO, 1998.
3 Dewey KG, Brown KH: Update on technical issues concerning complementary feeding of young children in developing countries and implications for intervention programs. Food Nutr Bull 2003;24:5–28.
4 Brown KH: Complementary feeding in developing countries: Factors affecting energy intake. Proc Nutr Soc 1997;56:139–148.
5 Hotz C: Assessment and Improvement of Complementary Diets in Rural Malawi with a Special Focus on Zinc; unpublished PhD thesis, University of Otago, 2000.
6 Gibson RS, Hotz C: Nutritional causes of linear growth failure during complementary feeding; in Martorell R, Haschke F (eds): Nutrition and Growth. Nestle Nutrition Workshop Series Pediatric Program. Nestec Ltd., Vevey, Nestec/Philadelphia, Lippincott Williams and Wilkins, 2001, vol 47, pp 159–196.
7 Bennett VA, Morales E, Gonzalez J, et al: Effects of dietary viscosity and energy density on total daily energy consumption by young Peruvian children. Am J Clin Nutr 1999;70:285–291.
8 Vieu MC, Traore T, Treche S: Effects of energy density and sweetness of gruels on Burkinabe infant energy intakes in free living conditions. Int J Food Sci Nutr 2001;52:213–218.
9 Underwood BA: Weaning practices in deprived environments: The weaning dilemma. Pediatrics 1985;75:194–198.
10 Brown KH, Sanchez-Griñan M, Perez F, et al: Effects of dietary energy density and feeding frequency on total daily intakes of recovering malnourished children. Am J Clin Nutr 1995;62:13–18.
11 Golden MHN: The nature of nutritional deficiency in relation to growth failure and poverty. Acta Paediatr Scand Suppl 1991;374:95–110.
12 Gibson RS, Ferguson EL, Lehrfeld J: Complementary foods for infant feeding in developing countries: Their nutrient adequacy and improvement. Eur J Clin Nutr 1998;52:764–770.
13 Onyango A, Koski KG, Tucker KL: Food diversity versus breastfeeding choice in determining anthropometric status in rural Kenyan toddlers. Int J Epidemiol 1998;27:484–489.
14 Perlas L: Nutrient Adequacy of Complementary Diets in Cebu, Philippines, and Laboratory Evaluation of Household Methods for Their Improvement; unpublished MSc thesis, University of Otago, 2002.
15 Allen LH, Black AK, Backstrand JR, et al: An analytical approach for exploring the importance of dietary quality versus quantity in the growth of Mexican children. Food Nutr Bull 1991;13:95–104.

16 Soh P, Ferguson EL, McKenzie JE, et al: Dietary intakes of 6–24-month-old urban South Island New Zealand children in relation to biochemical iron status. Public Health Nutr 2002;5: 339–346.
17 Skinner JD, Carruth BR, Houck KS, et al: Longitudinal study of nutrient and food intakes of infants aged 2 to 24 months. J Am Diet Assoc 1997;97:496–504.
18 Krebs NF: Dietary zinc and iron sources, physical growth and cognitive development of breastfed infants. J Nutr 2000;130(suppl):358S–360S.
19 Hurrell RF, Reddy MB, Juillerat M-A, Cook JD: Degradation of phytic acid in cereal porridges improves iron absorption by human subjects. Am J Clin Nutr 2003;77:1213–1219.
20 Mendoza C, Viteri FE, Lönnerdal B, et al: Effect of genetically modified, low-phytic acid maize on absorption of iron from tortillas. Am J Clin Nutr 1998;68:1123–1127.
21 Adams C, Hambidge M, Raboy V, et al: Zinc absorption from a low-phytic acid maize. Am J Clin Nutr 2002;76:556–559.
22 Merhav H, Amitai Y, Palti H, Godfrey S: Tea drinking and microcytic anemia in infants. Am J Clin Nutr 1985;41:1210–1213.
23 Dewey KG, Romero-abal ME, de Serrano JQ, et al: Effects of discontinuing coffee intake on iron status of iron-deficient Guatemalan toddlers: A randomized intervention study. Am J Clin Nutr 1997;66:168–176.
24 Englemann MDM, Davidsson L, Sandstrom BM, et al: The influence of meat on nonheme iron absorption in infants. Pediatr Res 1998;443:768–773.
25 Jalla S, Westcott J, Steirn M, et al: Zinc absorption and exchangeable zinc pool sizes in breast-fed infants fed meat or cereal as first complentary food. J Pediatr Gastroenterol Nutr 2002;34: 35–41.
26 Murphy SP, Beaton GH, Calloway DH: Estimated mineral intakes of toddlers: Predicted prevalence of inadequacy in village populations in Egypt, Kenya, and Mexico. Am J Clin Nutr 1992;56:565–572.
27 Hotz C, Gibson RS: Complementary feeding practices and dietary intakes from complementary foods amongst weanlings in rural Malawi. Eur J Clin Nutr 2001;55:841–849.
28 Miller M, Humphrey J, Johnson E, et al: Why do children become vitamin A deficient? J Nutr 2002;132(suppl):2867S–2880S.
29 Bhutta ZA: Iron and zinc intake from complementary foods: Some issues from Pakistan. Pediatrics 2000;106:1295–1297.
30 World Health Organization: Trace Elements in Human Health and Nutrition, ed 2. Geneva, World Health Organization, 2002.
31 Heiskanen K, Siimes MA, Salmenpera L, Perheentupa J: Low vitamin B6 status associated with slow growth in healthy breast-fed infants. Pediatr Res 1995;38:740–746.
32 Michaelson KF, Samuelson G, Graham TW, Lönnerdal B: Zinc intake, zinc status and growth in a longitudinal study of healthy Danish infants. Acta Paediatr Scand 1994;83:1115–1121.
33 Lartey A, Manu A, Brown KH, et al: Predictors of micronutrient status among six- to twelve-month-old breast-fed Ghanaian infants. J Nutr 2000;130:199–207.
34 Dijkhuizen MA, Wieringa FT, West CE, et al: Concurrent micronutrient deficiencies in lactating mothers and their infants in Indonesia. Am J Clin Nutr 2001;73:786–791.
35 Thu BD, Schultink W, Dillon D, et al: Effect of daily and weekly micronutrient supplementation on micronutrient deficiencies and growth in young Vietnamese children. Am J Clin Nutr 1999;69:80–86.
36 Rivera JA, Gonzalez-Cossio T, Flores M, et al: Multiple micronutrient supplementation increases the growth of Mexican infants. Am J Clin Nutr 2001;74:657–663.
37 Skeaff S, Ferguson EL, McKenzie JE, et al: Are breast-fed infants and toddlers in New Zealand at risk of iodine deficiency? Nutrition 2004, in press.
38 Brown KH, Peerson JM, Allen LH, Rivera J: Effect of supplemental zinc on the growth and serum zinc concentrations of pre-pubertal children: A meta-analysis of randomized, controlled trials. Am J Clin Nutr 2002;75:1062–1071.
39 Zinc Investigators' Collaborative Group: Prevention of diarrhea and pneumonia by zinc supplementation in children in developing countries: Pooled analysis of randomized controlled trials. J Pediatr 1999;135:689–697.
40 Lartey A, Manu A, Brown KH, Dewey KG: A randomized, community-based trial of the effects of improved centrally processed complementary foods on growth and micronutrient status of Ghanaian infants from 6 to 12 mos of age. Am J Clin Nutr 1999;70:391–404.

41 Lui D, Bates CJ, Yin T, et al: Nutritional efficacy of a fortified weaning rusk in a rural area near Beijing. Am J Clin Nutr 1993;57:506–511.
42 Haskell MJ, Santizo MC, Begin F, Torun B: Effect of supplementation with multiple micronutrients and/or bovine serum concentrate on the growth of low-income, peri-urban Guatemalan infants and young children (abstract). FASEB J 2000;14:543.
43 Dijkhuizen MA, Wieringa FT, West CE, et al: Effects of iron and zinc supplementation in Indonesian infants on micronutrient status and growth. J Nutr 2001;131:2860–2865.
44 Dewey KG: Success of intervention programs to promote complementary feeding; in Black RE, Fleisher K (eds): Public Health Issues in Infant and Child Nutrition Nestle Nutrition Workshop Series Pediatric Program. Vevey, Nestec/Philadelphia, Lippincott Williams & Wilkins, 2002, vol 48, pp 199–216.
45 Dewey KG: The challenges of promoting optimal infant growth. J Nutr 2001;131:1879–1880.

Discussion

Dr. Tolboom: Thank you for your crystal clear presentation. I have a question about appetite. I know nutritionists have been very keen to cut that out, to see what is causing a decreased appetite. As a pediatrician I would always think that it is caused because a child is not feeling well, and feeling well in most of the settings you have been researching show with a high incidence of the infections, the weanlings in Malawi are I presume in a highly malarial region. Did you look at infections per se in your Malawian population in terms of COP or other infectious parameters?

Dr. Gibson: No unfortunately we weren't able to collect blood samples in this particular trial in Malawi so we weren't able to examine infections. One of the things I didn't discuss in this presentation, which we all know is also very important in terms of appetite, is daily care practice, and we need to be much more attentive to caring practice. It became clear to us during our study in Malawi that also mothers need to be more proactive in terms of feeding sometimes.

Dr. Tolboom: There was a point at which the frequency of feeds was increased. But how practical is that for an African mother who is already overburdened, has to get the shaving water for the husband in the morning, collect firewood, etc?

Dr. Gibson: I recognize that that might be a problem and having worked in Malawi I realize how busy the mothers are. However, before any of these strategies were actually implemented we carried out a lot of qualitative research to find out whether or not the strategies that we were proposing would be acceptable to the mothers, so none of these strategies were used unless they were acceptable to the mothers before we started, that is very important.

Dr. Abrams: I have a comment about calcium. You made it sound as if most weaning foods are calcium deficient. This points out that the British Recommended Nutritional Index of 520 mg for 9- to 11-month-olds is considerably greater than the US, i.e. 270, and the British number goes down to 350 at 12 months of age. If you look at some of the data collected since the British Recommended Nutritional Index was developed, 520 mg/day is a very high estimate of what most infants of 9–11 months of age need. So I am not sure if the amount of calcium in infant weaning foods may not be as far off. Now I recognize that bioavailability is a problem, but there is a huge calcium gap and the US recommendations are, I think, the more current understanding of the bone growth in 9- to 11-month-old infants.

Dr. Gibson: Thank you very much for the comment. I agree, and it is actually reassuring to hear that the gap is probably not as bad as it looks from the data available.

Dr. Guesry: I am a bit confused by one of the aspects of your presentation which is not related to micronutrient but to energy because up to now all of what I have read about energy density and food intake show that when you increase energy density you reduce the overall amount of food, although insufficiently to reduce the energy intake. You said that when energy density is increased the quantity of food is increased as if there was no satiation effect of the energy density. Could you explain how you came to this conclusion?

Dr. Gibson: There have been very elegant experimental control trials to investigate this effect. The earlier literature was quite confusing because it was very difficult to separate the changes in energy density and feeding frequency. In fact more recent studies have clearly shown that you can in fact increase energy intake if you increase energy density [1], and in Malawi one of the things that we did to ensure that the increased energy density food, which was 16% dry matter, was acceptable for the infants was actually to use some germinated cereal so that the viscosity of the porridge prepared as 16% dry matter was similar to that of 7% dry matter.

Dr. Specker: With regard to the calcium recommendations for infants, in the US the adequate intake levels of calcium for 0–6 months were based on the calcium content of human milk and the average amount of human milk consumed per day in the exclusively breast-fed infant. The recommended intake for 6–12 months was based on intakes from human milk and what the normal US infant receives from complementary foods. The recommendations were not based on any functional indicator for calcium.

Dr. Neufeld: I have two comments. One is methodological really. You reported that poor appetite as perceived by the mother was predictive of intake, and I have to ask what would be the possible role of maternal responsive feeding? If we assume that the mother perceives and interacts with her child in a certain way, then she would perceive the lower appetite of the child. In terms of measuring this we must find a way to classify a mother's interaction with her child, the whole caregiving, in order to really understand that relationship. We have just recently finished a trial in Mexico, a multiple micronutrient supplementation trial, comparing multiple micronutrients and iron and vitamin A, and the results are not encouraging. We finished the trial in September and we are analyzing results, but I think we are really going to need to think about how to deal with multiple deficiencies in these countries because it looks as though supplementation with multiple micronutrients is not going to be the answer, at least not in our settings.

Dr. Gibson: That is very true and this is one of the reasons why in the final slide I suggested that we look at the multiple micronutrients specific for the setting. But perhaps in fact it would be preferable to use additional micronutrients as fortificants rather than supplements, which is probably a much more promising way to proceed. Even better in my view is to try and ensure that mothers have available to them foods that meet nutrient needs without even having to fortify. But from our study in Malawi even with our interventions which involved 4 different strategies, although we achieved an increase in intake of most nutrients in many cases, it was still not sufficient to meet the estimated needs. So we came to the conclusion that in this setting in Malawi, particularly for iron and zinc, there would be a problem. This was partly because the mothers had such limited access to flesh foods; their only source of animal protein was fish and that really constrained our efforts to try and produce a complementary food that would meet all the estimated needs of those infants.

Dr. Gebre-Medhin: One of the striking points you made is the very high occurrence of micronutrient deficiency in Sweden with the complementary feeding, if I understood you correctly. If that is the case this must be looked at in relation to the fact that we have the best growth ever published anywhere in Sweden, lowest mortality, lowest morbidity, highest quality of life, and the rest, and the figure that you gave very clearly put Sweden among the highest examples of deficiency.

Dr. Gibson: I am glad you raised that point, and of course it is very much dependent on the cutoff that we use. In terms of hemoglobin there is a lot of doubt or discussion

100

about the cutoff that we should be using to classify infants with anemia. So that might be some of the reason. In terms of New Zealand, where we saw a large proportion of children with urinary iodine deficiency, this is certainly a reemerging problem, as it is in Tasmania. In New Zealand one of the reasons for this is because dairy industries have stopped using iodine so that the iodine content of foods, dairy products particularly, has decreased, and although there is iodized salt in the country it is not mandated and mothers do not recognize the importance of using iodized salt and they are using less salt. This has just been presented to the Ministry of Health in New Zealand and they have a special committee to address this concern about the reemergence of iodine deficiency. In some developed countries, certainly in New Zealand and Tasmania, iodine deficiency is going to become a reemerging problem.

Dr. Tolboom: I looked at your figures on the weanlings aged 6–8 and then 9–11 months old in Malawi. I am a bit confused about the definition of weanling.

Dr. Gibson: I may have been responsible for that confusion. In fact those infants that I showed you were still being breast-fed, so all the data that I showed you were for infants who were still being breast-fed.

Dr. Tolboom: Then you assume the breast milk intake on data from the literature. Are there any ways that we can increase breast-feeding because in Zambia we found that in the 2nd year of life breast milk still contributes about 45% of the energy needs of children and protein about 40%. So is there any way apart from good complementary food to improve lactational performance regarding micronutrients?

Dr. Gibson: I am afraid I really can't answer that question. I know that a fully breast-fed infant after 6 months still cannot meet its estimated needs for all nutrients. After 6 months there are certain nutrients that they do require even if they are breast-fed fully. So breast milk itself does not meet the requirements for certain nutrients after 6 months of age. In New Zealand unfortunately most mothers go back to work so breast-feeding frequently actually drops off dramatically by 3 months.

Dr. Tolboom: Do you think the mother is a good vehicle to increase the micronutrient intake of her infant? We have said that mothers should be supplemented with vitamin A, giving all the supplements to a lactating mother rather than to putting it in a fortified food?

Dr. Gibson: I think that it is very unlikely that mothers in New Zealand are vitamin A-deficient.

Dr. Tolboom: I mean the mothers in Malawi.

Dr. Gibson: That may well be the case, but I think in addition we still need to ensure that there is vitamin A in a complementary food.

Dr. Zlotkin: I would like to discuss the concept of using meat as a complementary food. You showed that the group with the highest meat intake still had a significantly inadequate intake of iron and zinc. In Canada, in the communities one would expect to be the least likely to be iron-deficient are our native communities where in fact hunting is of major importance and deer and moose meat are major components of the diet. Yet if you look at the prevalence of iron deficiency among infants between 6 and 12 months of age in Canada in that population, it is around 35% compared to the rest of the country where it is around 5 or 6%. I looked at this a bit more carefully and in fact the populations do use meat, but they use it either as a dilute broth or, among the Inuit population, the mother actually chews the food and provides the chewed food to her infant, and I imagine that actually as the mother chews and swallows the juices of the meat the infant actually receives very little meat. The only studies that I have ever seen that actually demonstrated that meat as a complementary food can prevent anemia are those in which commercial meat products were fortified with iron. In fact we did a study that was published in the *Canadian Journal of Public Health* which showed that the combination of jar meat products and infant cereal could prevent anemia [2]. So my question is do you really think that a recommendation to include more meat in a complementary food strategy is actually going to work to prevent iron deficiency anemia?

Dr. Gibson: That is a very important question. In fact we are about to embark on a study in New Zealand looking exactly at that question. And indeed when we looked closely in the literature we could not find any study in which they had set out to try to encourage meat consumption that showed a positive effect on reducing iron-deficiency anemia either [3, 4]. I still think, however, that meat certainly might have an impact on the zinc status of the children. In New Zealand the amount of meat given to infants after 6 months is incredibly small, in fact negligible. In New Zealand most of the cereals that are given to infants are not infant cereals at all; Weatabix is given which until recently has not been fortified with iron. So we have a problem with iron deficiency in New Zealand weanlings and toddlers [5]. One of the arms of our study does include a meat group, so we will see.

Mr. Parvanta: Just to follow up on this point, I don't think that we are saying that meat is not a food to recommend. I think the problem is that a young infant just cannot eat enough meat to be able to consume the needed amount of iron from meat. Last year, as you recall, Gleason [6] did some modeling of different types of diets, looking at what the iron intake should be for a child less than 12 months. Essentially the bottom line was that, depending on the combination but assuming the children were to consume meat as the main source of their iron intake, they would have to eat approximately 150 g meat/day to meet their iron needs. So it is basically not feasible for children to consume that much meat in a day, not to say that they shouldn't consume meat, it is just how much they can consume.

Dr. Gibson: I would just like to elaborate on that. In fact Dr. Ferguson is the principal investigator for this study on meat we are doing in the toddlers. She has worked with Dr. Briend's group in Paris, so she is very aware of the problems associated with meeting the iron needs of infants. Her group has spent about 9 months developing special recipes, testing them with toddlers, to find recipes that they actually will eat. They have measured the amounts of meat that they are willing to consume in this pilot study, and at the beginning of next year we will embark on this study using the piloted recipes on these toddlers to see whether or not we can find a positive effect.

Dr. Specker: Since it appears that it is so hard to get this much iron into an infant's diet, what is the functional indicator for iron deficiency? It seems that if it is so unreasonable to get it in their diet, it might be that the requirement is set too high?

Dr. Gibson: Dr. Lozoff will talk about that tomorrow morning.

Dr. Barclay: I would like to underline your statement that it is very important not to assume that micronutrient deficiencies are all the same. We hear a lot about iron, vitamin A and iodine, but we have done studies in West Africa showing that in fact these three micronutrients are not major problems. The major micronutrient deficiencies in this area are calcium, zinc and B vitamins [7]. The data you presented show a difference in the response in girls and boys. We have also done a study on zinc fortification and shown that in boys the growth response is greater than in girls [8]. Do you think this is because boys have a greater requirement for growth or is there another explanation?

Dr. Gibson: One of the explanations in the literature suggests that it may be associated with the fact that males have a higher percentage of total body weight comprised of muscle, which in turn contains a greater content of zinc than fat [9]. Additionally, the growth rate of males is generally higher than females, so their zinc requirements are probably greater.

Dr. Gebre-Medhin: I would like to come back to this issue of the assessment of iron status using hemoglobin and the Swedish material that you showed. The Swedish children have a high prevalence of exclusive breast-feeding, iron-enriched or iron-supplemented formula, follow-on formula, porridges, and they even get meat from about

4–5 months, they grow well, have a very good morbidity and no mortality, and yet we have these figures that you showed us today. Unless that issue is resolved I think we are going to be in very serious trouble. I think this cutoff point that you mentioned will have to be taken into account before we go ahead. Don't you agree?

Dr. Gibson: I think we need to validate the cutoff points that we can use for designating anemia in infancy, and as Dr. Lönnerdal discussed earlier today there is a lot of discussion going on about what levels we should use and also the immaturity of the infants in the first 6 months. At that age it changes a lot so I think we have to bear that in mind when we are looking at these sorts of interpretation.

Dr. Lozoff: A couple of factors may be relevant to the discussion of the right amount of iron for babies. Even though we say that babies were well nourished during human evolution, babies in countries like the US or Sweden are bigger, and they grow more rapidly. It is possible that they are exceeding the capacity of breast milk iron to keep up. The other factor is the introduction of cereal due to agriculture. Although this was a big advance for humans, it may have worsened the situation with regard to iron. So you can think of some circumstances in which breast milk, despite tremendous advantages, might not totally meet iron needs. There are other considerations as we talk about the functional effects of iron deficiency. Different things may be required for good function now, compared to previous times. Thus, the behavioral benefits of good iron status might not have had a major impact under other conditions. These are hesitations before accepting the argument that because anemia was commonly observed in breast-fed infants in Sweden, the cutoffs might be wrong.

References

1   Bennett VA, Morales E, Gonzalez J, et al: Effects of dietary viscosity and energy density on total daily energy consumption by young Peruvian children. Am J Clin Nutr 1999;70:285–291.
2   Yeung GS, Zlotkin SH: Efficacy of meat and iron-fortified commercial cereal to prevent iron depletion in cow milk-fed infants 6 to 12 months of age: A randomized controlled trial. Can J Public Health 2000;91:263–267.
3   Engleman MD, Sandstrom B, Michaelsen KF: Meat intake and iron status in late infancy: An intervention study. J Pediatr Gastroenterol Nutr 1998;26:26–33.
4   Westcott JL, Simon NB, Krebs NF: Growth, zinc and iron status and development of exclusively breastfed infants fed meat vs. cereal as a first weaning food (abstract). FASEB J 1998;12:A847.
5   Soh P, Ferguson EL, McKenzie JE, et al: Dietary intakes of 6–24 month-old urban South Island New Zealand Children in relation to biochemical iron status. Publ Health Nutr 2002;5:339–346.
6   Gleason GR: Iron deficiency anemia finally reaches the global stage of public health. Nutr Clin Care 2002;5:217–219.
7   Barclay D, Mauron J, Bondel A, et al: Micronutrient intake and status in Democratic Republic of Congo. Nutr Res 2003;23:659–671.
8   Dirren H, Barclay D, Ramos JG, et al: Zinc supplementation and child growth in Ecuador. Adv Exp Med Biol 1994;352:215–222.
9   Iyengar GV: Reevaluation of the trace element content in reference man. Radiat Phys Chem 1998;51:545–560.

Pettifor JM, Zlotkin S (eds): Micronutrient Deficiencies during the Weaning Period and the
First Years of Life. Nestlé Nutrition Workshop Series Pediatric Program, vol 54, pp 105–118,
Nestec Ltd., Vevey/S. Karger AG, Basel, © 2004.

Micronutrient Malnutrition and Poverty

Martin W. Bloem and Saskia de Pee

Asia Pacific, Helen Keller Worldwide, Singapore

Introduction

In September 2000, the world's leaders adopted the UN Millennium Declaration committing their nations to stronger global efforts to reduce poverty, improve health and promote peace, human rights and environmental sustainability [1]. The Millennium Development Goals, enshrined in the Declaration, consist of 7 specific goals: (1) eradicate extreme poverty and hunger; (2) achieve universal primary education; (3) promote gender equality and empower women; (4) reduce child mortality; (5) improve maternal health; (6) combat HIV/AIDS, malaria and other diseases, and (7) ensure environmental sustainability. The last goal also reflects the commitment of the richer countries to the success of these goals by developing a global partnership for development.

The recognition that each country must pursue a development strategy that meets its specific needs should be the starting point of every attempt to reach the Millennium Goals. The national strategies should be based on good data from proper monitoring and evaluation. Helen Keller International (HKI) has always put a lot of emphasis on monitoring and evaluation; since 1990 it has developed surveillance and data-collection systems in Bangladesh, Vietnam, Cambodia and Indonesia [2, 3]. These surveillance systems have led to a much greater understanding of the interdependence of the various causes of undernutrition.

This article will discuss the importance of defining the indicators of undernutrition in a very specific way and determine the best possible strategies to combat the various forms of undernutrition. It will also highlight the importance of micronutrient undernutrition both as an important cause of childhood and maternal mortality as well as a very sensitive indicator of changes in poverty.

Famine

It has long been recognized that inadequate food intake leads to weight loss and growth retardation and, when severe and long lasting, proceeds to wasting and emaciation. Famines are among the most dramatic causes of inadequate food intake on a large scale and have been reported since the 4th millennium BC in ancient Egypt. Throughout history, famine has struck at least one area of the world every few years.

The causes of famine are many, but they are usually divided into human and natural categories. Natural causes destroy crops and food supplies and include: (1) drought (prolonged lack of rain); (2) too much rainfall and flooding, and (3) plant diseases and pests. Human causes of famine are primarily political in nature, e.g., war, economic boycotts, etc. Although this division between man-made and natural causes has widely been accepted, a recent discussion questioned whether natural causes for a lack of crop production necessarily lead to famine, or that governments were responsible for not taking the right actions during those times. Sen [4], the winner of the 1998 Nobel Memorial Prize in Economic Science, stated 'no famine has ever taken place in the history of the world in a functioning democracy'. He explained this by stating that democratic governments have strong incentives to undertake measures to avert famines and other catastrophes in order to gain public popularity and be re-elected into government [4].

Undernutrition

We can say that famines are responsible for major fluctuations in the prevalence of undernutrition throughout the world. However, millions of people, including 6 million children, die each year as a result of hunger. Of these millions, only a few are victims of famine but far more die from chronic hunger [5].

Although undernutrition has been known for centuries, it was only since the early 1900s that more scientific research has been carried out on this topic. In the beginning, most of the physicians were studying the phenomenon, and health workers in Latin America identified a clinical syndrome 'distrofia pluricarencial' [6]. In the mid 1930s in Africa, Williams [7, 8] identified two diseases: kwashiorkor and marasmus. Kwashiorkor literally meant 'deposed from the mother's breast by a newborn sibling' and turned out to be caused by a lack of protein [7, 8]. Marasmus was a classic form of undernutrition mainly caused by a lack of energy and therefore all other nutrients. These diseases were clinical entities and the public health people were struggling when they wanted to have a better insight on the magnitude of undernutrition in various countries and regions in the world. Therefore, anthropometry was developed, based on measuring weight and height and assessing age. Data from a reference population were used to construct tables to which data from individual children were compared in order to assess whether they were undernourished, based on how much they deviated from the norm. Undernutrition was divided into three forms: stunting (low height-for-age); underweight (low weight-for-age), and wasting (low weight-for-height) [9].

The next question was how anthropometry was associated with the clinical signs of undernutrition. Various studies in the 1960s and 1970s examined this. Then, various studies assessed the relationship between anthropometric indicators of undernutrition and the risk of morbidity and mortality. Those studies were fascinating as they found that the various indicators (weight-for-age, height-for-age, and weight-for-height) had their own specific relationships with mortality and morbidity. Undernutrition was no longer defined by clinical signs but by anthropometry. Each indicator had its specific use and, although this was very useful for the nutritional scientists, it became more and more complicated to understand what undernutrition really meant [10, 11].

Initially, protein deficiency was recognized as a cause of undernutrition, but it became clear in the following years that a lack of energy was the main cause of undernutrition defined by anthropometric indicators. Based on these findings, Jelliffe introduced the term 'protein-calorie malnutrition', which evolved into 'protein-energy malnutrition' [11]. The green revolution, however, increased the global production of staple foods, and this is one of the reasons why the level of protein-energy malnutrition has decreased dramatically in the past two decades, specifically in Asia and Latin America.

Micronutrient Undernutrition

Since the beginning of the 20th century, many researchers developed knowledge about the importance of vitamins and minerals. Diseases like beri beri, pellagra, xerophthalmia and other deficiency diseases had been known for centuries, and careful laboratory and epidemiological studies revealed the causes of these diseases. The role of these 'micronutrients' in preventing infectious diseases was elucidated, and large-scale prevention programs were developed [12]. These programs ranged from large-scale home gardening programs to intervention with cod-liver oil in households and factories [13]. After the Second World War, antibiotics were developed and many of these preventive nutrition programs collapsed.

However, since the work of Sommer and West [14] on the effect of vitamin A on mortality, many researchers have re-searched the role of micronutrients in morbidity and mortality [15]. There is more and more evidence that micronutrients may play a critical role as one of the strategies to reach the millennium goal of reducing childhood and maternal mortality.

Definitions of Undernutrition

So undernutrition is defined in various ways, which sometimes leads to the notion that nutritionists do not have clear ideas about the problem of undernutrition. A report from the World Bank entitled 'Does undernutrition respond to incomes and prices?' stated in its introduction the following: 'The attainment of adequate nutrition is an important criterion for evaluating the success of development policies. However, such evaluations have often been hampered by the fact that the measurement of undernutrition is fraught with both conceptual and technical problems. Most importantly, the nutritional requirements needed for good health vary across individuals and over time in generally unknown ways, and their intakes are typically also measured with error' [16]. Although many nutritionists will disagree with this statement, it is absolutely true that it is very important for nutritionists to define its various indicators for undernutrition specifically so that there is no confusion among other professions who have to work with these definitions.

The problem of definitions goes further than clinical signs and anthropometric indicators; the Food and Agriculture Organization is using the term 'undernourishment' for its definition of world hunger. The percentage of a population that is undernourished provides information on the number of people within a population whose dietary energy intake lies below their minimum requirements. Although this indicator is a valuable indicator, it confuses the discussion about undernutrition even more [5].

Causes of Undernutrition

The discussion about the causes of undernutrition has always been and is a difficult one. The first and most important question is, what indicators are we using to define undernutrition? Then, it also depends on the profession dealing with the analysis. To tackle this problem, UNICEF developed a model, which includes many of the various causes that contribute to undernutrition [17]. It distinguishes the following levels of causes: the immediate causes; the underlying causes, and the basic causes of undernutrition. The immediate causes are lack of food intake and diseases. The underlying causes are fourfold: access to food; caring practices; access to health services, and the environment. The basic causes are the political and economic circumstances.

This model has contributed much to the understanding of the interdependence of the various causes of undernutrition. Traditionally, the nutritionists have always put a lot of emphasis on the caring practice component, which includes 'lack of knowledge' as one of the causes of undernutrition; the economists have put much more emphasis on food prices and the availability of staple food; the public health authorities and experts on the primary health care services, and the social scientists on the socio-political background.

Analysis of the problem has consequences for the proposed intervention programs. A good lesson can be learned from the evolution of the education programs to reduce vitamin A deficiency. Vitamin A deficiency is considered to be one of the major public health problems in the world, specifically in the countries where rice is the main staple food. While xerophthalmia has been known since the time of the ancient Egyptians, the fact that vitamin A deficiency leads to increased mortality has only been established and accepted since the 1980s, after the important work of Sommer and West [14]. However, one of the first public health scientists in the field of vitamin A deficiency control, Oomen et al. [18] stated in one of their publications that it was very peculiar that vitamin A deficiency was endemic in those areas where vegetables, considered as major source of vitamin A, were abundant. The lack of knowledge among mothers was considered the major cause of vitamin A deficiency, because they did not feed their children the right amount of vegetables. Many campaigns were set up in the 1980s to improve the intake of vegetables by children and women in areas where vitamin A deficiency was endemic. Some of them have claimed to be successful in reducing vitamin A deficiency among its target group. In 1995, de Pee et al. [19] published an interesting paper, which has been confirmed since then by other studies that found that vegetables are a much less good source of vitamin A than previously thought. In fact it is impossible to provide children aged 6–23 months with enough vitamin A by giving them mainly vegetables as a source of vitamin A [20, 21]. Because of the much lower bioavailability of vitamin A from vegetables and fruits, animal products have become more essential as a dietary source of vitamin A than was thought before [20, 22]. This also explains the early observations from Oomen et al. [18]. These findings had consequences for the strategies to combat vitamin A deficiency throughout the world. Animal products are expensive and poor people can hardly afford any of these products. Vitamin A deficiency became a problem of poverty and not of ignorance. Home gardening programs are still considered effective strategies because they also increase the income of women of poor households, but more emphasis is now being put on animal husbandry components of these home gardens. Supplementation and fortification programs are now seen as the most cost-effective strategies to combat vitamin A deficiency in the short and medium term [23].

Therefore, the bioavailability of vitamin A in vegetables is a problem at the immediate cause level, and had consequences for the shift in emphasis on causes from 'caring practices' to 'access to food'. The role of home gardening in reducing vitamin A deficiency has shifted from addressing the underlying cause to addressing a basic cause by providing more income. However, despite the fact that vitamin A deficiency and other micronutrient deficiencies are clearly a poverty problem, many agencies still carry out programs that have behavior change as its key strategy [24].

Rice Prices and Undernutrition

In 1994, Bloem et al. [25] showed in an early analysis, using the Helen Keller International (HKI) nutrition surveillance data of Bangladesh, that there was a strong association between rice prices and undernutrition defined by weight-for-age. A follow-up analysis by Torlesse et al. [26] showed similar results after 10 years of data collection. The intake of rice during the period 1992–2000 did not change and the main fluctuations in the prevalence of low weight-for-age could be explained by the changes in the expenditure and consumption of non-grain food items. Expenditure on these items was higher when rice prices were lower and the prevalence of low weight-for-age during such periods was found to be lower. These reports thus describe the relationship between the basic (economic) causes of undernutrition and the outcome (underweight), and have hypothesized the following mechanism of the relationship. The immediate cause of undernutrition, measured by a low weight-for-age, is a lack of intake and/or diseases, e.g. diarrhea, respiratory diseases, etc. In countries where seasonal food shortages exist as in Bangladesh, women and children have a chronic or periodic lack of energy in their diet. When the total food intake lacks in quantity it also lacks in quality, which means a shortage of micronutrients. The main cause of this is that these women and children have limited access to food mainly because they cannot afford it for economic reasons or because of natural or man-made disasters. It is very interesting to observe that households always try to maintain their energy intake in the sense that they try to maintain the same intake of their staple food. When there is economic distress, they will reduce consumption of all other products so that they can consume the same amount of their staple food in order to maintain the most optimal energy intake. However, this still results in a lower energy intake as well as in a lower micronutrient intake, which results in a lower weight-for-age among children. This lower weight-for-age can thus be due both to a lower weight gain due to the lower energy intake, mainly from non-staple foods, as well as to less linear growth because of the poorer quality of the diet.

There are, however, also countries and regions where there is nearly no chronic or regular periodic lack of energy in the diet and where the quality of the food is the main bottleneck to further reducing undernutrition. Indonesia, Thailand, and many Latin American countries are good examples. Under the circumstances in these countries, undernutrition defined by low weight-for-age is mainly determined by lack of linear growth, also called stunting. Linear growth is much more dependent on the right mix of micronutrients and it is interesting to see that the progress in the reduction of stunting has stagnated in those countries where animal products are still not consumed by all strata in the society. The immediate cause is a lack of quality food, such as animal products and fortified foods, in the diet of women and children. However, the role of 'caring' practices becomes more important because households can now make decisions about the best mix of quality foods within reach of their budgets. While people have a good feel for maintaining energy intake as long it is possible, it is a much more difficult task for people to achieve or maintain consumption of an adequate mix of quality foods. Furthermore, food taboos and foods forbidden because of religious reasons make these choices even more complicated and limit the possibilities of further increasing the quality of the diet. While a right mix of micronutrients is important for linear growth and a stagnation in the reduction of stunting indicates a lack of micronutrients, such trends only become visible after a while because linear growth does not respond quickly to changes in diet. A more sensitive indicator to a sudden lack of micronutrients in the diet is the hemoglobin concentration, or the prevalence of anemia, especially among children.

Asian Economic Crisis

In September 1997, the Thai Baht was devaluated and it was the beginning of the Asian Economic crisis and the fall of the Asian Tigers. Although many economic indicators in the region have shown improvement since then, the effects of September 11, 2001, and the global recession have not helped the region either. In 1998, HKI reacted in Indonesia by setting up a continuation of a surveillance system which had been in place between 1995 and 1996. Using these data, HKI was able to compare health and economic household indicators before and during the crisis in one province, Central Java in Indonesia. Central Java is a province with about 50 million inhabitants.

Bloem and Darnton-Hill [27] reported the early results and showed similar results to those found in Bangladesh. The rice prices increased as a result of the crisis and the effect was that the expenditure on non-grain food items decreased, resulting in an increase in micronutrient deficiencies, indicated by an increase in the prevalence of anemia [27]. They showed an increase in maternal malnutrition but did not observe an increase in undernutrition measured by weight-for-age [28]. The urban poor were more affected than the rural poor but later analysis showed that the rural poor were also suffering but to a lesser extent [29]. Despite these results there were many debates in 1999 on whether the Asian economic crisis had an impact on health and nutritional status among the poor populations.

The HKI Health and Nutrition Surveillance System in Indonesia expanded to 12 sites in 1999, and is still in operation. The follow-up data between 1999 and 2003 showed that both childhood anemia and maternal malnutrition are very sensitive indicators of economic change.

Conclusions

Undernutrition is a major problem in the world, independent of the indicator that is used to define it. Millions of children, women, and men are affected by a lack of food resulting in many forms of undernutrition, including micronutrient malnutrition. The problem of micronutrient malnutrition is not only restricted to the developing countries but is also prevalent among the poor in the richer countries including the USA [30].

While child anthropometry has traditionally been used as the most sensitive indicator for food distress, micronutrient deficiencies such as iron deficiency anemia and vitamin A deficiency, seem to be more sensitive indicators during economic distress, specifically in those countries where energy deficiency is no longer the bottleneck of the food problem.

It is therefore recommended that hemoglobin levels should be routinely measured in surveillance systems in both developing as well as developed countries to measure the potential impact of economic changes on health and nutrition.

References

1 United Nations Development Programme: Human Development 2003: Millennium Goals: A Compact among Nations to End Human Poverty. Oxford, Oxford University Press, 2003.
2 Helen Keller International: The Nutritional Surveillance Project in Bangladesh in 1999. Towards the Goals of the 1990 World Summit for Children. Dhaka, Helen Keller International, 2001.
3 Helen Keller International/Indonesia: Monitoring the Economic Crisis: Impact and Transition 1998–2000. Nutrition and Health Surveillance System. Jakarta, Helen Keller International/ Indonesia, 2000.
4 Sen A: Development as Freedom. New York, Anchor Books, 1999.
5 Food and Agriculture Organization: The State of Food Insecurity in the World. Rome, FAO, 2002.
6 Schroeder DG: Malnutrition; in Semba RD, Bloem MW (eds): Nutrition and Health in Developing Countries. Totowa, Humana Press, 2001, pp 393–426.
7 Williams CD: A nutritional disease of childhood associated with a maize diet. Arch Dis Child 1933;8:423–428.
8 Williams CD: Kwashiorkor, a nutritional disease of children associated with a maize diet. Lancet 1936;ii:1151–1152.
9 World Health Organization: Physical status: The use and interpretation of anthropometry. Report of a WHO Expert Committee. World Health Organ Tech Rep Ser 1995;854:1–452.
10 Pelletier DL, Frolingo EA, Shroeder DG, Habicht JP: The effects of malnutrition on child mortality in developing countries. Bull World Health Organ 1995;7:443–448.
11 De Onis M: Child growth and development; in Semba RD, Bloem MW (eds): Nutrition and Health in Developing Countries. Totowa, Humana Press, 2001, pp 71–91.
12 Semba RD: Nutrition: Epidemiology and public health overview; in Ward JW, Warren C (eds): A Safer and Healthier America: Public Health in the 20th Century. New York, New York Academy of Medicine, in press.
13 American Red Cross: Relief Work in the Drought of 1930–31: Official Report of the Relief Operations. Washington, American Red Cross, 1931.
14 Sommer A, West KP Jr: Vitamin A Deficiency: Health, Survival, and Vision. New York, Oxford University Press, 1996.
15 Ramakrishnan U, Huffman SL: Multiple micronutrient malnutrition; in Semba RD, Bloem MW (eds): Nutrition and Health in Developing Countries. Totowa, Humana Press, 2001, pp 365–391.

16 Ravallion M: Does Undernutrition Respond to Incomes and Prices. Living Standards Measurement Study Working Papers. Washington, World Bank, 1991, vol 82.
17 Jonsson U: Towards an improved strategy for nutrition surveillance. Food Nutr Bull 1995; 16:102–111.
18 Oomen HAPC, McLaren DS, Escapine H: Epidemiology and public health aspects of hypovit-aminosis A. A global survey of xerophthalmia. Trop Geogr Med 1964;4:271–315.
19 De Pee S, West CE, Muhilal, et al: Lack of improvement in vitamin A status with increased consumption of dark-green leafy vegetables. Lancet 1995;346:75–81.
20 Miller M, Humphrey J, Johnson E, Marinda E, Brookmeyer R, Katz J: Why do children become vitamin A deficient? J Nutr 2002;132:2867S–2880S.
21 West CE, Eilander A, van Lieshout M: Consequences of revised estimates of carotenoid bio-efficacy for dietary control of vitamin A deficiency in developing countries. J Nutr 2002;132: 2920S–2926S.
22 De Pee S, West CE, Permaesih D, et al: Orange fruit is more effective than are dark-green, leafy vegetables in increasing serum concentrations of retinol and beta-carotene in school-children in Indonesia. Am J Clin Nutr 1998;68:1068–1074.
23 Bloem MW, de Pee S, Darnton-Hill I: New Issues in developing effective approaches for the prevention and control of vitamin A deficiency. Food Nutr Bull 1998;19:137–148.
24 Pachon H, Schroeder DG, Marsh DR, et al: Effect of an integrated child nutrition intervention on the complementary food intake of young children in rural north Vietnam. Food Nutr Bull 2002;23(suppl):70–77.
25 Bloem MW, Hye A, Gorstein J, et al: Nutrition surveillance in Bangladesh: A useful tool for policy planning at local and national levels. Food Nutr Bull 1994;16:131–138.
26 Torlesse H, Kiess L, Bloem MW: Association of household rice expenditure with child nutri-tional status indicates a role for macroeconomic food policy in combating malnutrition. J Nutr 2003;133:1320–1325.
27 Bloem MW, Darnton-Hill I: Micronutrient deficiencies. First link in a chain of nutritional and health events in economic crisis; in Bendich A, Deckelbaum RJ (eds): Primary and Secondary Preventive Nutrition. Totowa, Humana Press, 2000, pp 357–373.
28 De Pee S, Bloem MW, Sari M, et al: Indonesia's crisis causes considerable weight loss among mothers and adolescents. Mal J Nutr 2000;6:203–214.
29 Block SA, Kiess L, Webb P, et al: Did Indonesia's Crisis in 1997/98 Affect Child Nutrition? A Cohort Decomposition Analysis of National Nutrition. Surveillance Data CID Working Paper No. 90, April 2002.
30 Karp R: Malnutrition among children in the United States: The impact of poverty; in Shils M, Olson JA, Shike M, Ross AC (eds): Modern Nutrition in Health and Disease. Baltimore, Williams & Wilkins, 1999, pp 989–1001.

Discussion

Dr. Abrams: You mentioned child mortality as a marker of the overall situation. How does it follow the same trends as in Indonesia and in Bangladesh? It is one of the things that public policy makers always look to as an end point because it is very easy. It doesn't follow these trends as closely, is that true?

Dr. Bloem: In Bangladesh child mortality has reduced quite dramatically. The Banks have said that the progress Bangladesh made is great, though still far from enough. Actually that is the message, both for child mortality as well as looking at the malnutrition rates. In Indonesia we didn't have data on mortality at this particular time, and I think this is a pity but we didn't collect the data. What we have seen in Indonesia besides these data is that there was an increase in severe malnutrition in pockets – not like Bangladesh – which we hadn't seen. So suddenly we saw these children who were severely malnourished, and if that is the tip of the iceberg, there may have been increased mortality during that particular time, but I don't have the data.

Dr. Pettifor: You made a throw away line very early on in your statements saying that these effects seen with the crisis had no relationship to all the UNICEF-type programs of immunization and growth monitoring and all those programs which are built into the health systems. What you are saying is that we have to fix food prices because that is the major determinant of the things that you were looking at, and then we get into the system of saying fixing food prices is an untargeted global sort of event that should be taken within a country, which in fact costs or could cost governments considerable amounts of money. They eventually get to the stage where food prices are being kept so low that when they lift these fixed food prices there are suddenly major calamities within a country. Would you comment on that?

Dr. Bloem: It is always good to put that in so that people will react. Talking about rice prices for example, I don't know what happens in Africa or in Latin America, but I know that rice prices, global rice prices, are lower than the rice prices in Indonesia. In most of the countries, the government puts a tariff on it, so they pay more to the farmers, they subsidize the farmers. They don't in fact subsidize the poor; they have subsidized programs to support the poor. So on one hand they put a tariff on it and on the other hand they have that system. Again, I am not a food economist, I don't want to go into that, but I know there is a big discussion in Indonesia. For example some people are saying lower the food tariff and another group for political reasons says no, we have to support the farmers. One argument about this is that, for example in Bangladesh, only 15% of these farmers are net producers of rice, so when I show you the data from Bangladesh, that makes a lot of sense because most of these people are landless. In Indonesia the percentage is a little bit higher, about 30%. So you support 30% but most of the poor are actually not net consumers of rice. The issue of our health programs is a little more complicated because in fact what I am saying is not true. The relationship that I show is the better one which you have to look at. Within the better relationship of course there are health programs and health interventions, so this relationship is based on economic situations. But at the same time you can make optimal use of what is available, if you are allowed. That is why the last part of my presentation is about whether the countries, the International Monetary Fund and the World Bank allow you to do that. Kerala, Sri Lanka and even China are great examples. The difference between India and China was during the time when economic development was not very great in both countries. India invested a lot of money in a very highly qualified, top level of schooling so they have great scientists and great top people. As a consequence of course there is a brain drain because people would move to the United States or to England or to Western Europe, where they are relatively cheap to hire. But they didn't invest much in the schooling of the poor. China did it differently. They invested in schooling at all the different levels, when the economy was not very great, but the moment they started to switch to an open economy they were ready for it, and that is why you can see that they have moved quite dramatically. In India they are improving a lot of course, but not in similar way as China. The Kerala situation shows clearly that in fact when you invest in education and in health care, despite the fact that your gross national product is relatively low, you can still have a very dramatic effect. One of the issues is the transfer money. If you look at the total income of a country, there is a certain amount which is funded back to the population. For example in Holland, we pay a lot of taxes and a lot of funding goes back into social policies. In other countries, where they believe much more in private decision making on welfare issues, the level is much lower. So that is a factor which influences outcome. Programs like those of UNICEF take part in this transfer money, and I think it is a philosophical difference between, for example, Europe and the Unites States, and of course that reflects in how we support certain countries in this policy.

Dr. Tolboom: I am impressed and confused because urbanization is a process we can't stop and you said we get locked in cities, winners and losers, so everyone loses.

You showed that if populations are poor then the diversity of food is decreased and staple uses increase. So there is perhaps some promise if we fortify staple foods, because diversity is impossible for the poor who depend on staples. The food price must be guaranteed. We are not economists so perhaps we are not asking ourselves the right questions.

Dr. Bloem: As I showed in Bangladesh, it is the green revolution which increased the amount of rice produced per square meter. That is part of globalization if you follow the global market, and the next step in this is of course biotechnology. I am not going into that because there is a lot controversy about this issue, but at least it is something which people are discussing. So following an open market most probably helps the cost. It is not the lack of staple food in the whole world at this particular time, but the countries defend themselves by saying that they are in a situation in which they would like to support their own systems. So I don't know the answer to that question. But I see the tension in Indonesia between people saying just open the market and see that will help and people saying no, it must be done in sequence. For example, the financial market is still closed, but the market for rice is open. So these are the issues which people are discussing and I don't have the answer for that. To look at the solutions we have to offer, let's go back to our field. We have food fortification, we have supplementation and we have horticulture to a certain extent because in urban areas that would be quite difficult. Those are great solutions. Fortification is one way to go. However, we have to think this through very carefully because it doesn't fit all that is one of the main problems. In Bangladesh you can't find the food. A lot of these experiments worked in Latin America because they have wheat as a main staple food; in Africa maybe that is possible, but rice fortification has not been successful yet so we must put a lot of effort into these technologies to do these kinds of things. I am not pessimistic, I am just saying that we should not forget what is the reality today and how can we fit our work into this reality. That is the message, the fact that we have only one economist in the world who tries to translate the work we are doing in micronutrients for the World Bank, that is actually not a very positive sign. When Dr. Semba and I were working on our book (Nutrition and Health in Developing Countries) we had to find someone doing this work. Dr. Horton was not able to do this part, but we could not find anyone else. That means we need more people who can translate what we are doing, not only to the Minister of Finance but at the top level. I think we have a moral obligation to do so because the work we are doing is in principle to support these kinds of activities. So I am not pessimistic, I am just saying don't be unrealistic, don't be like an ostrich.

Dr. Horton: There are a lot of very interesting data and big ideas in your presentation but I will ask you a question about a smaller topic. I was very struck by the data on anemia and the urban rural differences for Indonesia and I was actually very surprised, I wouldn't have predicted that. I wanted to ask you if you have seen that same trend where the urban areas are worse in other countries during normal times, not in conditions of crisis, and secondly why do you think it is, is it primarily lack of dietary diversity in urban foods or is it health issues or what do you think causes this surprising finding?

Dr. Bloem: Many different urban areas have been analyzed and in fact the stunting levels are always lower than in the rural areas in most places. Only in Bangladesh the opposite was found. So Indonesia is not an exception to that rule. The only point is that, what I showed are the anemia levels which are still very high. We know that they consumed a lot of fortified food. Before the crisis, there were fortified noodles. They used processed food for the children. Suddenly because of the crisis they couldn't afford it anymore so they went back to some traditional food like rice, and didn't use fortified or processed products anymore. In urban areas the food is not the same as in rural areas; more processed food is eaten in urban areas. I think most of the time it is better than the food they eat in rural areas. So that is the explanation for why you see such an increase. There is still not much investment in Indonesia since the crisis, hardly any. Because it is a big country there is a kind of internal economy coming up, but of course it is a different form of economy. So there is an improvement but the improvement is not as dramatic as what we have seen in the past 10 years.

Dr. Guesry: In your presentation you spoke about rice price and availability and vitamin A deficiency, but you did not mention even a word about the golden rice project. In your answer to Dr. Tolboom you very briefly alluded to genetically modified organisms (GMO) and said that you didn't want to discuss it. Everybody knows that GMO would be a way to improve productivity, to decrease cost, to improve the nutritional value of these products, and many countries like China, India, Brazil have understood this. I do not understand why are you so shy, what is taboo about genetic engineering. If we can't discuss it in this type of setting where we are all open and scientists, then how can we discuss this issue?

Dr. Bloem: First of all, I am not an expert in this field but I believe that if you are realistic, there is no other way to go. However, I know there is a lot of discussion about it and since I am not an expert in this field I don't want to touch it because I would then have to defend or attack a certain policy on this. But I know it is a big topic. At the last INS meeting in Austria, it was a topic and thousands of people are discussing it. When I look at the data I think we have hardly any other way to go. I don't see any other solution than improve the quality of our products because, as we said yesterday, supplementation at this scale is almost impossible, so you have to do it through food and then we have this solution.

Mr. Parvanta: I suppose in any economic situation it is a matter of making choices, and you showed that obviously there was a difference. During the crisis there was a change in dietary patterns or at least in the selection of foods that people consumed. Do you know if there are any data on non-food products such as cigarettes or what I would consider non-essential consumer goods that people would still use in many ways, whether there are any patterns on that? I feel that there is some work to be done on making consumer choices, influencing consumer choice with regard to food and nutrition.

Dr. Bloem: That is a good question. We have looked at all these issues because one of the principles is, when you use the UNICEF conceptual framework, you look at food access, caring practices, health infrastructure, and socioeconomic issues. In Indonesia there is an incredible tobacco industry. It is one of the places where you can still see the most beautiful advertisements and you would love to smoke at the end when you see all those advertisements. So we looked at that and in fact after the crisis it was very interesting. Among the poor, the people who normally would buy a pack of cigarettes moved away from that. Ten years ago in Indonesia, you didn't have to buy a whole pack, you could buy 1 cigarette, and you pay for the cigarette and you smoke, or you buy 2 cigarettes. And that happened again. So people didn't stop smoking but they didn't buy whole packs. So it is true that even that had its effect. But we looked at this for policy reasons, and we said if you don't smoke at all and you spend that on the consumption of health products, you would save your child. But realistically people also like to enjoy life; even when they are poor they make choices not only based on the fact that they want to survive. There are a lot of other things in life.

Dr. Zlotkin: Thank you for taking on a difficult topic, quite related to what we were talking about in terms of the implications in ideology of micronutrient deficiencies. If I understood you correctly a lot of what you were saying had to do with food security, and the four components which influence food security to a large extent are economy, war, the weather and political instability. No matter how much we want stability in terms of those four conditions, we can't influence them very much and I think that no matter what we want, these things are going to continue in our lifetime. But with regard to micronutrients, at least we do have the opportunity to invest, if I can use that analogy, and possibly put some of the investment in a bank, and for some of the micronutrients like the fat-soluble vitamins, iron, vitamin A, we can in fact increase our stores and put it into the bank. The only way that we can increase our stores, recognizing that there is going to be a time of food insecurity, is in fact by either a major emphasis on food fortification during times of stability and maybe in fact thinking more about increasing the value of our plant crops possibly through GMO. Can you make any further comments and perhaps mention something about GAIN or the other international initiatives to bank some of the micronutrients in light of the food insecurity that is likely going to occur.

Dr. Bloem: When I was preparing this presentation, I looked through one of the text books of nutrition and there was a chapter by Carp, from Columbia University in New York, and he presented a very interesting story about micronutrient deficiencies among the urban poor in the US. I thought that was very interesting because in the countries we live in, for example the Netherlands or the States, although we have fortified products, supplementation, all the support of the health care system, we still find micronutrient deficiencies among the poor. Coming back to your question, yes, GAIN is a fantastic initiative. I think GAIN is the exception and it is really interested in making a difference in the lives of poor people. Whether GAIN is the most optimal group, I think it is a great initiative and I think it is good something has started. The danger of this initiative is that we always work only with governments. What we need to do is also to involve the private sectors in countries. It is very important. For example, there are two fortification projects we do with Heinz and a Western university, and the counterpart in the country itself is a non-government organization (NGO) involving technicians. So all these people have been brought together and that is actually very important. So I think GAIN is a great initiative and I hope they will involve all the different parties in it.

Dr. Gebre-Medhin: I am quite sure you are aware that these issues of food supply assistance, nutrition, etc., have been very eloquently discussed by Sen in his monumental work. He has also taken up the issue of urban rural dichotomy. In fact I very strongly believe that one of the interesting things with these analyses is that the increases in food price are very insignificant. These nations are nearly all net exporters of food. I think in this presentation governments are getting off very easily; I think we must get back to this issue very strongly. You mentioned Ethiopia and the World Bank. The main reason for the World Bank not giving Ethiopia the money was not because they didn't believe in their program but because nearly all of the NGO work and international support were used for very destructive wars, extremely destructive wars. Your main message was that in crisis micronutrient intake goes down. You also said food intake generally goes down in special groups. Is the solution fortification with micronutrients?

Dr. Bloem: I personally believe that we have to explore this further. Biotechnology is extremely important and I don't think that fortification itself is the solution alone. I don't believe in a single solution. All these activities are important. Let me give you one example about iodization of salt which is a success story. Looking at the data from Indonesia, you can see that even before the crisis – I am not talking about after the crisis because it is collapsing now – but before the crisis, we had an extremely successful program which almost went to 95% coverage in certain places; of course not in every place but a lot of places. But then if you analyze who is not receiving iodized salt, we are talking about the 5–10% of the poorest in that population. In a place like Indonesia, where you have over 200 million people, it is quite a dramatically large group. So the Indonesian government also thought we need to do something else, we also need another form, injections or capsules or whatever, to supplement this activity. But because all the driving forces were only looking at iodization of salt and there was hardly any interest in supporting any other type of activity. That is one of the dangers when you say fortification is the solution. I think fortification is a major strategy, however supplementation has a role to play and also all the other potential strategies. We have to be open minded to really solve a problem with many differences in different places, even in different ecological situations. A solution that fits all doesn't work in the world, but it doesn't mean that we should neglect these important global strategies and those are very important to support.

Dr. Villalpando-Carrión: In Mexico we also have very long periods of instability, but if we don't look at the nutritional problem as a stepwise problem, if you cannot try or make an attempt to modify the micronutrient status, if you haven't solved a first issue like severe malnutrition, it would be naïve at some point to try to do both things, both steps at one time. I don't know what you think about having different programs or different offers to different organizations, having a government subsidizing staple foods and NGO doing micronutrient fortification, could this happen?

Dr. Bloem: Let me state again, I am not supporting subsidized staple food. In fact it is the opposite, I believe that we need to open up so I am not for that at all. I don't think that you can say let's first solve severe malnutrition and then we will go to micronutrient malnutrition. They are happening at the same time. The data I showed you in Bangladesh, there is more severe malnutrition because there is an energy problem on top of the micronutrient problem; while in Indonesia the energy problem is much less than the micronutrient problem because there already is a different economic status level. But these problems are happening at the same time. I believe that we have to have comprehensive strategies, and the talk I gave today is actually to hopefully open the mind of the medical field, saying you have to communicate with other fields, bankers, economists, because if you don't we are working in isolation. It is nice because by still publishing papers we can still have a career in our field, but it doesn't solve the problems which we are facing. That is actually the message.

Pettifor JM, Zlotkin S (eds): Micronutrient Deficiencies during the Weaning Period and the First Years of Life. Nestlé Nutrition Workshop Series Pediatric Program, vol 54, pp 119–135, Nestec Ltd., Vevey/S. Karger AG, Basel, © 2004.

Impact of Micronutrient Deficiencies on Behavior and Development

Betsy Lozoff[a] *and Maureen M. Black*[b]

[a]Center for Human Growth and Development and Department of Pediatrics and Communicable Diseases, University of Michigan, Ann Arbor, Mich., and
[b]Department of Pediatrics, University of Maryland School of Medicine, Baltimore, Md., USA

Introduction

A variety of micronutrients affect infant behavior and development [for a recent review see, 1]. Here we focus on deficiencies of iron or zinc, which are among the most common single nutrients disorders in the world.

Iron Deficiency

A comprehensive review of studies on the behavioral and developmental effects of iron deficiency was published in 2001 [2]. That article and a Cochrane review [3] concluded that the association between iron deficiency in infancy and poorer behavioral/developmental outcome is strong, but causal connections remain to be proved. Thoughtful cautions have also been noted about interpretation [4]. Though still not definitive, some recent studies strengthen the causal link, and the results are consistent with current understanding of iron's role in the developing brain. We will emphasize these studies, summarizing previous research only briefly to lay the foundation. Unless otherwise indicated, studies assessed iron status by multiple measures in addition to hemoglobin. Most studies used case-control designs, comparing infants with iron-deficiency anemia to those with better iron status, and some included controlled trials of iron treatment. Most included reasonable

Supported in part by grants from the National Institutes of Health (R01 HD33487, R01 HD31606 and P01 HD39386), Betsy Lozoff, Principal Investigator, and (R01 HD37430) Maureen Black, Principal Investigator.

assessments of environmental and potentially confounding factors. The very few randomized trials of preventing iron deficiency will be specifically identified. It is important to note that most studies have focused on healthy full-term infants without other health or nutritional problems. Researchers have studied such populations by design in order to assess the effects of iron deficiency without the confounding effects of malnutrition, infectious diseases, etc.

Mental Development

Mental outcomes in most studies have been global tests of development, such as the Bayley Scales of Infant Development [2]. In almost all the case-control studies, mental development test scores averaged 6–15 points lower among iron-deficient anemic infants, even after control for background factors, an important consideration since iron-deficient anemic infants may have a variety of disadvantages in background. In general, iron therapy did not correct the lower test scores in the majority of iron-deficient anemic infants. A major exception was a study in Indonesia [5] in which iron-deficient anemic infants dramatically improved in test scores after iron therapy. Despite the consistency of finding lower pretreatment scores, global test scores provide little indication of what iron deficiency might be doing to the developing brain.

Of the few available preventive trials, a recent large study in Chile was the only one to find effects of iron supplementation specifically on mental functioning. Infants supplemented with iron between 6 and 12 months (n = 1,123) were compared to a no-added-iron group (n = 534) [6]. There were no differences in overall mental or motor test scores, but infants in the no-added-iron group showed differences on the Fagan Test of Infant Intelligence. On this test of visual recognition memory and novelty preference, there were no differences in novelty preference but the infants in the no-added-iron group looked longer. Longer looking times are considered to be an indicator of less efficient high-speed information processing and predict later IQ better than global tests of infant development [6].

One recent case-control study also examined specific cognitive processes. This study used event-related potentials to assess recognition memory among infants of diabetic mothers, who are at high risk for being born with brain iron deficiency [7]. These infants showed poorer recognition memory than control babies on age-appropriate measures, from birth to 8 months [8]. This study is unique in its use of neuroimaging with event-related potentials and a strong developmental cognitive neuroscience perspective.

There is evidence that differences associated with iron-deficiency anemia in infancy are long-lasting. Most follow-up studies have been at early school age (4–8 years), with generally uniform results: children who had iron-deficiency anemia in infancy tested lower than peers in overall mental functioning [2]. In the longest follow-up to date [9], 11- to 14-year-old children in Costa Rica who had been treated for severe, chronic iron deficiency in infancy still tested lower in arithmetic and writing achievement than their peers who had had good iron status in infancy. Twice as many had repeated a grade, and 3 times as many had been referred for special education or tutoring. They also had poorer performance on some tests of specific cognitive functions (tachistoscopic threshold, spatial memory, and selective attention).

Another important study of long-term outcome was conducted statewide in Florida [10]. Anemia in infancy, based on hemoglobin screening in the Women, Infant, and Children program, was associated with special education placement at age 10 years, based on the criteria used by the Florida Department of Education for mild or moderate mental retardation. Although this study was limited in that hemoglobin was the sole measure of iron status, it is exceptional in relating anemia in infancy (presumably due to iron deficiency) to mental retardation or special education placement among school-aged children in an entire population.

The above long-term follow-up studies involved infants who were identified as having iron deficiency in the infant/toddler period. Only one study has related a measure of iron status at birth (cord ferritin level) to later development (at 5 years) [11]. Children with cord ferritin levels in the lowest quartile received lower scores for language ability, fine-motor skills, and tractability.

Social/Emotional Development

Virtually every study that has examined infant affect or social/emotional behavior has found differences in iron-deficient anemic infants compared to those with better iron status [2]. In case-control studies, infants with iron-deficiency anemia were typically rated as being more wary/hesitant, fearful, unreactive to usual stimuli, solemn, unhappy, and/or easily fatigued during developmental testing. In studies in Guatemala and Costa Rica, infant behavior was also coded and rated from videotape during play and developmental testing. Infants with iron-deficiency anemia stayed closer to their mothers, made fewer attempts at task items, showed less pleasure and delight, were less playful, were more wary/hesitant, etc. [12]. In the Costa Rica study, the only study to date that included observations in the home, daily spot observations over a 3-month period showed that iron-deficient anemic infants were more likely to be asleep, irritable, carried, doing nothing, in bed, not interacting with anyone, etc. [12].

Two of the preventive trials reported differences in the affective domain as well. In a study in the UK in which infants were supplemented with iron from 7 to 18 months [13], there were no differences between supplemented and unsupplemented infants at the conclusion of the trial. However, at 24 months, supplemented infants did not show the decline in global development quotient that was observed in babies who did not receive iron. An examination of the test's subscales revealed that the only significant difference was the personal/social subscale. In the preventive trial in Chile [6], a greater proportion of infants who did not receive iron showed no social interaction, no positive affect, and no social referencing throughout a 45-min test session. Among the few babies who cried, more of the no-added-iron group could not be soothed by words or objects; they had to be held or they could not be soothed at all. Fewer of them were considered to be 'unadaptable'. In this rating, being 'unadaptable' means protesting when a toy is taken away. Since this is quite normal behavior for infants who are engaged with an object, it appears that the babies who did not get iron were less involved with test objects.

Affective and social/emotional differences were still observed in former iron-deficient children in the Costa Rica follow-up at 11–14 years [8]. Their parents and teachers rated their behavior as more problematic in several areas, agreeing in increased concerns about anxiety/depression, social problems, and attention problems.

Motor Development

Among studies that included an assessment of motor development, most found that infants with iron-deficiency anemia received lower motor test scores, averaging 9–15 points lower [2]. An important population study in the UK found that a hemoglobin level of <95 g/l at 8 months predicted poorer locomotor development at 18 months [14]. Several studies have observed little or no improvement in motor test scores after iron therapy or improvements only in a minority of iron-deficient anemic children who showed the most dramatic hematologic response to iron. The above-mentioned study in Indonesia was again an exception – motor score deficits were completely corrected with iron therapy [5].

Among the preventive trials, one conducted in Canada [15], with iron supplementation between 2 and 15 months, showed lower motor scores in the unsupplemented group at 9 and 12 months. In the preventive trial in Chile [6], infants who did not receive iron crawled somewhat later, on average, than iron-supplemented infants. At 12 months, a greater proportion of the unsupplemented group was rated as tremulous.

In long-term follow-up studies, differences in motor test scores have been observed, up to more than 10 years after iron treatment [9, 16, 17]. Differences in visual-motor integration years after the period of iron-deficiency anemia have also been observed in 2 studies that have included such a measure [16, 17].

Spontaneous Motor Activity and the Sleep/Wake Cycle

Despite compelling reasons from animal studies to expect differences in spontaneous motor activity in the iron-deficient anemic infant, only one project has assessed this directly. Using activity meters on the baby's ankle, spontaneous motor activity was compared between Chilean infants with iron-deficiency anemia and a non-anemic group. In the course of a year of iron treatment, the formerly iron-deficient anemic infants showed reduced motor activity during waking before and after a nap in a neurophysiology laboratory [18]. A different pattern was observed in the home. During the period of iron deficiency, there was increased motor activity (leg movement) in virtually every phase of the sleep/wake cycle throughout a 24-hour period [19]. Most differences in the home disappeared after iron therapy.

In the same Chile study, polysomnographic recordings were obtained during a spontaneous daytime nap in the laboratory in infancy and an overnight sleep study at 4 years. There were multiple differences in measures of the sleep/wake cycle in infancy and/or at follow-up. Findings included differences in REM latency, duration of REM episodes and their pattern through the night, the duration of slow wave sleep episodes early in the night, both the isolated REMS and non-isolated REMS indices and inter-REM intervals [20, 21]. Thus, iron-deficiency anemia appears to alter key components of the internal temporal order within the 24-hour cycle.

Sensory Development
A few recent studies have examined sensory development in iron-deficient anemic infants [22]. In the neurophysiology component of the study in Chile, 6-month-old infants with and without iron-deficiency anemia were studied with auditory brainstem responses (ABRs) during a spontaneous nap in the laboratory [23]. There was slower transmission throughout the auditory pathway (longer latency for the wave I–V interval) among the babies with iron-deficiency anemia. The differences became even bigger after a year of iron therapy and correction of anemia. Children who had participated in the study as infants were assessed at 4–5 years of age with ABRs and visual evoked potentials [22]. The formerly iron-deficient anemic group showed longer ABR and visual evoked potential latencies. The magnitude of effects was large: 1–1.2 SD.

Effects among Infants and Toddlers Who Are Not Healthy and Well-Nourished
One recent study of undernourished infants in Indonesia found that those who received an energy supplement plus iron-containing micronutrients walked at an earlier age, had higher mental and motor test scores, were more motorically active, and showed more mature social-cognitive and emotional regulatory behaviors. This multifaceted project, although involving a relatively small sample, was noteworthy in its comprehensive approach and development of a model that encompassed affective, motor, and mental effects [24].

A large double-blind, placebo-controlled trial of iron supplementation and anthelminthic treatment was conducted in Zanzibar, where malnutrition was widespread and malaria omnipresent [25]. Infants and preschoolers assigned to iron for a 12-month period improved more in language development than those assigned to placebo. Among children 12–36 months of age, iron supplementation also improved motor development, but the effect was apparent only in children with baseline hemoglobin concentrations of <90 g/l. Since so many of the world's children live in settings where generalized undernutrition and infectious diseases occur along with iron deficiency, more research in such settings is urgently needed.

Postulated Mechanisms

Some of these findings can be interpreted in light of the current understanding of iron's role in the developing brain. Iron is required by every cell in the body and is thus involved with many processes. So far, the most relevant to behavior and development are iron's role in myelination, neurotransmitter function, and neuronal metabolism [26, 27]. The findings most tightly linked to alterations in myelination are slower transmission in the auditory and visual systems. Both of these sensory systems are rapidly myelinating during the period of iron deficiency, and they are sensory systems critical for learning and social interaction. It is also likely that there are other intracerebral effects, given that so many brain systems are myelinating during this period. Thus, impaired myelination could underlie other poorer outcomes. For instance, longer looking times on the Fagan Test, long-lasting differences in visual-motor integration, and later crawling/walking might be consistent with altered myelination.

With regard to alterations in neurotransmitter functioning, the dopamine system has been best studied [26]. Among many functions, dopamine plays a major role in systems of behavioral activation and inhibition and the degree to which individuals experience inherent reward. The affective changes in iron-deficient anemic infants (wariness, hesitance, absence of positive affect), their lack of social referencing, and the observation that toys can be taken away from them without protest all seem to make sense in this context.

Dopamine's role in extraneous motor movement is also well-established, and the observations of tremor would fit. In addition, there is a strong association between iron deficiency and periodic leg movements or restless leg syndrome in older children and adults. The increased leg movements observed in the Chilean infants during the period of iron-deficiency anemia might be an infant equivalent or precursor [19]. In addition, differences between home and laboratory suggest that the iron-deficient anemic children respond differently to context – with a reduction in motor activity after the stress or unfamiliarity of the laboratory.

Recent work in the animal model has documented iron's role in neuronal metabolism and shown that there are differential effects on the developing hippocampus and other parts of the brain required for cognitive functioning [27]. The findings of poorer recognition memory in infants at high risk for iron deficiency (due to maternal diabetes) appear to fit with an effect of iron deficiency on the hippocampus and related components of the central nervous system [7]. However, the findings need to be replicated among infants with dietary iron deficiency.

To summarize, there seems to be delayed or mistimed sensory input in at least 2 sensory systems in early iron-deficiency anemia. These changes, together with other cognitive, motor, and affective differences, may mean that the iron-deficient baby seeks and/or receives less stimulation. Over time this may result in reduced input from the physical and social environment, which, in animal models, has been shown to have secondary effects on brain structure and function.

Zinc Deficiency

There are no clear biomarkers to identify zinc deficiency [28]. Therefore, investigators rely on responses in randomized zinc supplementation trials among children thought to be zinc-deficient. In contrast to studies of iron deficiency, most of which involved well-nourished, healthy babies, research on zinc deficiency has generally focused on children at risk of poor growth. Recent studies among nutritionally at-risk infants have demonstrated the beneficial effects of zinc supplementation on infant mortality [29] and on multiple indicators of health, including growth [30], diarrhea [31, 32], and pneumonia morbidity [31]. An early observational study from Egypt reported an association between maternal micronutrient intake and infants' developmental skills at 6 weeks and 6 months of age [33, 34], suggesting that zinc may play a critical role in the development of infants' mental and motor skills. However, reviews of the randomized trials of zinc supplementation conducted in the past decade have concluded that there are inconsistent findings regarding the relationship between zinc supplementation and child development [35, 36].

Mental Development
Mental development has been examined in at least 6 randomized trials of zinc supplementation. They were conducted among very low-birth-weight infants in Canada [37], small-for-gestational age infants in India [35], and low-income infants in Chile [38], Brazil [39], and Bangladesh [40, 41]. In the Bangladesh trials, zinc-supplemented infants had mental scores that were 3–6 points higher than unsupplemented infants at 12 months, regardless of whether zinc supplementation was administered to mothers during pregnancy [41] or directly to the infants [40]. None of the other trials found differences in mental development related to zinc supplementation.

Social/Emotional Development
Two trials assessed infants' social/emotional development related to zinc supplementation. Zinc-supplemented infants in Brazil were more cooperative than unsupplemented infants, based on behavioral observations conducted by examiners [39]. In a trial among infants born small-for-gestational age in

India, there were no differences in orientation or emotional regulation related to zinc supplementation [35]. However, when mothers were asked about their infants' behavior, mothers of zinc-supplemented infants with a birth weight of <2,500 g were more likely to report that their infants were irritable than were mothers of unsupplemented infants [35].

Motor Development

Very low-birth-weight infants in Canada who received formula with a higher concentration of zinc (11 versus 6.7 mg/l) for the first 5 months of life had better scores in motor development than those who received the lower concentration of zinc [37]. In Chile, low-income infants who received zinc daily for 1 year had higher scores in motor quality (gross and fine motor movement and control), but there were no differences in the children's overall motor scores [38]. In India, infants born small-for-gestational age who received zinc supplements for the first 9 months of life had marginally higher motor scores at 6 months [35], but there were no differences at 10 months.

Spontaneous Motor Activity

Three trials that examined infant activity all found increases related to zinc supplementation. In Peru, fetuses of mothers who received zinc supplementation during pregnancy were more active during prenatal sonograms, in comparison to fetuses of control mothers [42]. In India, low-income toddlers who received zinc daily for 6 months had more vigorous activity during play compared with control toddlers [43]. In Guatemala, stunted toddlers who received zinc daily for 7 months had more functional activity during play compared with control toddlers [44]. Thus, findings related to zinc supplementation and spontaneous motor activity among infants at high risk for zinc deficiency are relatively consistent.

Methodological Considerations

Most of the studies examining the impact of zinc supplementation on child development used global measures of development (e.g., Bayley Scales of Infant Development) and were conducted with careful controls for environmental and potentially confounding variables. Although the Bayley Scales are well-standardized and include explicit instructions for administration, they may not capture subtle differences in information processing.

Infants who experience intrauterine growth retardation are likely to become zinc-deficient, because they have limited hepatic stores of zinc and increased requirements for catch-up growth [45]. Children with low consumption of bioavailable sources of zinc (e.g., animal products) are also at risk for zinc deficiency. However, undernourished children are also at risk for other micronutrient deficiencies that have been associated with developmental delays, especially iron and B_{12} [46], emphasizing the importance of examining the interrelationships among micronutrients.

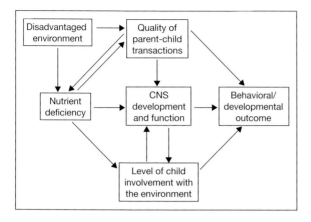

Fig. 1. Functional isolation. Modified from Wachs, 2002 [50].

Postulated Mechanisms

Zinc deficiency may be particularly relevant to early development because zinc is present in all cells, playing fundamental roles in cell division and maturation and in the growth and function of many organ systems, including the central nervous system [47]. In the central nervous system, zinc is concentrated in the synaptic vesicles of specific glutaminergic neurons. Zinc serves as a neurotransmitter, passing into postsynaptic neurons during synaptic events. Zinc is thought to be essential for nucleic acid and protein synthesis, processes that may be disrupted by zinc deficiency [48]. However, none of the measures used in studies of human infants/toddlers can be easily or directly linked to these central nervous system processes.

Conceptual Framework for Developmental/Behavioral
Effects of Early Nutrient Deficiencies

There is ample evidence that nutrient deficiencies are more likely to occur in disadvantaged environments, which themselves have adverse effects on children. There is also clear indication that nutrient deficiencies have direct effects on central nervous system development. Research examining the impact of iron and/or zinc deficiencies on children's development has often hypothesized a direct effect, through changes in neuroanatomy or neurotransmission, for example. However, it is also possible that behavior changes associated with micronutrient deficiencies alter the caregiving that the child receives, thereby compromising the child's development even further. For example, if a micronutrient-deficient child is unable to elicit or to benefit from nurturant interactions from a caregiver, that child may be denied the enrichment that is known to promote early development. The result could be a child who experiences the brain changes that have been associated with micronutrient deficiency, together with limited environmental input. Over time, these combined influences may result in poorer behavioral and developmental outcomes (fig. 1). This process, whereby poorer outcomes in infants and toddlers with nutritional deficiencies are partially mediated through caregiving behavior, is known as functional isolation [49]. Future research should consider how the caregiving system is related to child development and whether it mediates the effects of micronutrient deficiencies.

References

1 Georgieff MK, Rao R: The role of nutrition in cognitive development; in Nelson CA, Luciana M, (eds): Handbook of Developmental Cognitive Neuroscience. Boston, MIT Press, 1999.
2 Grantham-McGregor S, Ani C: A review of studies on the effect of iron deficiency on cognitive development in children. J Nutr 2001;131:649S–668S.
3 Martins S, Logan S, Gilbert R: Iron therapy for improving psychomotor development and cognitive function in children under the age of three with iron deficiency anaemia (Cochrane Review). The Cochrane Library. Oxford, Update Software, 2003.
4 Pollitt E: Developmental sequel from early nutritional deficiencies: Conclusive and probability judgments. J Nutr 2000;130:350S–353S.
5 Idjradinata P, Pollitt E: Reversal of developmental delays in iron-deficient anaemic infants treated with iron. Lancet 1993;341:1–4.
6 Lozoff B, De Andraca I, Castillo M, et al: Behavioral and developmental effects of preventing iron-deficiency anemia in healthy full-term infants. Pediatrics 2003;112:846–854.
7 Nelson CA, Wewerka SS, Borscheid AJ, et al: Electrophysiologic evidence of impaired cross-modal recognition memory in 8-month-old infants of diabetic mothers. J Pediatr 2003;142:575–582.
8 Nelson CA, Wewerka S, Thomas KM, et al: Neurocognitive sequelae of infants of diabetic mothers. Behav Neurosci 2000;114:950–956.
9 Lozoff B, Jimenez E, Hagen J, et al: Poorer behavioral and developmental outcome more than 10 years after treatment for iron deficiency in infancy. Pediatrics 2000;105:E51.
10 Hurtado EK, Claussen AH, Scott KG: Early childhood anemia and mild or moderate mental retardation. Am J Clin Nutr 1999;69:115–119.
11 Tamura T, Goldenberg RL, Hou J, et al: Cord serum ferritin concentrations and mental and psychomotor development of children at five year of age. J Pediatr 2002;140:165–170.
12 Lozoff B, Klein NK, Nelson EC, et al: Behavior of infants with iron deficiency anemia. Child Dev 1998;69:24–36.
13 Williams J, Wolff A, Daly A, et al: Iron supplemented formula milk related to reduction in psychomotor decline in infants for inner city areas: Randomised study. BMJ 1999;318:693–698.
14 Sherriff A, Emond A, Bell JC, et al: Should infants be screened for anaemia? A prospective study investigating the relation between haemoglobin at 8, 12, and 18 months and development at 18 months. Arch Dis Child 2001;84:480–485.
15 Moffatt MEK, Longstaffe S, Besant J, Dureski C: Prevention of iron deficiency and psychomotor decline in high risk infants through iron fortified infant formula: A randomized clinical trial. J Pediatr 1994;125:527–534.
16 Lozoff B, Jimenez E, Wolf AW: Long-term developmental outcome of infants with iron deficiency. N Engl J Med 1991;325:687–694.
17 De Andraca I, Walter T, Castillo M, et al: Iron Deficiency Anemia and Its Effects upon Psychological Development at Preschool Age: A Longitudinal Study. Nestle Foundation Nutrition Annual Report 1990. Vevey, Nestec, 1991, pp 53–62.
18 Angulo-Kinzler RM, Peirano P, Lin E, et al: Spontaneous motor activity in human infants with iron-deficiency anemia. Early Hum Dev 2002;66:67–79.
19 Angulo-Kinzler RM, Peirano P, Lin E, et al: Twenty-four-hour motor activity in human infants with and without iron deficiency anemia. Early Hum Dev 2002;70:85–101.
20 Garrido M, Peirano P, Algarin C, Lozoff B: Early iron deficiency anemia affects the modulation of motor activity in sleeping infants. J Sleep Res 2002;11(suppl 1):172S–173S.

21 Algarin C, Peirano PD, Garrido MI, et al: Iron deficiency anemia (IDA) in infancy alters the temporal organization of sleep states in childhood (abstract). Sleep 2001;24(suppl):A13.

22 Algarin C, Peirano P, Garrido M, et al: Iron deficiency anemia: Long-lasting effects on auditory and visual systems functioning. Pediatr Res 2003;53:217–223.

23 Roncagliolo M, Garrido M, Walter T, et al: Evidence of altered central nervous system development in infants with iron deficiency anemia at 6 mo: Delayed maturation of auditory brain stem responses. Am J Clin Nutr 1998;68:683–690.

24 Pollitt E, Schurch B (eds):Developmental pathways of the malnourished child: Results of a supplementation trial in Indonesia. Eur J Clin Nutr 2000;54(suppl 2):S1–S119.

25 Stoltzfus R, Kvalvig J, Chwaya H, et al: Effects of iron supplementation and anthelminthic treatment on motor and language development of preschool children in Zanzibar: Double blind, placebo controlled study. BMJ 2001;323:1389–1393.

26 Beard J: Iron deficiency alters brain development and functioning. J Nutr 2003;133:1468S–1472S.

27 DeUngria M, Rao R, Wobken JD, et al: Perinatal iron deficiency decreases cytochrome c oxidase (CytOx) activity in selected regions of neonatal rat brain. Pediatr Res 2000;48:169–176.

28 Hambidge M: Biomarkers of trace mineral intake and status. J Nutr 2003;133:948S–955S.

29 Sazawal S, Black RE, Menon VP, et al: Zinc supplementation in infants born small for gestational age reduces mortality: A prospective, randomized, controlled trial. Pediatrics 2001;108: 1280–1286.

30 Brown KH, Peerson JM, Rivera J, Allen LH: Effect of supplemental zinc on the growth and serum zinc concentrations of prepubertal children: A meta-analysis of randomized controlled trials. Am J Clin Nutr 2002;75:1062–1071.

31 Bhutta ZA, Black RE, Brown KH, et al: Prevention of diarrhea and pneumonia by zinc supplementation in children in developing countries: Pooled analysis of randomized controlled trials. Zinc Investigators' Collaborative Group. J Pediatr 1999;135:689–697.

32 Bhutta ZA, Bird SM, Black RE, et al: Therapeutic effects of oral zinc in acute and persistent diarrhea in children in developing countries: Pooled analysis of randomized controlled trials. Am J Clin Nutr 2000;72:1516–1522.

33 Kirksey A, Rahmanifar A, Wachs TD, et al: Determinants of pregnancy outcome and newborn behavior of a semirural Egyptian population. Am J Clin Nutr 1991;54:657–667.

34 Kirksey A, Wachs TD, Yunis F, et al: Relation of maternal zinc nutriture to pregnancy outcome and infant development in an Egyptian village. Am J Clin Nutr 1994;60:782–792.

35 Black MM: The evidence linking zinc deficiency with children's cognitive and motor functioning. J Nutr 2003;133:1473S–1476S.

36 Bhatnagar S, Taneja S: Zinc and cognitive development. Br J Nutr 2001;85:S139–S145.

37 Friel JK, Andrews WL, Matthew JD, et al: Zinc supplementation in very-low-birth-weight infants. J Pediatr Gastroenterol Nutr 1993;17:97–104.

38 Castillo-Duran C, Perales CG, Hertrampf ED, et al: Effect of zinc supplementation on development and growth of Chilean infants. J Pediatr 2001;138:229–235.

39 Ashworth A, Morris SS, Lira PI, Grantham-McGregor SM: Zinc supplementation, mental development and behaviour in low birth weight term infants in northeast Brazil. Eur J Clin Nutr 1998;52:223–227.

40 Hamadani JD, Fuchs GJ, Osendarp SJ, et al: Randomized controlled trial of the effect of zinc supplementation on the mental development of Bangladeshi infants. Am J Clin Nutr 2001;74: 381–386.

41 Hamadani JD, Fuchs GJ, Osendarp SJ, et al: Zinc supplementation during pregnancy and effects on mental development and behaviour of infants: A follow-up study. Lancet 2002;360:290–294.

42 Merialdi M, Caulfield LE, Zavaleta N, et al: Adding zinc to prenatal iron and folate tablets improves fetal neurobehavioral development. Am J Obstet Gynecol 1999;180:483–490.

43 Sazawal S, Bentley M, Black RE, et al: Effect of zinc supplementation on observed activity in low socioeconomic Indian preschool children. Pediatrics 1996;98:1132–1137.

44 Bentley ME, Caulfield LE, Ram M, et al: Zinc supplementation affects the activity patterns of rural Guatemalan infants. J Nutr 1997;127:1333–1338.

45 Zlotkin SH, Cherian MG: Hepatic metallothionein as a source of zinc and cysteine during the first year of life. Pediatr Res 1988;24:326–329.

46 Grantham-McGregor SM, Ani CC: The role of micronutrients in psychomotor and cognitive development. Br Med Bull 1999;55:511–527.

47 Sandstead HH, Frederickson CJ, Penland JG: History of zinc as related to brain function. J Nutr 2000;130:496S–502S.

48 Frederickson CJ, Suh SW, Silva D, et al: Importance of zinc in the central nervous system: The zinc-containing neuron. J Nutr 2000;130:1471S–1483S.
49 Levitsky DA, Barnes RH: Nutritional and environmental interactions in the behavioral development of the rat: Long-term effects. Science 1972;176:68–71.
50 Wachs TD: Nutritional deficiencies as a biological context for development; in Hartup W, Silbereisen R (eds): Growing Points in Developmental Science. Dove, UK, Psychology Press 2002, pp 64–84.

Discussion

Dr. Pettifor: I have a question about the preventive trial in Chile in which there were some subjects on iron and others without iron. What percentage of those who were not on iron actually developed clinical iron deficiency? If one looks at iron deficiency as being a continuum was there a cutoff point where it could be said that a certain level of iron status was needed before they develop any of the changes that you noted, or was it a continuous progression from those who were severely iron deficient to those who were quite iron replete?

Dr. Lozoff: In the Chile study [1], the unsupplemented group was given milk or vitamins in identically marked cans or bottles, so the study was double-blind. There was no added iron. Chile and Costa Rica at the time and Brazil are countries where babies are often given unmodified cow's milk quite early. Even mixed with breast-feeding, there is a lot of iron deficiency under those conditions. Like other studies, we found that 23% of the unsupplemented group had iron deficiency anemia and an additional 31% or so had iron deficiency without anemia. Overall more than 50% of the unsupplemented group had iron deficiency by the strict criteria of at least 2 of 3 abnormal iron measures, and all iron parameters were worse. This means that the entire unsupplemented group had a poorer iron status. We looked for a continuum of effects but didn't observe any. What we found was that the whole unsupplemented group did worse in behavior and development. Thus, in a study where infants were randomly allocated, there was no suggestion of a cutoff point.

The earlier community study in Costa Rica [2] had been designed to try to answer that question in a non-experimental study. With children at every level of iron deficiency, we analyzed the Bayley test scores. In that study we concluded, and Walter et al. [3] in Chile reached pretty much the same conclusion, that iron deficiency needed to be severe enough to cause anemia before lower mental and motor test scores were seen. I was comfortable with that for a long time, but I think this could be revisited for the following reasons. These were effects on a global test of development. As we move into more sensitive measures, such as nerve conduction and other things, it is an open question whether there are effects of iron deficiency without anemia. In fact we are looking at that right now in a program project grant from the US National Institutes of Health (I should add that all of the work I reported was supported by the National Institutes of Health). What is this program project grant? It is a cross-species project with human infants, two developing monkey projects, and a rodent model. Across these species we are trying to develop behavioral measures that link them and then go progressively to the brain in the animal models. We are also specifically looking for effects of iron deficiency without anemia using very sensitive measures and also trying to identify which behaviors can be corrected by iron treatment and which not.

Dr. Pettifor: Looking at all the factors that influence the development of children in early life and trying to relate the percentage effect of genetics, of assessing data on iron deficiency, etc., how much do you think is the overall effect of iron deficiency on mental development?

Dr. Lozoff: All of the results I showed are statistically significant after controlling for everything that we could. We measured mothers' IQ, the home environment, socioeconomic status, child's growth, etc. and controlled for all these factors. But that is statistical control. One of the very special things about the Chilean study, the preventive trial, is that children were randomly assigned to receive high or low iron or no added iron. By that design the children of mothers with lower IQs and worse environments were equally likely to be in the different groups, and they were. In addition, we controlled for all of those things statistically. So the behavioral differences are most likely due to lack of iron.

In the analysis of the Costa Rica study, we gave all these factors a chance to account for variability and then asked how much variance was left over that could be attributed to iron deficiency anemia. Background factors accounted for 3–8% of the variance, and iron deficiency anemia accounted for an additional 5–8%. That doesn't fully answer the question, however, because these things co-occur. By statistical control, for instance, you remove the shares effects.

Dr. Endres: As you described this relationship almost too beautifully to be believed, I just have a very simple question. Were the psychologists blinded to the study?

Dr. Lozoff: Absolutely, neither the parents nor the psychologists knew the child's iron status. In fact, the mothers were not told the baby's blood results until the end of the study, so it was always double-blind. Even though the results are dramatic and I think they are important, it is not as though you would see a child in your waiting room and say that there is something wrong with that baby. They are very carefully screened so that nobody was sick, and in fact if you look at the developmental test scores, there was virtually nobody below the normal range. So we are finding differences within the normal range. This relates to another point. Much research on iron deficiency has carefully focused on such otherwise healthy children. We don't know much about the effects of iron deficiency among children in less optimal health. Yet around the world in developing countries many children have a variety of health problems. Studies with otherwise healthy infants help us understand the effects of iron deficiency apart from generalized undernutrition or other illnesses or infections, so it gives a conservative estimate of what iron is doing.

Dr. Gebre-Medhin: I think we have no doubt about the fact that iron deficiency anemia in an infant is a very serious matter. A child with verified iron deficiency is a very sick child so this is a very important area for discussion. Now my question is partly a follow-up on Dr. Endres' question, what about the parents: do they communicate with the psychologist; do they tell them whether the child has been iron medicated or not? Was this an experimental study in which you were responsible for the distribution of iron and treatment, or was this an observational retroactive prospective study? The reasons that lead children to iron deficiency anemia may be one thing, but seeking care in the hospital will dramatically disaggregate them into very different groups. How was that issue controlled?

Dr. Lozoff: The first question is could mothers have alerted the testers in some way or the other. There are a couple of observations here. I don't agree that most children with iron deficiency anemia are very sick. I don't know if you noticed the percentages of those showing altered behavior, but the highest percentage was for 'no social referencing': 18% of the unsupplemented group compared to 8% of the children who received iron [1]. That means that over 80% of the children who were in the unsupplemented group did check in with their mothers. So it is not that every iron-deficient child or every child who is not getting iron shows this behavior. We have no indication from available studies that there is something affecting every baby or something easy for the mothers to report. In Costa Rica, I asked the pediatrician to indicate who she thought was iron deficient based on her interaction and examination, and it was about 50–50 whether she could guess. That is my most direct indication that even a highly skilled pediatrician, when asked to pick out these children, could not do it, let alone the mothers.

Your second question is were the studies observational or intervention. The earlier studies I talked about are almost universally case-control studies. However, children were identified not in a clinic setting but in neighborhoods. The studies tested the children and then compared those with iron deficiency anemia with those with better iron status. In Costa Rica, it was a door-to-door study: knock on the door and ask whether there was a child between 12 and 23 months. If the baby was completely healthy and full-term, they were invited to enter the study. So they did not come to the doctor seeking attention. We closely supervised the iron therapy and have continued to follow them. Nonetheless, Costa Rica was an observational study in that whatever factors might go along with iron deficiency were there. We statistically controlled them but nonetheless they are there.

Now we come to the Chile study and why the Chilean study had its design. We made sure no child with iron deficiency anemia went into the preventive trial, and then they were randomly allocated to get high iron or low iron, or high or no added iron. So this study is different from most earlier ones. The children were not simply turning up with iron deficiency later on. Rather, iron status was a result of randomization. I told you that 23% of the children in the no-added-iron group had iron deficiency anemia. The figure for the iron-supplemented group was 3%. There is no question that the study design produced groups with extremely different iron status.

Dr. Abrams: I want to put my hand up as a neonatologist here. What we do every day in the nursery is we care for premature infants who would otherwise be in utero and allow them to have hemoglobins of 7–10 without problems and leave them that way for several months without transfusing them. In this general change over the last 10 years in neonatology, I was wondering if you have any data or any comments about whether or not this is a very good idea from a developmental perspective and if any one has ever looked at this issue in in utero terms?

Dr. Lozoff: The question relates to the premature infant and the low hemoglobins we allow them to have. Dr. Georgieff is a neonatologist very involved with iron deficiency these days, and he would be a wonderful person to address this question. A concern around the premature infant and the perinatal period is that iron regulation is not fully developed. This means that iron toxicity may be more of a risk then that it is later on. Iron deficiency is not good for babies' brains, but excess iron might also occur in the very immature brain. We certainly need more research on these issues.

Dr. Guesry: Could you say something about the critical age threshold because earlier studies seem to say that if one wants to avoid neurological sequelae the correction of iron deficiency anemia should take place before 1 year of age. The latest study, the one that you mentioned in Indonesia, seems to say that, even after 1 year of age [4], correction of the anemia could also correct neurological symptoms.

Dr. Lozoff: The Costa Rican children averaged 17 months of age; in that study the children were between 12 and 23 months. So all of them were after the first year of life. In Chile, the period of supplementation was between 6 and 12 months. You have brought up an important point that I can't emphasize enough: when looking at different studies, attention must be paid to the age at which they are performed. Timing questions are very challenging in the human: timing, duration and severity of iron deficiency are intimately intertwined. A baby who gets iron deficient earlier is likely to have iron deficiency longer and more severely. Thus, from observational studies in the human it is almost impossible to separate timing, duration and severity. Now in the Chile study we know with confidence that no baby had iron deficiency anemia for longer than 6 months, because we tested their blood at 6 months and those with iron deficiency anemia were pulled out. Then we tested their blood again at 12 months. So the maximum duration of iron deficiency anemia can only have been 6 months. In fact, it is probably less. Infants started on the different supplements at 6 months, and so it was probably not until 8, 9, 10 months that some developed iron deficiency anemia.

This is a very short time period. I actually think this is why we did not see differences in the Bayley test in the Chilean study: the babies had iron deficiency for such a short time. Timing is a question that we are looking at in the program project grant using animal models, because timing, duration and severity can be controlled experimentally. So again it is humbling how long it takes to get answers to some of these very important questions.

Dr. Bloem: Were these studies carried in the urban or rural areas?

Dr. Lozoff: All of the studies I'm involved in have been in urban settings. They involved working class communities – lower to lower middle class. The mothers in Chile and Costa Rica averaged about 9 years of education. Everybody was literate, and health was excellent in both these countries with national health care systems. So they are in much better conditions than most children in the world.

Dr. Bloem: How much do you think lead toxicity has influenced your results?

Dr. Lozoff: Both of these countries have used unleaded paint for many decades. In Costa Rica we measured lead in all the children; the lead levels averaged about $10\,\mu g/dl$. This was in the early 1980s, when the US cutoff was $25\,\mu g/dl$. Lead levels were controlled in all of the results. It is very interesting that in Costa Rica there was no negative correlation between lead and child development at those levels [5]. In Chile we didn't have enough money to do lead levels on everybody. With the good graces of the CDC we were able to test for lead in a sub-sample. We sent bloods from infants with the very highest erythrocyte protoporphyrin values and some of the normal values. Then one of my colleagues, Dr. Pino, got a grant in Chile that covered more lead testing. All combined, we were able to do leads on about 330 children. Again, for Chile there was no negative relation between lead and poor development [1], but we couldn't control for lead levels in all analyses because we didn't have them for everybody. The mean lead level was about 8. Chile was in the process of implementing unleaded gasoline at the time. We found that there was a further drop in the lead level of infants over the last 18 months of the study. At the start of that time the average was about $8.3\,\mu g/dl$ and at the end it was $5.9\,\mu g/dl$ [6]. So the lead levels of infants seem incredibly sensitive to an environmental intervention like the switch to unleaded gasoline.

Mr. Parvanta: How do children who are somewhat delayed in development, like this second child who was not really reacting, impact on what is the reaction of the mothers of these children?

Dr. Lozoff: The nature of child development is transactional. An alteration in the child's behavior will have an effect on caregivers and vice versa, and there are cascades of transactional effects. What was interesting to me is that these testers, who just met these babies, modified their behavior. That seems appropriate. If you see a baby who is looking hesitant, you back off. I presume that the mothers would have that same kind of reaction and appropriately and adaptively buffer their children from unhappier reactions to the world. So it may not be that the mothers are responding inappropriately. However, if the caregiver behavior is sustained over time, there could be an adverse impact in terms of the baby's experiences of the world. In another unpublished study involving Indian children at about 3 years of age, the children came into an observational room in a familiar neighborhood clinic. A mat was placed on the floor, and toys were given to the child. The initial few minutes were only for the mother, the child, and the toys, and there were no differences in behavior in children with iron deficiency anemia. Then an examiner came in with a new toy covered by a box, removed the box, and walked out. That is all that happened, and under these conditions children with iron deficiency anemia were less likely to touch the toy or smile. So it appears that the simple perturbation of something unfamiliar happening was sufficient to alter behavior. These results allow me to make another point. In the familiar environment I am not sure that the altered behavior would be very obvious.

In developmental research, you often have to push the system, you have to stress the child a bit before you will see whatever is going on. The India study is an example. It was just the tiniest push – a little unfamiliarity of a box covering a toy or a new person coming in – was sufficient to make the behavioral differences apparent. So I completely agree with you that we must consider not only the babies' behavior but also what impact that has on the caregiving environment or we will not be really understanding how poorer outcome happen and might be sustained.

Dr. Pettifor: About the issue of the global problem of iron deficiency and ways of trying to address the problem: if one looks at the major problems of infants from 6 months to 2.5 years in many developing countries, they are huge, yet iron supplementation programs are poor basically as far as implementation and compliance are concerned. If you were going to look at this problem, how would you attempt to address it on a global scale, and is it something that should be placed up there right at the top with all the other problems in the developing world?

Dr. Lozoff: I know others are going to be talking about this. Asking mothers to give babies iron drops for months may not work very well, even though under controlled circumstances, a benefit can be shown. The United States is an example of tremendous success in improving the iron status in the population in a different way [7, 8]. Up until about 1970, 20–25% of poor children in the United States also had iron deficiency anemia. At that point a number of things started happening: infant formula became fortified with iron; infant cereals became fortified with iron; breast-feeding was encouraged; a lot more ascorbic acid was added to the infant diet. And iron deficiency anemia went down to 3%. Canada now does the same, as does Chile. Although these are examples of effective interventions, the challenge for the developing world is how to improve infant iron status without interfering with breast-feeding. I am going to defer this to other speakers. I will just simply say that this is a problem that can be solved, but I am not saying that improving iron status is easy or simple.

Dr. Barclay: From the data currently available, is it possible to say which would be a most effective strategy in preventing the type of deficiencies you are talking about? Would iron supplementation or fortification of food be the best way to go?

Dr. Lozoff: My role in this area has been on the 'why does it matter' side of things. Other speakers are better for answering these questions.

Dr. Lönnerdal: Considering the strong interaction between the caregiver and the infant, I have a question concerning the findings of Murray-Kolb et al. [9] regarding the behavior and emotional scale of pregnant women. The worst case here would be an iron-deficient anemic mother interacting with an iron-deficient anemic child where this interaction could be seriously affected. Have you looked at the iron status of the women?

Dr. Lozoff: In Costa Rica and Chile we measured mothers' iron status. In Costa Rica it is absolutely amazing, there were only about 2 mothers with iron deficiency anemia and 8 with iron deficiency. Thus, at least 20 years ago, the diet in Costa Rica was perfectly good for the adult. But the mothers' blood was obtained when the children averaged 17 months of age. We don't have the mothers' blood during pregnancy. For Chile we have mothers' blood only for some infants and only at 12 months of age.

Typically the peak period for iron deficiency is 6–24 months. However, an increasing number of people are interested in the prenatal iron deficiency question. Dr. Lönnerdal is referring to a new study by Corwin et al. [10] in which they looked at maternal depression and mood and found a relationship with the mother's iron status. In the adult literature there have been no consistent findings about iron deficiency and mood, but such a link makes sense. Of course, as Dr. Lönnerdal points out, having a mother who is iron deficient and depressed is unlikely to be good for the baby.

Dr. Specker: Did you find any infants who didn't respond to the iron supplementation?

Dr. Lozoff: In Costa Rica, we went into the home at least 5 days/week and placed the medication into the child's mouth. 93% of the children responded to iron with an increase in hemoglobin of 10 gl or more or normalization of all iron measures. No child had iron deficiency anemia after 3 months, none. In some cases, however, the biochemistry indicators were vastly improved but not fully corrected. Thus, in that study I can say that non-response was not a problem. In Chile, there were 2–3 children who did not respond to iron and it seemed that something else was going on.

References

1 Lozoff B, De Andraca I, Castillo M, et al: Behavioral and developmental effects of preventing iron-deficiency anemia in healthy full-term infants. Pediatrics 2003;112:846–854.
2 Lozoff B, Brittenham GM, Wolf AW, et al: Iron deficiency anemia and iron therapy: Effects on infant development test performance. Pediatrics 1987;79:981–995.
3 Walter T, De Andraca I, Chadud P, Perales CG: Iron deficiency anemia: Adverse effects on infant psychomotor development. Pediatrics 1989;84:7–17.
4 Idjradinata P, Pollit E: Reversal of developmental delays in iron-deficient anemic infants treated with iron. Lancet 1993;341:1–4.
5 Wolf AW, Jimenez E, Lozoff B: No evidence of developmental ill effects of low-level lead exposure in a developing country. J Dev Behav Pediatr 1994;15:224–231.
6 Pino P, Walter T, Oyarzun M, et al: Rapid drop in infant blood lead levels during change to unleaded gasoline. In press.
7 Yip R, Binkin N, Fleshood L, Trowbridge F: Declining prevalence of anemia among low-income children in the United States. JAMA 1987;258:1619–1623.
8 Vazquez-Seoane P, Windom R, Pearson H: Disappearance of iron-deficiency anemia in a high-risk infant population given supplemental iron. N Engl J Med 1985;313:1239–1240.
9 Murray-Kolb LE, Beard JL, Perez E, et al: Maternal iron status is associated with maternal cognitive functioning and behavior. FASEB J 2003;17:A1149.
10 Corwin EJ, Murray-Kolb L, Beard JL: Low hemoglobin level is a risk factor for postpartum depression. J Nutr 2003;133:4139–4142.

Pettifor JM, Zlotkin S (eds): Micronutrient Deficiencies during the Weaning Period and the First Years of Life. Nestlé Nutrition Workshop Series Pediatric Program, vol 54, pp 137–152, Nestec Ltd., Vevey/S. Karger AG, Basel, © 2004.

Impact of Micronutrient Deficiencies on Immune Function

Richard D. Semba

Ocular Immunology Division, Department of Ophthalmology, Johns Hopkins School of Medicine, Baltimore, Md., USA

Micronutrients such as vitamin A and zinc play a major role in immunity to infectious diseases during the weaning period and the first years of life. In the last two decades, clinical trials have shown that vitamin A or zinc supplementation reduces morbidity and mortality from infectious diseases among infants and children in developing countries [1, 2]. The underlying assumption from these clinical observations is that vitamin A and zinc improve immunity to certain infectious diseases, an observation that is corroborated by extensive observations from experimental animal models and in vitro studies [3, 4]. Iron supplementation has been shown to reduce anemia and improve cognitive development among infants and young children, but less is known about the role of iron in immunity to infectious diseases in humans [5]. The immunologic consequences of micronutrient malnutrition among infants and young children are far-reaching and include greater morbidity and mortality from diarrheal disease, pneumonia, measles, and human immunodeficiency virus infection, reduced vaccine responses, and impaired growth and development. The purpose of this article is to highlight the role of three micronutrients, vitamin A, zinc, and iron, in immune function among infants and young children and to identify major gaps in knowledge that remain to be addressed regarding the role of these micronutrients and others in immune function.

Supported in part by the National Institutes of Health (HD32247, HD30042, AI41956), the Fogarty International Center, and the United States Agency for International Development (Cooperative Agreement HRN A-0097–00015–00).

137

Historical Background

Early empirical observations on the use of vitamin A in individuals with tuberculosis, puerperal sepsis, and measles, led to the idea that vitamin A was the 'anti-infective vitamin' in the 1920s and 1930s [6]. In London Joseph Bramhall Ellison made the seminal discovery in 1932 that vitamin A supplementation reduced mortality in young children with acute complicated measles [3, 6]. In the first half of the 20th century, studies showed that vitamin A deficiency affected the growth and survival of experimental animals, and a large series of clinical trials was conducted using vitamin A as prophylactic or therapeutic treatment for a variety of infections [6]. Vitamin A was thought to be essential for the development of the lymphoid system and for the maintenance of mucosal surfaces of the gastrointestinal, respiratory, and genitourinary tracts. By the 1960s, a great deal of evidence had accumulated that vitamin A was essential for normal immune function [7], and further large clinical trials of vitamin A supplementation were conducted in the last two decades which showed that vitamin A supplementation or fortification could reduce diarrheal disease morbidity and mortality in preschool children [1, 3].

Zinc was used empirically for treating diseases, including diarrhea, during the 19th century. By the 1930s, zinc was considered to be essential for the growth of animals and low zinc levels were described among adults in China, but a syndrome of human zinc deficiency was not described until the 1960s by Prasad and colleagues. The recommended dietary allowance for zinc was not established by the National Academy of Sciences until 1974, which belies the relatively recent recognition of zinc as an essential nutrient. Zinc supplementation was evaluated as a therapeutic intervention for diarrheal disease by Sachdev and colleagues in 1988, and during the 1990s, many studies were conducted to evaluate zinc supplementation for diarrheal disease, pneumonia, malaria, and child growth and development [8]. Experimental animal studies conducted in the last two decades have shown that zinc-deficient animals are more susceptible to a wide variety of infections [4] and that zinc is required for many aspects of immune function [4, 9].

Iron has long been recognized to play a role in anemia, but the role of iron in immunity to infectious diseases has been less clear. Since the 1920s, the data have been inconsistent: there have been studies that suggest that iron supplementation reduces the incidence of diarrheal and respiratory diseases among infants, and others that suggest that iron supplementation may worsen the morbidity from infections. Side effects of parenteral iron were reported, and studies from developing countries suggested that there might be a deleterious effect of iron on malaria and on respiratory infections [10]. There is still much speculation about iron supplementation being a 'double-edged sword' in iron deficiency, but harmful effects of iron supplementation may be more relevant to the situation of excess iron stores or in situations where iron supplementation is given to children with malaria without any concomitant treatment for malaria.

Immune Function in Infants and Young Children

The immune system is often functionally divided into innate and adaptive immunity, the former consisting of nonspecific immune defenses such as phagocytosis, natural killer (NK) cells, antimicrobial substances in mucosal secretions, etc., with the latter consisting of specific immune responses to certain pathogens that involve immunologic memory and rapid expansion of immune effector cells. The mucosal surfaces of the body include the respiratory, gastrointestinal, and genitourinary tracts as well as the cornea and conjunctiva. NK cells play a role in antiviral and antitumor immunity that is not major histocompatibility complex (MHC)-restricted, and NK cells are involved in the regulation of immune responses. Neutrophils play an important role in nonspecific immunity because they phagocytize and kill bacteria, parasites, virus-infected cells, and tumor cells. Macrophages are involved in the inflammatory response and in the phagocytosis of viruses, bacteria, protozoa, fungi, and tumor cells.

The adaptive immune system consists of antigen-specific responses that are mediated by T and B cells, and this includes humoral and cell-mediated immunity. Immunoglobulins, or antibodies, are secreted by after B-cell proliferation into plasma cells. Immunoglobulins contain antigen-binding sites that bind to specific antigenic sites on microorganisms or toxins. The binding of antibodies can neutralize pathogens by inhibiting them from binding to cell surfaces or by promoting phagocytosis. T lymphocytes can be divided into two major sublineages, CD4+ and CD8+ T cells. CD4+ T cells are major regulatory cells that provide help for B-cell activation through MHC class-II-restricted responses. CD8+ T cells can develop into cytotoxic T cells that play an important role in defense against viral infections through recognition of virus-infected cells that express MHC class-I molecules.

Infants are also a special case in that they are protected by maternal antibodies that cross the placenta during pregnancy, and by immunologically active substances in breast milk, such as antibodies, lactoferrin, lysozyme, cytokines, and chemokines that may protect the gut from pathogens and play a role in gut development.

Micronutrient malnutrition can affect various aspects of the immune response, and there is a great challenge in linking specific micronutrient deficiencies with certain immune compartments. Multiple micronutrient deficiencies may occur together, making it difficult to conclude from cross-sectional studies that particular defects in immunity are associated with specific micronutrient deficiencies. Clinical trials with single micronutrients may provide more definitive data regarding specific immune compartments, but investigators are usually limited to studies of peripheral blood, mucosal secretions, breast milk, and skin testing. Much more data have been derived from experimental animal models in which the immune system is more accessible for investigation.

Micronutrient Deficiencies and Immune Function

Vitamin A

Vitamin A modulates both innate and adaptive immunity [3]. Some immune compartments are not affected by vitamin A deficiency. Vitamin A deficiency is associated with loss of cilia in the respiratory tract, loss of microvilli in the gastrointestinal tract, loss of mucin and goblet cells in the respiratory, gastrointestinal, and genitourinary tracts, squamous metaplasia with abnormal keratinization in the respiratory tract, alterations in antigen-specific secretory IgA concentrations, impairment of alveolar monocyte/macrophage function, and decreased integrity of the gut. Vitamin A is involved in the expression of both mucins and keratins, and lactoferrin, an iron-binding glycoprotein involved in immunity to bacteria, viruses, and fungi, appears to be modulated in mucosal secretions.

In the respiratory tract, pathogens are constantly trapped and removed by the mucociliary elevator in the normal tracheobronchial tree, but the loss of ciliated epithelial cells and mucus and replacement by stratified, keratinized epithelium in vitamin A deficiency may increase susceptibility to respiratory infections [3]. Vitamin A deficiency also appears to affect the linings of the inner ear and eustachian tube, making children more susceptible to otitis media.

Vitamin A deficiency reduces the number of NK cells and impairs their activity [11]. The function of neutrophils appears to be impaired during vitamin A deficiency [12]. Impaired phagocytosis and decreased complement lysis activity may occur during vitamin A deficiency. During vitamin A deficiency, the hematopoiesis of some lineages, such as CD4+ lymphocytes, NK cells, and erythrocytes, appears to be impaired. In humans, clinical vitamin A deficiency has been characterized by lower total lymphocyte counts and decreased CD4+ lymphocytes in peripheral blood, and CD4+ lymphocyte counts or percentage increased after vitamin A supplementation [13, 14]. Vitamin A supplementation does not appear to have any long-term effect on CD4+ or CD8+ lymphocyte subsets among infants without clinical vitamin A deficiency [15].

Vitamin A deficiency has been linked with reduced phagocytic function by macrophages. Vitamin A deficiency may influence T-lymphocyte-related immunocompetence through modulation of numbers or distribution of T cells, changes in phenotype, alterations in cytokine production, or decreased expression or function of cell surface molecules involved in T-cell signaling [3]. In a trial in Bangladesh, vitamin A supplementation improved responses to delayed-type hypersensitivity skin testing among infants who were supplemented to higher vitamin A levels [16]. In experimental animals, vitamin A appears to modulate the balance between T-helper type-1-like responses and T-helper type-2-like responses, but there is less evidence to support this model for human vitamin A deficiency [3]. Observations from clinical trials are not consistent with this model, as vitamin A supplementation has been shown to enhance immunity to a wide variety of infections such as tuberculosis, measles, malaria, HIV infection, and diarrheal diseases, where the specific immune protective immune responses have been characterized as either T-helper-1-like or T-helper-2-like responses.

Vitamin A deficiency impairs the growth, activation, and function of B lymphocytes. The hallmark of vitamin A deficiency is an impaired capacity to generate an antibody response to T-cell-dependent antigens [17, 18] including tetanus toxoid [19] and diphtheria antigens in humans [20], and T-cell-independent type-2 antigens such as pneumococcal polysaccharide [21]. These findings suggest that vitamin A deficiency may compromise immunity to many types of infections where the main immune defense is dependent upon antibody responses.

Controlled studies of vitamin A supplementation and aspects of immunity in infants and young children are summarized in table 1. Several trials have addressed the issue of vitamin A supplementation with measles vaccine at either 6 [22, 23], or 9 months of age [23–27]. When vitamin A supplementation is given simultaneously with live measles vaccine in 6-month-old infants who have maternal antibodies present, there appears to be an inhibitory effect upon antibody titers to measles [22]. In 9-month-old infants who have lower levels of maternal antibodies, vitamin A supplementation has been reported to have either no overall effect on antibody titers [24, 26] or to enhance antibody titers [23, 25]. Long-term follow-up among children who were previously immunized at 9 months of age shows that those who received vitamin A supplementation had higher geometric mean antibody concentrations against measles at age 6–8 years [27].

Vitamin A supplementation appears to improve gut integrity among hospitalized infants [28] and among infants whose mothers were supplemented with vitamin A/β-carotene during pregnancy [29]. Vitamin A supplementation, when integrated with oral poliovirus vaccination at 6, 10, and 14 weeks, did not influence seroconversion rates or geometric mean antibody titers to poliovirus types 1, 2, and 3 [30], although a study in India suggested that a slightly higher proportion of infants had protective antibody to poliovirus type 1 with no differences in antibody titers to types 2 and 3 [31]. A large trial from India recently showed that infants who received vitamin A at birth had reduced nasopharyngeal colonization by pneumococcus [32].

Zinc

Zinc plays a role in both innate and adaptive immunity. Zinc deficiency impairs the function of neutrophils [33], NK cells [34], and chemotactic responses of monocyte/macrophages [4]. In preschool children, zinc

Table 1. Controlled studies of vitamin A and aspects of immunity in infants and young children

Location	n	Subjects	Intervention	Effects of vitamin A supplementation	Reference
Indonesia	236	Preschool children	30 mg RE vs. placebo	Enhanced IgG response to tetanus toxoid 3 weeks later; increase in circulating CD4%	13, 19
Indonesia	336	6-month-old infants	15 mg RE vs. placebo with measles vaccine	Reduced antibody titers to measles at 7 and 12 months; fewer infants with vaccine-related rash in vitamin A group	22
Indonesia	394	9-month-old infants	15 mg RE vs. placebo with measles vaccine	No impact of vitamin A on antibody titers to measles; antibody titers to measles at 10 and 15 months	24
Guinea Bissau	312	9-month-old infants	15 mg RE vs. placebo with measles vaccine	Enhanced antibody titers to measles at 18 months; higher antibody titers at 6–8 years	23, 27
Guinea Bissau	150	6-month-old infants	15 mg RE vs. placebo with measles vaccine	Higher antibody titers to measles after repeat vaccination at 9 months	23
India	100	9-month-old infants	15 mg RE vs. placebo with measles vaccine	Enhanced antibody titers to measles at 10 months	25
India	618	9-month-old infants	15 mg RE vs. placebo with measles vaccine	No impact on antibody titers to measles at 12 months; enhancement of antibody response in subgroup of malnourished infants	26
India	56	Infants	15 mg RE vs. placebo with DPT vaccine	Enhanced IgG response to diphtheria toxoid	20

Country	N	Subjects	Intervention	Outcome	Ref.
India	120	Infants	15 mg RE/month with DPT vaccine	Increased skin test responses among subgroup of those supplemented to higher vitamin A levels	16
India	144	Hospitalized infants	(1) 60 mg RE at admission, (2) 60 mg RE at discharge, or (3) placebo at discharge	Improved gut integrity in groups 1 and 2 vs. group 3	28
India	80	Infants	16,700 IU/week vs. placebo	No difference in gut integrity	28
South Africa	238	Infants	1.5 mg RE and 30 mg β-carotene/day to mothers during pregnancy	Improved gut integrity	29
Indonesia	467	Infants	7.5 mg or 15 mg RE, vs. placebo at 6, 10, 14 weeks with oral poliovirus vaccine	Seroconversion rates of 98–100% in all three treatment groups, no differences in mean antibody titers to types 1, 2, or 3 between treatment groups	30
India	399	Infants	7.5 mg RE vs. placebo at 6, 10, and 14 weeks with oral poliovirus vaccine	Higher proportion with protective antibody titer to poliovirus type 1; no differences in antibody titers to poliovirus types 2 and 3	31
India	464	Infants	7 mg RE vs. placebo at birth	Reduced nasopharyngeal colonization by pneumococcus	32

supplementation was associated with an increase in delayed-type hypersensitivity skin responses to multiple antigens [35]. Another trial among low birth weight infants showed that zinc supplementation had no effect on delayed-type hypersensitivity skin responses to phytohemagglutinin [36]. The investigators noted that phytohemagglutinin is a strong antigen, and the test may have been insensitive to detect more subtle differences in immunity. Another study that used a multiple antigen skin test to several antigens (tetanus, diphtheria, tuberculin, *Candida*, *Trichophyton*, and *Proteus*) showed that zinc supplementation reduced anergy by skin testing [37].

The number of circulating CD4+ and CD8+ lymphocytes decreases during zinc deficiency [4, 34, 38]. The number of circulating CD8+ CD73+ T cells, which are mostly precursors for cytotoxic T lymphocytes, are reduced during zinc deficiency [38]. A decrease in CD8+ CD73+ T cells could possibly increase the susceptibility of zinc-deficient individuals to viral, parasitic, and bacterial infections [38]. Zinc deficiency plays a role in thymic atrophy and may modulate maturation of T lymphocytes [4, 39].

Zinc deficiency is associated with impaired antibody responses to T-cell-dependent and T-cell-independent antigens [4]. In experimental human zinc deficiency, peripheral blood mononuclear cells showed a decrease in interferon-γ and interleukin (IL)-2 production, but no change in IL-4, IL-6, and IL-10 production, suggesting that there may be a depression of Th1-like responses during zinc deficiency [40].

Many studies have shown that zinc supplementation reduces the morbidity from infectious diseases [8]. Among the more recent studies are investigations among infants in Ethiopia [41], infants in Bangladesh [42], and infants and young children in India [43], which show that zinc supplementation is associated with reductions in infectious disease morbidity. A few controlled trials have addressed the effect of zinc supplementation on aspects of immunity in infants and young children, and these are summarized in table 2. A recent trial among preschool children shows that oral zinc supplementation increases the antibody response to killed oral cholera vaccine [44]. Among infants and young children, zinc supplementation was associated with increases in CD3+ and CD4+ T cells, and an increase in the CD4/CD8 ratio [38].

Iron

In contrast to vitamin A deficiency and zinc deficiency, less is known about the role of iron in immune function in humans, and much of the available data are inconsistent [5] (table 3). Iron deficiency appears to affect neutrophil function [45], impair NK cell function, and reduce delayed-type hypersensitivity skin testing [5, 46]. It is not clear whether iron deficiency affects lymphocyte proliferation responses to mitogens or the composition of T-cell subsets in peripheral blood, as results from various studies have been inconsistent [5, 10]. Iron deficiency does not appear to impair antibody responses following immunization in children [46, 47]. There are few solid data

Table 2. Controlled studies of zinc and aspects of immunity in infants and young children

Location	n	Subjects	Intervention	Effects of zinc supplementation	Reference
Ecuador	50	Children 12–59 months	10 mg/day vs. placebo	Higher delayed type hypersensitivity responses at day 60	35
India	66	Children 6–35 months	10 mg/day vs. placebo	Higher delayed type hypersensitivity responses at day 120; increase in CD3, CD4, and CD4/CD8 ratio	37
Brazil	134	Low birth weight infants	5 mg/day vs. placebo birth to 8 weeks	No differences in phytohemagglutinin skin tests at 8 weeks; reduction in diarrhea and cough	36
Bangladesh	256	Children	20 mg/day vs. placebo; 60 mg RE vitamin A in 2 × 2 factorial design	Improved seroconversion to vibriocidal antibody of killed oral cholera vaccine	44

Table 3. General influence of selected micronutrient deficiencies on immunity

Immune component	Vitamin A	Zinc	Iron
Phagocyte function	↓	↓	↓
Natural killer cell function	↓	↓	↓
T-cell subsets (CD4+, CD8+), circulating	↓	↓	↔
Lymphocyte proliferation	↓	↓	↔
Delayed-type hypersensitivity	↓	↓	↓
Cytotoxic T-cell function	↓	↓	↔
Antibody responses	↓	↓	↔
Monocyte function	↓	↓	?
Mucosal surfaces	↓	?	↔
Apoptosis	?	↓	?
Breast milk immune factors	?	?	?

↓ = Decreased; ↑ = increased; ↔ = no effect; ? = unknown or not well characterized.

from observational studies that show that iron deficiency increases the morbidity and mortality of infectious diseases [10], and it appears to be fairly clear that increased infectious disease morbidity is not part of the syndrome of iron deficiency [46]. Oral iron supplementation has not been associated with a reduction in the morbidity of infectious diseases [10], and a recent systematic review of 28 controlled clinical trials shows that iron supplementation has no apparent effect on the incidence of infectious diseases, including malaria, except for a slightly increased risk of diarrhea [48].

Other Micronutrients

Iodine deficiency is highly prevalent in certain areas of the world among infants and young children, yet iodine deficiency remains one of the most promising, yet neglected areas for investigation in nutritional immunology. Iodine supplementation has been shown to reduce infant mortality [49], but little has been done to examine the relationship of iodine to immune function in humans. Vitamin D deficiency has been associated with immune abnormalities and may influence macrophage function [50], and further studies are needed to characterize the relationship between vitamin D status and immune function in infants and children.

Future Directions

There are several general areas that merit attention in future studies of the effects of micronutrient status on immune function in humans. Controlled clinical trials of single micronutrient supplementation may provide the most valid data for assessing the effects of single micronutrients on specific immune compartments, provided that there is sufficient statistical power to examine the immunological endpoint being addressed and that there is evidence that individuals with marginal or deficiency micronutrient status are being supplemented to a replete state. Of all the micronutrients, the relationship of vitamin A to immune function is the best characterized, but there are still notable gaps in knowledge relevant to infants and children, such as the possible effects of vitamin A deficiency on immunological modulators in breast milk and on transfer of maternal antibodies from mother to infant. Much work remains to be done with regard to zinc deficiency, especially on the relationship between zinc deficiency to antibody responses following immunization, and the effect of zinc deficiency on mucosal immunity in humans. Studies using newer methods such as fluorescence in situ hybridization (flow FISH), more complex flow cytometry, single cell gel electrophoresis, and microarrays could be used to study the effects of micronutrient deficiencies upon telomere shortening, clonal expansion of T cells, DNA damage in lymphocytes, and cytokine and chemokine expression by specific immune effector cells. Such new data could provide insights into the overall role of micronutrients in the maturation of the immune system in infants and children.

References

1 Beaton GH, Martorell R, L'Abbe KA, et al: Effectiveness of Vitamin A Supplementation in the Control of Young Child Morbidity and Mortality in Developing Countries. ACC/SCN State-of-the-Art Nutrition Policy Discussion Paper No. 13, United Nations, 1993.
2 Black RE: Zinc deficiency, infectious disease and mortality in the developing world. J Nutr 2003;133(suppl 1):1485S–1489S.
3 Semba RD: Vitamin A; in Hughes DA, Bendich A, Darlington LG (eds): Dietary Enhancement of Human Immune Function. Totowa, Humana Press, 2003, in press.
4 Shankar AH, Prasad AS: Zinc and immune function: The biological basis of altered resistance to infection. Am J Clin Nutr 1998;68(suppl):447S–463S.
5 Kuvibidila S, Baliga BS: Role of iron in immunity and infection; in Calder PC, Field CJ, Gill HS (eds): Nutrition and Immune Function. Oxon, CABI International and Nutrition Society, 2002, pp 209–228.
6 Semba RD: Vitamin A as 'anti-infective' therapy, 1920–1940. J Nutr 1999;129:783–791.
7 Scrimshaw NS, Taylor CE, Gordon JE: Interactions of nutrition and infection. Monogr Ser World Health Organ1968;57:3–329.
8 Bhutta ZA, Black RE, Brown KH, et al: Prevention of diarrhea and pneumonia by zinc supplementation in children in developing countries: Pooled analysis of randomized controlled trials. J Pediatr 1999;135:689–697.
9 Fraker PJ, King LE, Laakko T, et al: The dynamic link between the integrity of the immune system and zinc status. J Nutr 2000;130:1399S–1406S.
10 Oppenheimer SJ: Iron and its relation to immunity and infectious disease. J Nutr 2001;11: 616S–635S.
11 Zhao Z, Murasko DM, Ross AC: The role of vitamin A in natural killer cell cytotoxicity, number and activation in the rat. Nat Immun 1994;13:29–41.
12 Twining SS, Schulte DP, Wilson PM, et al: Vitamin A deficiency alters rat neutrophil function. J Nutr 1996;127:558–565.
13 Semba RD, Muhilal, Ward BJ, et al: Abnormal T-cell subset proportions in vitamin A-deficient children. Lancet 1993;341:5–8.

14 Hussey G, Hughes J, Potgieter S, et al: Vitamin A status and supplementation and its effects on immunity in children with AIDS (abstract). 17th International Vitamin A Consultative Group Meeting, Guatemala City. Washington, International Life Sciences Institute, 1996, p 6.
15 Benn CS, Lisse IM, Bale C, et al: No strong long-term effect of vitamin A supplementation in infancy on CD4 and CD8 T-cell subsets. A community study from Guinea-Bissau, West Africa. Ann Trop Paediatr 2000;20:259–264.
16 Rahman MM, Mahalanabis D, Alvarez JO, et al: Effect of early vitamin A supplementation on cell-mediated immunity in infants younger than 60 mo. Am J Clin Nutr 1997;65:144–148.
17 Wiedermann U, Hanson LA, Kahu H, et al: Aberrant T-cell function in vitro and impaired T-cell dependent antibody response in vivo in vitamin A-deficient rats. Immunology 1993;80: 581–586.
18 Smith SM, Hayes CE: Contrasting impairments in IgM and IgG responses of vitamin A-deficient mice. Proc Natl Acad Sci USA 1987;84:5878–5882.
19 Semba RD, Muhilal, Scott AL, et al: Depressed immune response to tetanus in children with vitamin A deficiency. J Nutr 1992;122:101–107.
20 Rahman MM, Mahalanabis D, Hossain S, et al: Simultaneous vitamin A administration at routine immunization contact enhances antibody response to diphtheria vaccine in infants younger than six months. J Nutr 1999;129:2192–2195.
21 Pasatiempo AMG, Bowman TA, Taylor CE, et al: Vitamin A depletion and repletion: Effects on antibody response to the capsular polysaccharide of *Streptococcus pneumoniae*, type III (SSS-III). Am J Clin Nutr 1989;49:501–510.
22 Semba RD, Munasir Z, Beeler J, et al: Reduced seroconversion to measles in infants given vitamin A with measles vaccination. Lancet 1995;345:1330–1332.
23 Benn CS, Aaby P, Balé C, et al: Randomised trial of effect of vitamin A supplementation on antibody response to measles vaccine in Guinea-Bissau, West Africa. Lancet 1997;350:101–105.
24 Semba RD, Akib A, Beeler J, et al: Effect of vitamin A supplementation on measles vaccination in nine-month-old infants. Public Health 1997;111:245–247.
25 Bhaskaram P, Rao KV: Enhancement in seroconversion to measles vaccine with simultaneous administration of vitamin A in 9-months-old Indian infants. Indian J Pediatr 1997;64: 503–509.
26 Bahl R, Kumar R, Bhandari N, et al: Vitamin A administered with measles vaccine to nine-month-old infants does not reduce vaccine immunogenicity. J Nutr 1999;129:1569–1573.
27 Benn CS, Balde A, George E, et al: Effect of vitamin A supplementation on measles-specific antibody levels in Guinea-Bissau. Lancet 2002;359:1313–1314.
28 Thurnham DI, Northrup-Clewes CA, McCullough FS, et al: Innate immunity, gut integrity, and vitamin A in Gambian and Indian infants. J Infect Dis 2000;182(suppl 1):S23–S28.
29 Filteau SM, Rollins NC, Coutsoudis A, et al: The effect of antenatal vitamin A and beta-carotene supplementation on gut integrity of infants of HIV-infected South African women. J Pediatr Gastroenterol Nutr 2001;32:464–470.
30 Semba RD, Muhilal, Mohgaddam MEG, et al: Integration of vitamin A supplementation with the Expanded Program on Immunization does not affect seroconversion to oral poliovirus vaccine in infants. J Nutr 1999;129:2203–2205.
31 Bahl R, Bhandari N, Kant S, et al: Effect of vitamin A administered at Expanded Program on Immunization contacts on antibody response to oral polio vaccine. Eur J Clin Nutr 2002;56: 321–325.
32 Coles CL, Rahmathullah L, Kanungo R, et al: Vitamin A supplementation at birth delays pneumococcal colonization in South Indian infants. J Nutr 2001;131:255–261.
33 Briggs WA, Pedersen MM, Mahajan SK, et al: Lymphocyte and granulocyte function in zinc-treated and zinc-deficient hemodialysis patients. Kidney Int 1982;21:827–832.
34 Allen JI, Perri RT, McClain CJ, et al: Alterations in human natural killer cell activity and monocyte cytotoxicity induced by zinc deficiency. J Lab Clin Med 1983;102:577–589.
35 Sempertegui F, Estrella B, Correa E, et al: Effects of short-term zinc supplementation on cellular immunity, respiratory symptoms, and growth of malnourished Equadorian children. Eur J Clin Nutr 1996;50:42–46.
36 Lira PIC, Ashworth A, Morris SS: Effect of zinc supplementation on the morbidity, immune function, and growth of low-birth-weight, full-term infants in northeast Brazil. Am J Clin Nutr 1998;68(suppl):418S–424S.
37 Sazawal S, Jalla S, Mazumder S, et al: Effect of zinc supplementation on cell-mediated immunity and lymphocyte subsets in preschool children. Indian Pediatr 1997;34:589–597.

38 Beck FWJ, Kaplan J, Fine N, et al: Decreased expression of CD73 (ecto-5′-nucleotidase) in CD8+ subset is associated with zinc deficiency in human patients. J Lab Clin Med 1997;130:147–156.
39 Ibs KH, Rink L: Zinc-altered immune function. J Nutr 2003;133:1452S–1456S.
40 Prasad AS: Effects of zinc deficiency on Th1 and Th2 cytokine shifts. J Infect Dis 2000;182(suppl 1):S62–S68.
41 Umeta M, West CE, Haidar J, et al: Zinc supplementation and stunted infants in Ethiopia: A randomised controlled trial. Lancet 2000;355:2021–2026.
42 Osendarp SJM, van Raaij JMA, Darmstadt GL, et al: Zinc supplementation during pregnancy and effects on growth and morbidity in low birthweight infants: A randomised placebo controlled trial. Lancet 2001;357:1080–1085.
43 Bhandari N, Bahl R, Taneja S, et al: Effect of routine zinc supplementation on pneumonia in children aged 6 months to 3 years: Randomised controlled trial in an urban slum. BMJ 2002;324:1358–1362.
44 Albert MJ, Qadri F, Wahed MA, et al: Supplementation with zinc, but not vitamin A, improves seroconversion to vibriocidal antibody in children given an oral cholera vaccine. J Infect Dis 2003;187:909–913.
45 Murakawa H, Bland CE, Willis WT, et al: Iron deficiency and neutrophil function: Different rates of correction of the depressions in oxidative burst and myeloperoxidase activity after iron treatment. Blood 1987;69:1464–1468.
46 Farthing MJG: Iron and immunity. Acta Paediatr Scand Suppl 1989;361:44–52.
47 Bagchi K, Mohanram M, Reddy V: Humoral immune response in children with iron-deficiency anemia. Br Med J 1980;280:1249–1251.
48 Gera T, Sachdev HPS: Effect of iron supplementation on incidence of infectious illness in children: Systematic review. BMJ 2002;325:1142–1151.
49 Cobra C, Muhilal, Kusnandi, et al: Infant survival is improved by oral iodine supplementation. J Nutr 1997;127:574–578.
50 Hayes CE, Nashold FE, Spach KM, Pedersen LB: The immunological functions of the vitamin D endocrine system. Cell Mol Biol 2003;49:272–300.

Discussion

Dr. Tolboom: Thank you for a very clear and comprehensive presentation. I have a question related to gut integrity. You mentioned that vitamin A supplementation improves gut integrity. How was that checked? Were permeability studies done? How could, e.g., effects on villous atrophy be differentiated?

Dr. Semba: The lactose/mannose ratio was analyzed. So these are permeability studies.

Dr. Albar: Nephrotic syndrome, especially minimal chain nephrotic syndrome, is thought to be caused by T-cell dysfunction. You mentioned that zinc plays a role in T-cell function. If zinc deficiency is repaired in the neonate, can this syndrome be prevented in infants and children? Some treatments, for example levamisol, have been tried to stimulate T-cell functions in children with minimal change nephrotic syndrome as well as prednisone therapy. So if zinc is routinely given to neonates, perhaps we can also prevent children from developing minimal chain nephrotic syndrome. Any comment?

Dr. Semba: I missed the first part of the question. What kind of syndrome?

Dr. Albar: Minimal chain nephrotic syndrome, is one of the renal diseases which mostly occurs in children presenting with generalized edema, massive albuminuria, and heavy albuminemia.

Dr. Semba: You think zinc supplementation can correct that?

Dr. Albar: The supplementation of zinc may correct minimal change nephrotic syndrome in children if zinc has a similar T-cell-activating effect as levamisol. A clinical study is necessary to make any conclusions.

Dr. Semba: I am not aware of any data.

Dr. Albar: Levamisol, as a stimulator of T-cell function, has been tried based on the hypothesis that T-cell dysfunction is a cause of minimal change nephrotic syndrome

149

in children [1–6]. If we can prevent zinc deficiency in neonates, this may stimulate T-cell function normally, and subsequently we could also prevent the development of nephrotic syndrome in children. But a zinc supplementation trial seems to be necessary to support the role of zinc as a T-cell stimulator in this syndrome. So zinc deficiency has not only an impact on infections but also on the syndrome.

Dr. Semba: This is an interesting idea. I think someone needs to address this.

Dr. Pettifor: A nice cover of the immune situation. If I quote Moore et al. [7] correctly from studies in the Gambia, they showed that babies with intrauterine growth retardation didn't have an increased mortality in childhood. But there seemed to be significant effects on adult mortality once they were into adult life. Do you have any comments on this? It looks as though early infant malnutrition might well influence long-term immune function, mortality and morbidity, and infections in adult life.

Dr. Semba: This is an important phenomenon that needs to be addressed, and the first way to address this will be to look at T-cell subsets to see whether some markers are being altered. For example, in older adults immune dysfunction is associated with loss of the CD28 receptor which occurs earlier on in life and it is linked to cytomegalovirus infection. So one must ask what happens earlier in life that could cause the loss of CD28, for example, from CD8 and CD4 T cells. Now whether this is something that happens earlier on and influences immunity later, we don't know for certain. I hope I have answered your question.

Dr. Zlotkin: As a pediatrician I have always been taken by the fact that in order to assess immunologic status a lot of blood is needed because white blood cells are being measured, and in young infants that precludes a lot of studies that perhaps could be done in adults. My question has to do with indirect markers of immune function, and let me just give an example from vitamin A and from zinc. We can define vitamin A status based on the serum level, or below a serum level we say someone may be deficient in vitamin A. For zinc it is a bit harder because we really don't have super markers which could distinguish between severe zinc deficiency because of the clinical science, but for moderate zinc deficiency it is often difficult to define that population. Are there any indirect markers with regard to zinc or vitamin A that would help us to find the immunologic risk in an individual subject?

Dr. Semba: I don't know of any good marker that can be used for that. One thing that might be useful for looking at comorbidity that we can't observe very well, and we discussed this yesterday, would be to look at different acute phase proteins that have different dynamics of response to an acute phase reaction. That might tell us a little bit about what is going on, but it is not to say that there is a certain CD4/CD8 ratio where you see something like moderate deficiency. I don't think we have anything.

Dr. Zlotkin: About vitamin A specifically: there is a definition of vitamin A deficiency based on the serum level. Is that level actually related to immunological dysfunction or function?

Dr. Semba: Again that is hard to sort out because there is an effect when studying this in children. There can be children with low vitamin A levels, but a high proportion of them have elevated C-reactive protein and α_1-glycoprotein. It is hard to interpret. I don't know if anybody has actually done a dose-response study to find out at what vitamin A level T-cell subsets are altered.

Dr. Villalpando-Carrión: I am interested in the use of antioxidants not only for immunological purposes of this nutrient but also in fat metabolism, etc. What kind of dose and what type of vitamin A did you use for the HIV children, and did you have any antioxidant evidence or reactive oxygen species activity or levels in plasma or something like that?

Dr. Semba: The dose we used in the Uganda study was 60 mg RE, or 200,000 IU, which is the standard UNICEF capsule, and we gave that every 3 months. We don't have any indicators of antioxidant status.

Dr. Villalpando-Carrión: Do you have plasma?

Dr. Semba: Yes, we do.

Dr. Tolboom: I have a question on iron and malaria. You mentioned that there is no adverse effect of iron supplementation in a population of children living in malaria-endemic areas. But you gave a word of caution, you said that we have to be careful with untreated severe malaria. I would like you to elaborate a little bit on that in view of the fact that 80% of African children, in sub-Sahara Africa, if they die, die at home, and most probably die of malaria. So we don't know what the effect on severe illness is, and the mortality of supplementation programs. All the programs in which iron supplementation is used are connected to anti-malaria treatment or prophylactics, for example. Could you elaborate a little bit on that?

Dr. Semba: There is an unpublished meta-analysis by Shankar showing that iron supplementation is associated with a slight increase in malaria morbidity, and Oppenheimer [8] has also looked at this and published it in the *Journal of Nutrition*. I made this cautionary note because I have heard that there is an ongoing study in which the iron arm was dropped because of some apparent effect on malaria, but I don't know the details.

Dr. Endres: In this workshop we are mainly talking about deficiencies which occur in many infants, and apparently it is somewhat difficult to study the consequences of clinical micronutrient deficiencies, e.g. the impact on immune function. I would like to ask you whether in some human models of severe micronutrient deficiencies such as zinc, copper and selenium, acrodermatitis enteropathica, Menkes disease and Keshan disease would be wonderful human models to study the impact on the immune system. Are you aware of any studies in these diseases?

Dr. Semba: I think acrodermatitis enteropathic disease has been studied. What else did you mention?

Dr. Endres: The next one would be Keshan disease, a cardiomyopathy due to selenium deficiency, which has practically disappeared from China.

Dr. Semba: I am not aware of any immune studies that have been conducted with Keshan disease.

Dr. Guesry: We have been studying selenium deficiency in animal models in collaboration with Dr. Beck in conjunction with influenza virus infection, and it was shown that it was not the immune defense of the animal which was impaired by selenium deficiency or vitamin E deficiency, which gave the same effect, but the virulence of the virus [9]. In the presence of selenium deficiency or vitamin E deficiency, influenza virus, becomes more virulent.

Dr. Semba: I think that it is a very interesting model that has been developed and perhaps it raises some questions that we might be seeing viral mutations coming from areas where a large part of the population is micronutrient-deficient. That is something that people have been extrapolating from these animal studies.

Dr. Bloem: You showed a slide of a market with a lot of vegetables and fruits, and I have a question about β-carotene or carotenoids. If you look at a study on maternal mortality, one of the Hopkins studies [10], it shows a reduction in maternal mortality actually more by β-carotene than by vitamin A. It was not significant and that is why it is a vitamin A-related mortality. We also know from some studies that the β-carotene is not very effective in vegetables. So could you elaborate a little bit more on whether β-carotene in itself or other carotenoids perhaps have an effect on the immune status besides the vitamin A effect, so that vegetables could potentially have an effect on mortality reduction?

Dr. Semba: There is an excellent review on this by Bendich [11], and I think as far as β-carotene is concerned it goes beyond the pro-vitamin-A quality, and some of the properties of β-carotene in immune response relate to its property as an antioxidant, which is of course much stronger than that for retinol. But there is a lot we don't know

151

about the excentric cleavage of β-carotene. We don't know what happens with all these other excentric cleavage products. What role do they play in immunity, and I think that hasn't been well studied. But β-carotene has been shown to have similar effects on immune function as vitamin A.

Dr. Bloem: So why then don't they use β-carotene instead of vitamin A in supplements for example?

Dr. Semba: Cost has got to be the main thing.

Dr. Delgado: Pro- and anti-inflammatory cytokines can be released. Which specific supplementation could improve anti-inflammatory cytokines?

Dr. Semba: That was perhaps vitamin E, I think this has been shown in studies in Toronto [12].

Dr. Horton: I know the focus in the sessions here is on the weaning period in the first year of life, but another group where we might see the effects of micronutrient deficiencies on immune function would be in the elderly, and I wonder if you could comment on any of those studies.

Dr. Semba: There have been some studies looking at immune function in the elderly. A lot of these studies have come from Europe and we see some effects of micronutrient malnutrition on T-cell subsets. But I think that when we are dealing with older adults, the main deficiencies we are dealing with are vitamin D or low vitamin E and zinc. Some studies have been conducted by Bogden [13] in New Jersey looking at zinc and immune function in older adults. Meydani [14] showed that with lymphocyte proliferation, by supplementation you can increase these indicators of immune function.

References

1 Taki HN, Schwartz SA: Levamisole as an immunopotentiator for T cell deficiency. Immunopharmacol Immunotoxicol 1994;16:129–137.
2 Tanphaichitr P, Tanphaichitr D, Sureeratanan J, Chatasingh S: Treatment of nephrotic syndrome with levamisole. J Pediatr 1980;96:490–493.
3 Dayal R, Prasad R, Mathur P, et al: Effect of levamisole on T cell in minimal change nephrotic syndrome. Indian Pediatr 1988;25:1184–1187.
4 Mancini ML, Rinaldi S, Rizzoni G: Treatment of partially corticosteroid-sensitive nephrotic syndrome with levamisole. Pediatr Nephrol 1994;8:788.
5 La Manna A, Polito C, Del Gado R, Foglia AC: Levamisole in children's idiopathic nephrotic syndrome. Child Nephrol Urol 1988–89;9:200–202.
6 Tenbrock K, Muller-Berghaus J, Fuchshuber A, et al: Levamisole treatment in steroid-sensitive and steroid-resistant nephrotic syndrome. Pediatr Nephrol 1998;12:459–462.
7 Moore SE, Cole TJ, Collinson AC, et al: Prenatal or early postnatal events predict infectious deaths in young adulthood in rural Africa. Int J Epidemiol 1999;28:1088–1095.
8 Oppenheimer SJ: Iron and its relation to immunity and infectious disease. J Nutr 2001;131(suppl 2):616S–635S.
9 Beck MA, Nelson HK, Shi Q et al: Selenium deficiency increases the pathology of an influenza virus infection. FASEB 2001;15:1481–1483.
10 West KP Jr, Katz J, Khatry SK, et al: Double blind, cluster randomised trial of low dose supplementation with vitamin A or beta carotene on mortality related to pregnancy in Nepal. BMJ 1999;318:570–575.
11 Bendich A: Beta-carotene and the immune response. Proc Nutr Soc 1991;50:263–274.
12 Allard JP, Aghdassi E, Chau J, et al: Effects of vitamin E and C supplementation on oxidative stress and viral load in HIV-infected subjects. AIDS 1998;12:1653–1659.
13 Bogden JD, Oleske JM, Munves EM, et al: Zinc and immunocompetence in the elderly: baseline data on zinc nutriture and immunity in unsupplemented subjects. Am J Clin Nutr 1987;45:101–109.
14 Meydani SN, Meydani M, Blumberg JB, et al: Vitamin E supplementation and the in vivo immune response in health elderly subjects. J Am Med Assoc 1997;277:1380–1386.

Pettifor JM, Zlotkin S (eds): Micronutrient Deficiencies during the Weaning Period and the
First Years of Life. Nestlé Nutrition Workshop Series Pediatric Program, vol 54, pp 153–171,
Nestec Ltd., Vevey/S. Karger AG, Basel, © 2004.

Impact of Micronutrient Deficiencies
on Bone Growth and Mineralization

Bonny Specker

South Dakota State University, Brookings, S. Dak., USA

Introduction

The first 2 years of life are a period of significant bone growth and mineralization. Garn [1] was one of the first researchers who eloquently described
early bone growth based on over 25,000 radiographs of the metacarpals. He
measured the mid-shaft width (T) and medullary cavity width (M) of metacarpals and, assuming a cylindrical shape for tubular bones, estimated periosteal diameter, cortical area and cortical thickness (T–M) [1]. Changes in
mid-shaft width, or periosteal bone apposition, with age are shown in figure 1.
The pattern of periosteal expansion during childhood parallels that of growth
curves, with rapid apposition during the first year of life followed by a phase
of slower growth until the sex hormone-mediated growth spurt during adolescence occurs. Resorption at the endosteal surface, as measured by the
width of the medullary cavity (M), occurs from birth to the second decade of
life. The width of the medullary cavity is larger in males compared to females
and changes are more rapid during the first half of the first year of life compared to later in infancy. The increase in medullary cavity during the first year
of life exceeds that of periosteal formation leading to a transient decrease in
cortical thickness (fig. 2). Although the decrease in cortical thickness was
originally thought to be a result of protein-energy malnutrition, this decrease
has been observed in other pediatric studies in well-nourished infants and
children [1].

Single photon absorptiometry (SPA) measures bone mineral density
(BMD) at peripheral bone sites and was used extensively in pediatric nutritional intervention studies during the 1970s and 1980s. Since the early 1990s
dual energy X-ray absorptiometry (DXA) methods have been used to measure bone mineral content (BMC) in the total body or at a particular skeletal
site such as the lumbar spine, hip or radius. The DXA method has been shown

Bone Growth and Mineralization

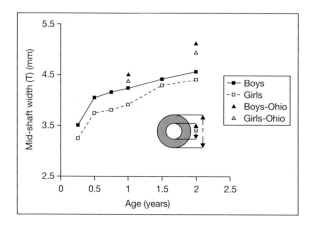

Fig. 1. Garn [1] measured mid-shaft width (T) and medullary cavity width (M) of the metacarpals to estimate sub-periosteal diameter and cortical area. Changes in metacarpal width, or periosteal bone apposition, with age among Central American infants and children are shown, as well as data obtained from young Ohio children.

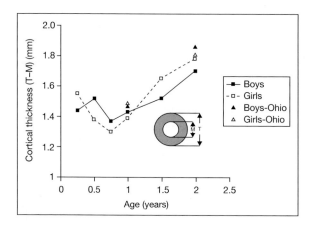

Fig. 2. The increase in medullary cavity width during the first year of life exceeds that of periosteal formation leading to a transient decrease in cortical thickness. Data are from Garn [1].

to be precise and accurate [2], and changes in total body BMC with growth provide data on bone mineral accretion. Areal BMD (aBMD) measured by DXA is BMC divided by the bone area of the scanned region and thus is not a measure of true volumetric density. There are concerns on the use of aBMD measures in children due to the artifact that larger bones may erroneously appear to have greater density. Figure 3 illustrates this phenomenon.

Peripheral quantitative computed tomography (pQCT) has been used in some pediatric studies and provides measures of bone size (periosteal and

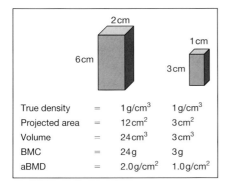

True density	=	$1\,g/cm^3$	$1\,g/cm^3$
Projected area	=	$12\,cm^2$	$3\,cm^2$
Volume	=	$24\,cm^3$	$3\,cm^3$
BMC	=	$24\,g$	$3\,g$
aBMD	=	$2.0\,g/cm^2$	$1.0\,g/cm^2$

Fig. 3. DXA measures BMD in 2 dimensions and is not a true volumetric density. Because it is an areal BMD measurement, it may be influenced by bone size.

endosteal circumferences) and volumetric BMD (vBMD) at peripheral sites. However, the current pQCT technology does not allow for accurate measurement of cortical vBMD when the cortical thickness is less than 1.5 mm (up to approximately age 8 years) [3]. However, accurate measures of bone size can be obtained and results confirm many of Garn's [1] original findings. It has been suggested that differences in bone size due to periosteal bone apposition and endosteal expansion is determined early in life and could explain some of the gender and ethnic differences in fracture risk [1]. Insulin-like growth factor-1 and growth hormone are also thought to influence periosteal expansion prior to puberty, while sex hormones are important regulators of periosteal expansion later in childhood. Androgens are thought to increase periosteal expansion while estrogens are thought to decrease endosteal expansion. Effects of vitamin D, calcium and phosphorus on these measures of bone size, as well as on total body and site-specific BMC are described below. Other factors that may influence bone growth or mineralization that are not discussed here include protein, vitamin C, magnesium, zinc, and other trace minerals.

Vitamin D

Vitamin D is either synthesized in the skin upon exposure to sunlight or is obtained from the diet. Vitamin D is converted to 25-OHD in the liver and further hydroxylated in the liver to $1,25\text{-}(OH)_2D$, the biologically active form of vitamin D. $1,25\text{-}(OH)_2D$ increases intestinal absorption of calcium and phosphorus, and along with parathyroid hormone (PTH) increases bone turnover. PTH also acts in the kidney to increase calcium reabsorption and increase phosphorus excretion. Thus, adequate vitamin D status is necessary to maintain blood calcium and phosphorus at sufficient concentrations that enable their deposition in bone as hydroxyapatite. Serum 25-OHD concentrations are used as the biochemical indicator of an individual's vitamin D status.

Breast-fed infants are at increased risk of vitamin D deficiency rickets due to the low amounts of vitamin D in human milk [4]. Conservative estimates of 2 h/week of sunlight exposure with only the face exposed, or 30 min/week with just a diaper on, are sufficient to maintain serum 25-OHD concentrations within the lower limit of the normal range [5]. Although sunlight exposure is a natural method for obtaining vitamin D, there are concerns on the long-term cancer risk associated with sunlight exposure early in life. Due to these concerns, and the recent resurgence of the numbers of cases of vitamin D deficiency rickets, the Centers for Disease Control in the United States has recommended that all infants receive vitamin D through the first year of age [6].

Serum PTH concentrations are high with vitamin D deficiency and the 25-OHD concentrations at which PTH concentrations begin to increase is considered the lower limit of normal in adults [7]. An observational study of 8-year-old children found that serum PTH increased when serum 25-OHD concentrations were below 8 ng/ml (20 nmol/l) [8]. Although there are numerous case reports and case studies on vitamin D deficiency and growth in the literature, few studies have systematically determined the relationship between vitamin D status and either linear growth or bone mineralization in infants or young children.

Linear Growth

There are few studies on the relationship between linear growth and vitamin D status during the weaning period and the first years of life. Vitamin D status theoretically may affect fetal growth, as well as linear growth during infancy. Several observational studies and vitamin D supplementation trials have reported associations between maternal vitamin D status during pregnancy and neonatal calcium homeostasis and fetal growth [9–15]. In general these studies have reported lower serum calcium concentrations in neonates of mothers who are vitamin D-deficient, along with decreased birth weight and birth size.

In 1936 Stearns et al. [16] summarized a series of longitudinal studies investigating the relationship between linear growth and vitamin D supplementation. They found that infants who were given 340 IU vitamin D/day (as either cod liver oil or via irradiated milk) in their whole milk feedings grew at a faster rate than infants who were given 60–135 IU/day. Exposure to sunlight increased the linear growth rate among those infants receiving 60–135 IU/day. Slyker et al. [17] analyzed linear growth rates among 414 infants and found that those infants who received between 250 and 810 IU/day appeared to have greater gains in length over the first year of life than those infants receiving 95–162 IU/day, which was greater than those infants not receiving vitamin D. The adverse effect of vitamin D deficiency on linear growth appeared to occur from 6 to 12 months of age. However, no results of statistical analyses were presented for either of these two studies. More recent studies on vitamin D supplementation in human milk-fed infants have found no differences in linear growth rates, but the infants were only studied until 6 months of age [18, 19].

Large amounts of vitamin D supplementation, in excess of 1,800 IU/day, have been shown to lead to decreased linear growth rates, similar to that of infants receiving no vitamin D [20]. In 1966 Fomon et al. [21] reported the results of a quasi-randomized trial among 60 newborn infants: 26 were breast-fed and received 300 IU/day in a vitamin preparation; 25 were alternatively assigned to receive either 400 (350–550 IU/day) or 1,600 (1,380–2,170 IU/day) IU vitamin D/can of evaporated milk. All infants were followed to 5.5 months of age and no differences in rates of gain in length were observed among the 3 groups. Whether decreased linear growth would be observed after longer periods of vitamin D supplementation is not known.

In summary, infants with vitamin D intakes between 250 and 810 IU/day have linear growth rates greater than infants with vitamin D intakes of <162 IU/day. Vitamin D intakes of >1,800 IU/day may lead to linear growth rates comparable to those observed in infants not receiving vitamin D. The effects of vitamin D on linear growth appear to occur after 6 months of age.

Bone Mineralization

Decreased bone mineral accretion in utero may be manifested as rickets or osteopenia in the newborn infant [22]. Although congenital rickets of the new-born are rare, case reports in newborn infants of mothers with severe nutritional osteomalacia associated with vitamin D or calcium deficiency have been reported [15, 23]. Results from several [12, 24, 25], but not all [10], observational studies have suggested an association between bone ossification and maternal vitamin D deficiency.

Vitamin D deficiency leads to increased serum PTH concentrations and theoretically should increase bone resorption and decrease bone density or bone mass accretion. Very few pediatric studies have correlated BMD with serum 25-OHD concentrations and the results are not consistent among those studies that have. The only studies that could be located among healthy infants or young children were conducted within the first 6 months of life. In 1981 Greer et al. [26] conducted a vitamin D supplementation trial and found that 25-OHD concentrations of human milk-fed infants not receiving supplemental vitamin D (n = 9) decreased during the winter months, whereas the 25-OHD concentrations did not change among the infants randomized to receive 400 IU/day (n = 9). By 12 weeks of age, BMC at the 1/3 distal radius (measured by SPA), was lower in infants randomized to placebo compared to infants randomized to 400 IU vitamin D/day. By 26 weeks of age the differences in radius BMC between those infants receiving vitamin D and those receiving placebo was no longer apparent [27]. These same investigators conducted an additional randomized vitamin D supplementation trial among 46 human milk-fed infants from birth to 6 months of age and found no difference in BMC at the 1/3 distal radius between supplemented and non-supplemented infants, despite significant differences in serum 25-OHD concentrations [28]. Park et al. [29] measured BMC of the lumbar spine (measured by DXA) in 2- to 5-month-old Korean infants who were either breast-fed without vitamin D supplementation or received infant formula containing 400 IU vitamin D/l. They found no significant difference in lumbar BMC between the 2 groups despite a greater serum 25-OHD concentration among the formula- vs. breast-fed infants. Lumbar BMC was not correlated with serum 25-OHD concentrations.

It is possible that these conflicting results are due to differences in the bone sites measured or the methodologies used. Greer et al. [26–28] measured BMD at a cortical bone site, whereas Park et al. [29] measured BMC at a predominantly trabecular bone site. Both SPA and DXA obtain areal measures of BMD and BMC and it is not possible to obtain separate measurements for both cortical and trabecular bone. Serum PTH concentrations are increased in vitamin D deficiency and the effect of PTH differs depending upon whether it is cortical or trabecular bone. Hyperparathyroidism (HPT) is one of the more prevalent diseases related to altered bone metabolism. Primary HPT is a disease condition caused by the parathyroid glands overproducing PTH, whereas vitamin D deficiency and the need to regulate blood calcium concentrations cause secondary HPT. Cortical and trabecular bone appear to be affected differently in patients with primary HPT. A selective reduction in cortical BMD and preservation of trabecular BMD in patients with primary HPT has been reported [30, 31]. Bilzekian et al. [32] reported significant cortical thinning, despite maintenance of trabecular architecture, based on the histomorphometric studies conducted in a subset of these patients. Not only was trabecular architecture maintained, there was a significant increase in trabecular volume that appeared to be due to increased trabecular number rather than thickness. Duan et al. [33] reported similar findings using CT measurements of the spine and suggested that assessment of BMD in relation to PTH requires separation of cortical and trabecular bone. Whether these disparate effects of elevated PTH concentrations on trabecular and cortical bone occur in infants and children with secondary hyperparathyroidism resulting from vitamin D deficiency is not known, but these differing effects may be why bone studies using SPA or DXA technology do not find a relationship between bone density and vitamin D status.

Although primary hyperparathyroidism in adults is associated with an increase in trabecular volume due to increased trabecular number, this is not what is observed in vitamin D deficiency rickets. In rickets histologically there is a thinning of the cortical width in the diaphyseal region, a widening of the epiphyseal plate, and a thinning out and loss of trabecular bone in the metaphyseal region. This thinning and loss of trabecular bone in rickets is not consistent with the histological findings in adult patients with secondary hyperparathyroidism described above.

Historically there have been hypotheses that vitamin D deficiency is not the sole cause of rickets. During the early 1920s it was thought that rickets was a result of overeating, was caused by an acidosis, was a manifestation of congenital syphilis, or was a result of infection. In 1923, Parks [34] presented a summary of the epidemiological findings and animal studies regarding the etiology of rickets and although vitamin D had not yet been identified he was able to deduce that the absence of 'Factor X' was necessary for the development of rickets. Parks further proposed, based on studies available during this period, that: (1) 'When the organism is deprived of the influence of X in the food and of radiant energy, defects in the diet become reflected in the blood'; (2) 'In the absence of X and of radiant energy, rickets can be made to develop by altering the composition of the diet in several ways'. He further described several conditions that could produce rickets, including decreasing the phosphorus content of the diet and administering calcium or decreasing the calcium content of the diet while maintaining the phosphorus content. (3) 'In the absence of X and radiant energy, rickets can be prevented by means of the diet'. Additionally, he described that the organic portion of the diet, if given correctly, could prevent the development of rickets. In 1976 Bronner [35] proposed that rickets was not the result of a simple vitamin D deficiency, but rather a combination of vitamin D and phosphate deficiency. He provided evidence from animal studies showing that simple vitamin D deficiency leads to biochemical alterations without the classical bone lesions that are observed in rickets. He also provided evidence that the bone lesions associated with phosphate deficiency are similar to those observed with classical rickets. These previous hypotheses of Parks [34] and Bronner [35] are supported by findings that vitamin D deficiency alone, as reflected by low serum 25-OHD concentrations, are not associated with BMD.

Calcium and Phosphorus

During the first 6 months of life the average calcium intake of breast-fed infants is used to define an adequate intake (AI) level (210 mg Ca/day and 100 mg P/day), while the average calcium intake from both human milk and foods define the AI at 7–12 months of age (270 mg Ca/day and 275 mg P/day) [36]. Breast milk calcium concentrations are fairly consistent with increasing length of lactation, while phosphorus concentrations decline. Beyond the first year, calcium and phosphorus intakes that maximize bone mass accretion are considered optimal. Total body calcium is approximately 30 g at birth [37] and mean net calcium retention during the first year of life is estimated at approximately 70 mg Ca/day [38]. Calcium retention at 1 and 2 years of age is approximately 85 mg/day and increases to approximately 110 mg/day in 3- and 4-year-olds; male children have greater calcium retention than female children [1]. Calcium and phosphorus are the most abundant minerals in bone and adequate intake of these minerals is essential for appropriate bone mineral accretion. DXA measurements provide reasonable estimates of total body bone mass in infants and young children and several studies have used this measure to assess the impact of micronutrients on bone mass accretion early in life.

Linear Growth

No studies specifically looking at the effect of calcium and phosphorus intake on linear growth were found. In a recent study by Kramer et al. [39], the growth of infants exclusively breast-fed for either 3 or 6 months differed: infants breast-fed for only 3 months had greater gains in length (20.3 ± 7.0 mm/month) between 3 and 6 months of age compared to infants exclusively breast-fed through 6 months (19.2 ± 6.4 mm/months). Once complimentary foods were introduced there was equalization in length so that by 12 months of age there was no difference. There are numerous differences in nutrient composition between human milk and infant formula other than mineral content, making it impossible to ascribe these differences to an influence of mineral intake on length. However, one randomized trial described in detail below did not find significant differences in length gain among infants receiving different formulas with varying mineral intake [40].

Bone Mineralization

In 1993, Lee et al. [41] reported the results of a longitudinal observational study of 128 children from Hong Kong for whom they had collected extensive dietary intake data during the first 5 years of life. They found that BMC at the 1/3 distal radius was associated with the cumulative calcium intake during the first 5 years of life. Calcium intake during the second year of life had the strongest correlation with BMC at 5 years.

In 1997 the results of a randomized trial of varying mineral intake in 101 infants during the first year of life were reported [40]. This trial was conducted in two phases: phase I was conducted during the first 6 months of life when infants were either breast-fed or randomized to one of two infant formulas containing different amounts of calcium and phosphorus (table 1). Phase II involved the same infants who were re-randomized at 6 months of age to 1 of 3 feeding groups that differed in mineral content (table 1). During the first 6 months the infants who received the moderate mineral containing formula had a greater bone mass accretion than the other 2 feeding groups (human milk and low mineral containing formula). Although there was no effect of the type of feeding on BMC gain during the second 6 months, there was a difference during the second 6 months by the first 6 month feeding groups: infants who received breast milk had a greater gain in BMC than either the low- or moderate-mineral formula groups. By 12 months of age there were no differences in BMC among either the first or second 6-month feeding groups. These results indicate that early mineral intake is associated with early bone mass accretion, but when mineral intake is increased later in infancy these differences disappear.

Table 1. Randomized trial of varying mineral intake during the first year of life (data from Specker et al. [40])

0–6 months of age	Human milk	Low mineral	Moderate mineral	Significance
Mineral content				
Ca, mg/l	300	430	510	
P, mg/l	150	240	390	
Changes in				
Length, cm	11.1 ± 1.7^a	12.5 ± 1.9^a	11.8 ± 2.9	0.05
BMC, g	$59 \pm 17^{a,b}$	66 ± 18^a	82 ± 25^b	<0.001
Gain in BMC at 6–12 months[1]	$81 \pm 16^{a,b}$	73 ± 15^a	71 ± 15^b	0.04

6–12 months of age	Moderate mineral	High mineral	Cow's milk	Significance
Mineral content				
Ca, mg/l	510	1,350	1,230	
P, mg/l	390	900	960	
Changes in				
Length, cm	8.4 ± 1.8	8.6 ± 1.6	8.6 ± 1.3	Not significant
BMC, g	72.9 ± 21.1	75.9 ± 24.9	71.7 ± 38.1	Not significant

Significance values are for group differences.
[a,b]Means with the same symbols on each row are different at $p < 0.05$.
[1]Gain in BMC after re-randomization to one of the three feeding groups at 6 months of age.

Nutrients may interact with other environmental factors in their effect on bone growth and mineralization. Increased bone loading through physical activity is one of the major factors influencing bone mass accretion during growth. Early studies found that physically active children had greater BMD or BMC than less active children [42]. A randomized trial on the effect of gross motor activities on bone mass accretion in infants found evidence that calcium intake during infancy may modify the bone response to activity [43]. Infants were randomly assigned to an intervention of either gross motor or fine motor activities for 5 days/week for 1 year. Gross motor activity had no effect on bone mass accretion among infants receiving moderately high calcium intakes, whereas among infants with moderate to low calcium intakes, gross motor activity actually resulted in less gain in BMC than the fine motor activity group (fig. 4). The results of this study lead to the hypothesis that calcium intake modified the bone response to physical activity in young children. This hypothesis was formally tested in a randomized trial using a factorial design.

The randomized trial to formally test for an interaction between calcium intake and physical activity involved 239 children aged 3–5 years [44]. Children

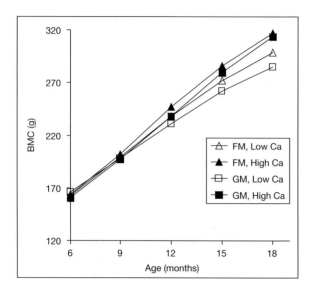

Fig. 4. Illustration of the effect of calcium intake on changes in total body BMC over the 12-month study period of infants in the gross motor (GM) and fine motor (FM) activity programs. The interaction term of age, activity group, and calcium intake was significant at p = 0.07. Reprinted from Specker et al. [43].

were randomized to participate in gross motor or fine motor activities for 30 min/day, 5 days/week for 1 year. Within each group, children were blindly assigned to receive either a placebo or 1,000 mg/day of calcium carbonate. Total body and regional BMC measurements using DXA and tibia cross-sectional measurements were obtained at baseline and study completion. Three-day diet records and accelerometer readings were obtained at 0, 6 and 12 months and showed a high baseline calcium intake among this population and a higher percent time in moderate plus vigorous activity among those children in the gross motor vs. fine motor group. Overall, calcium intake did not influence bone mass accretion. However, the difference in leg BMC gain between gross motor and fine motor was more pronounced in children receiving calcium vs. placebo (fig. 5; interaction, p = 0.05). At study completion, children in the gross motor group had greater periosteal and endosteal circumferences at the tibia compared to children in the fine motor group. There was also a significant interaction between the calcium intake and activity groups in both cortical thickness and cortical area: among children receiving placebo, thickness and area were smaller with gross motor vs. fine motor activity, but among children receiving calcium, thickness and area were larger with gross motor activity (fig. 5). These results indicate that the relationship of bone growth or mineralization and calcium intake is not simple and may depend upon other environmental factors that influence bone development, such as physical activity.

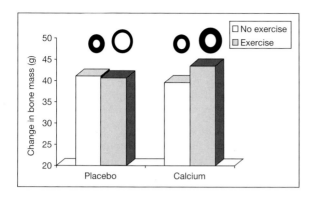

Fig. 5. Results showed a significant interaction between the calcium intake and physical activity groups in the gain in regional leg BMC measured by DXA. The figures above each mean are schematic illustrations showing the effect of both calcium intake and physical activity on a cross-section of the 20% distal tibia. Data are from Specker and Binkley [44].

Both low and high phosphorus intakes may theoretically lead to reduced bone mass accretion. A low phosphate intake will limit the substrate availability for bone formation, while a high phosphate may decrease serum calcium leading to an increase in serum PTH. A randomized trial tested whether the introduction of cereals between the ages of 16 and 26 weeks would lead to higher PTH and lower BMC [45]. Forty-one infants were randomized to either formula alone or formula plus infant cereal beginning at 16 weeks of age. Although serum PTH concentrations increased significantly in the cereal-fed group, there was no difference between groups in BMC changes (1/3 distal radius using SPA).

Early Diet and Bone Later in Life

While it is possible to increase bone mass accretion early in life, the long-term effect on bone health is not known. There are no studies showing that increasing bone mass in the first years of life is associated with greater bone mineralization later in childhood or adolescence. Bishop et al. [46] reported that preterm infants fed human milk with a high mineral fortifier in the neonatal period had lower bone mass at 5 years of age compared to preterm infants fed only human milk with its relatively low mineral content. These authors suggested that 'programming' may occur in the early neonatal period with infants who have low mineral intakes developing improved calcium retention later in life. However, this hypothesis has not been confirmed in other studies [47, 48], including one by the same authors involving a larger number of children who were aged 8–12 years [47].

Bone Growth and Mineralization

There are single studies that report both a positive relationship between childhood BMD and length of breast-feeding or infant vitamin D supplementation. Jones et al. [49] studied 330 eight-year-old children in Australia and found that total body, femoral neck and spine BMD was higher among prepubertal 8-year-old children who were breast-fed for more than 3 months compared to those children who were breast-fed for less than 3 months. These findings were only observed among the 245 children born at term and not among those born preterm (n = 85). Zamora et al. [50] reported the results of a retrospective study and found that the 91 prepubertal girls (median age 8 years) who received vitamin D supplements during the first of year of life had greater aBMD at the radius, femoral neck, and greater trochanter than the 15 girls who were not supplemented with vitamin D. Both of these studies used retrospective designs and the issue of bias needs to be considered, in particular recall bias and selection bias.

Conclusions

Vitamin D, calcium and phosphorus are the major micronutrients involved in bone growth and mineralization. There are few studies that have systematically determined the effect of vitamin D deficiency on either linear growth or bone mineralization. Maternal vitamin D deficiency during pregnancy is associated with fetal bone growth and ossification. Vitamin D supplementation of infants at high risk of vitamin D deficiency may improve linear growth, but this affect does not become apparent until the second half of the first year of life. There are no consistent findings of a relationship between BMC or BMD measured by DXA and vitamin D status of infants, possibly due to differences in the bone sites that have been measured. Calcium and phosphorus intakes early in life are associated with early bone mass accretion, but the long-term implications of early infant feeding on bone size and mass are not clear.

References

1   Garn SM: The Earlier Gain and the Later Loss of Cortical Bone. Springfield, Thomas, 1970.
2   Brunton JA, Wiler HA, Atkinson SA: Improvement in the accuracy of dual energy X-ray absorptiometry for whole body and regional analysis of body composition: Validation using piglets and methodologic considerations in infants. Pediatr Res 1997;41:590–596.
3   Binkley TL, Specker BL: pQCT measurement of bone parameters in young children: Validation of technique. J Clin Densitom 2000;3:9–14.
4   Specker BL, Tsang RC, Hollis BW: Effect of race and diet on human milk vitamin D and 25-hydroxyvitamin D. Am J Dis Child 1985;139:1134–1137.
5   Specker B, Valanis B, Hertzberg V, et al: Sunshine exposure and serum 25-hydroxyvitamin D concentrations in exclusively breast-fed infants. J Pediatr 1985;107:372.
6   Vitamin D Expert Panel Meeting: Atlanta, Centers for Disease Control, 2001: http://www.cdc.gov/nccdphp/dnpa/nutrition/pdf/Vitamin_D_Expert_Panel_Meeting.pdf
7   Krall EA, Sahyoun N, Tannenbaum S, et al: Effect of vitamin D intake on seasonal variations in parathyroid hormone secretion in postmenopausal women. N Engl J Med 1989;321:1777–1783.

8 Meulmeester JF, vandenBerg H, Wedel M, et al: Vitamin D status, parathyroid hormone and sunlight in Turkish, Moroccan and Caucasian children in The Netherlands. Eur J Clin Nutr 1990;44:461–470.
9 Marya RK, Rathee S, Lata V, Mudgil S: Effects of vitamin D supplementation in pregnancy. Gynecol Obstet Invest 1981;12:155–161.
10 Congdon P, Horsman A, Kirby PA, et al: Mineral content of the forearms of babies born to Asian and white mothers. Br Med J (Clin Res Ed) 1983;286:1234–1235.
11 Cockburn F, Belton NR, Purvis RJ, et al: Maternal vitamin D intake and mineral metabolism in mothers and their newborn infants. Br Med J 1980;231:1–10.
12 Brooke DG, Brown IRF, Bone CDM, et al: Vitamin D supplements in pregnant Asian women: Effects on calcium status and fetal growth. Br Med J 1980;280:751–754.
13 Delvin EE, Salle BL, Glorieux FH, et al: Vitamin D supplementation during pregnancy: Effect on neonatal calcium homeostasis. J Pediatr 1986;109:328–334.
14 Mallet E, Gugi B, Brunelle P, et al: Vitamin D supplementation in pregnancy: A controlled trial of two methods. Obstet Gynecol 1986;68:300–304.
15 Marya RK, Rathee S, Dua V, Sangwan K: Effect of vitamin D supplementation during pregnancy on foetal growth. Indian J Med Res 1988;88:488–492.
16 Stearns G, Jeans PC, Vandecar V: The effect of vitamin D on linear growth in infancy. J Pediatr 1936;9:1–10.
17 Slyker F, Hamil BM, Poole MW, et al: Relationship between vitamin D intake and linear growth in infants. Proc Soc Exp Biol Med 1937;37:499–502.
18 Chan GM, Robert CC, Folland D, Jackson R: Growth and bone mineralization of normal breast-fed infants and the effects of lactation on maternal bone mineral status. Am J Clin Nutr 1982; 36:438–443.
19 Feliciano ES, Ho ML, Specker B, et al: Seasonal and geographic variations in the growth rate of infants in China receiving increasing dosages of vitamin D supplements. J Trop Pediatr 1994;40:162–165.
20 Jeans PC, Stearns G: The effect of vitamin D on linear growth in infancy. II. The effect of intakes above 1,800 USP units daily. J Pediatr 1938;13:730–740.
21 Fomon S, Younoszai M, Thomas L: Influence of vitamin D on linear growth of normal full-term infants. J Nutr 1966;88:345–350.
22 Russell JGB, Hill LF: True fetal rickets. Br Radiol 1974;47:732.
23 Zhou H: Rickets in China; in Glorieux FH (ed): Rickets. New York, Raven Press, 1991, p 253.
24 Reif S, Katzir Y, Eisenberg Z, Weisman Y: Serum 25-hydroxyvitamin D levels in congenital craniotabes. Acta Paediatr Scand 1988;77:167–168.
25 Specker B, Ho M, Oestreich A, et al: Prospective study of vitamin D supplementation and rickets in China. J Pediatr 1992;120:733–739.
26 Greer FR, Searcy JF, Levin RS, et al: Bone mineral content and serum 25-hydroxyvitamin D concentration in breast-fed infants with and without supplemental vitamin D. J Pediatr 1981; 98:696–701.
27 Greer FR, Searcy JE, Levin RS, et al: Bone mineral content and serum 25-hydroxyvitamin D concentrations in breast-fed infants with and without supplemental vitamin D: One-year follow-up. J Pediatr 1982;100:919–922.
28 Greer F, Marshall S: Bone mineral content, serum vitamin D metabolite concentrations, and ultraviolet B light exposure in infants fed human milk with and without vitamin D2 supplements. J Pediatr 1989;114:204–212.
29 Park MJ, Namgung R, Kim DH, Tsang RC: Bone mineral content is not reduced despite low vitamin D status in breast milk-fed infants versus cow's milk based formula-fed infants. J Pediatr 1998;132:641–645.
30 Silverberg SJ, Shane E, Clemens TL, et al: The effect of oral phosphate administration on major indices of skeletal metabolism in normal subjects. J Bone Miner Res 1986;1:383–388.
31 Parisien M, Silverberg SJ, Shane E, et al: Bone disease in primary hyperparathyroidism. Endocrinol Metab Clin N Am 1990;19:19–34.
32 Bilzekian JP, Silverberg SJ, Shane E, et al: Characterization and evaluation of asymptomatic primary hyperparathyroidism. J Bone Miner Res 1991;6:S85–S89.
33 Duan Y, De Luca V, Seeman E: Parathyroid hormone deficiency and excess: Similar effects of trabecular bone but differing effects on cortical bone. J Clin Endocrinol Metab 1999;84:718–722.
34 Park EA: The etiology of rickets. Physiol Rev 1923;3:106–163.

35 Bronner F: Vitamin D deficiency and rickets. Am J Clin Nutr 1976;29:1307–1314.
36 Food and Nutrition Board SCotSEoDRI, Institute of Medicine: Dietary Reference Intakes for Calcium, Phosphorus, Magnesium, Vitamin D, and Fluoride. Washington, National Academy Press, 1997.
37 Widdowson EM, McCance RA, Spray CM: The chemical composition of the human body. Clin Sci 1951;10:113–125.
38 Abrams SA, Wen J, Stuff JE: Absorption of calcium, zinc and iron from breast milk by 5- to 7-month-old infants. Pediatr Res 1997;41:1–7.
39 Kramer MS, Guo T, Platt RW, et al: Infant growth and health outcomes associated with 3 compared with 6 mo of exclusive breastfeeding. Am J Clin Nutr 2003;78:291–295.
40 Specker BL, Beck A, Kalkwarf H, Ho M: Randomized trial of varying mineral intake on total body bone mineral accretion during the first year of life. Pediatrics 1997;99:e12.
41 Lee WT, Leung SS, Lui SS, Lau J: Relationship between long-term calcium intake and bone mineral content of children from birth to 5 years. Br J Nutr 1993;70:235–248.
42 Cassell C, Benedict M, Specker B: Bone mineral density in elite 7–9 year old female gymnasts and swimmers. Med Sci Sports Exerc 1996;28:1243–1246.
43 Specker BL, Mulligan L, Ho ML: Longitudinal study of calcium intake, physical activity, and bone mineral content in infants 6–18 months of age. J Bone Miner Res 1999;14:569–576.
44 Specker B, Binkley T: Randomized trial of physical activity and calcium supplementation on bone mineral content in 3–5 year old children. J Bone Miner Res 2003;18:885–892.
45 Bainbridge RR, Mimouni FB, Landi T, et al: Effect of rice cereal feedings on bone mineralization and calcium homeostasis in cow milk formula fed infants. J Am Coll Nutr 1996;15:383–388.
46 Bishop NJ, Dahlenburg SL, Fewtrell MS, et al: Early diet of preterm infants and bone mineralization at age five years. Acta Paediatr 1996;85:230–236.
47 Fewtrell MS, Prentice A, Jones SC, et al: Bone mineralization and turnover in preterm infants at 8–12 years of age: The effect of early diet. J Bone Miner Res 1999;14:810–820.
48 Backstrom MC, Maki R, Kuusela AL, et al: The long-term effect of early mineral, vitamin D, and breast milk intake on bone mineral status in 9- to 11-year old children born prematurely. J Pedatr Gastroenterol Nutr 1999;29:575–582.
49 Jones G, Riley M, Dwyer T: Breastfeeding in early life and bone mass in prepubertal children: A longitudinal study. Osteoporos Int 2000;11:146–152.
50 Zamora SA, Rizzoli R, Belli DC, et al: Vitamin D supplementation during infancy is associated with higher bone mineral mass in prepubertal girls. J Clin Endocrinol Metab 1999;84:4541–4544.

Discussion

Dr. Zlotkin: One of the characteristics of children in the developing world, especially rural children, which differentiate them perhaps from a typical American population, is the fact that the majority are breast-fed and don't receive any formula, and as they get older they exercise a lot. One of the groups you didn't talk about would be in terms of periosteal impact, decreased calcium and increased exercise. Could you postulate on what you think you would find for that group?

Dr. Specker: I think you will still find an increase in bone circumference with periosteal expansion from exercise, but it may not be as great if calcium is low. The body has to adapt to the low calcium intake, perhaps by removing calcium from bone. Exercise will increase both periosteal and endosteal expansion, low calcium intake is likely to increase endosteal expansion. If the cortical thickness is too small then periosteal expansion is going to slow down, so calcium must be going into the bone in order for it to expand. Therefore I would speculate that periosteal expansion will not be as large on a calcium-deficient diet, but there would still be some expansion.

Dr. Guesry: You selected to speak only on vitamin D, phosphate and calcium. We did animal studies 20 years ago on zinc deficiency, the elasticity module of the bone, and resistance to fracture. Do you know if there are new data on that, or human data related zinc deficiency and bone fragility?

Dr. Specker: I am not aware of any, but Dr. Abrams might.

Dr. Abrams: There are several animal studies suggesting that zinc supplementation improves bone strength. There was one control trial on zinc supplementation in adults suggesting an increasing bone mass, but that is an area that needs considerable more work.

Dr. Pettifor: A couple of issues, first of all just to pick up on what Dr. Zlotkin asked which is that one generally perceives children as being more active in less developed countries or in developing countries than in developed countries. We are busy doing a longitudinal study of children through puberty. At age 9 years our black children from a poor socioeconomic environment in fact exercised less than our white children, basically because they had no formal physical activity at school, which was a major component of the exercise that white children had. So the high socioeconomic group was going to schools that had organized physical activity with high stress and strain which is important for bone development. If we look at actual bone mineral density in those children, the black children showed no change in bone mass with quartiles of physical activity, while the white children did. So the children with the highest physical activity, the highest peak strain on the bone, had higher bone mineral density. It appears that the black children didn't get up to those physical activity levels that were seen in the last quartile of the white children, suggesting that perhaps it is the extent of exercise that is important, and again the issue of calcium intake. Our black children were on a significantly lower calcium intake than the white children, but the bone mass was similar in both groups, except at the hip where black children have a higher bone mass. We have seen this as well in adults, both pre- and postmenopausal adults, suggesting that a genetic difference rather than an environmental factor is influencing the hip change. A question I want to ask is about calcium intake and changes with exercise. You said the subjects were already on a very high calcium intake. Was there any evidence that if you looked at those on a low calcium intake that exercise had less effect on bone, or was there any effect of dietary calcium intake on bone at all?

Dr. Specker: No, there was no main effect of dietary calcium on bone. If calcium is interacting with physical activity that means that there is an effect of calcium, but it is through modifying the relationship between bone changes and physical activity. If we grouped all the children and looked at changes in leg bone mass by quartiles of calcium intake, based on both the supplement and the diet, there was a very nice dose-response relationship. The children in the exercise group had a greater increase in bone with increasing quartile of calcium intake. However, at the lowest quartile of calcium intake there was no benefit, it was actually detrimental, and the children in the gross motor group had less bone accretion than the fine motor group. This may explain part of your findings. The other thing I just want to mention is when looking at bone mass using DXA, as in our study, we didn't see any difference in the change in leg bone mass between the calcium and the no calcium groups among the children in the fine motor group who had similar changes as the gross motor, no calcium group. It wasn't until bone geometry was looked at that differences in bone size were actually found, which explains those findings, or lack of findings, a little bit better. If there is this expansion of bone and a smaller cortical thickness then mass can be the same. I am trying to make the point that bone size itself is a very important outcome parameter that needs to be looked at in pediatric studies.

Dr. Mogrovejo: What is the relation among other nutrients like protein, energy, vitamin C or copper in bone accretion?

Dr. Specker: Protein deficiency should have an effect on bone through the IGF system. IGF is important for this periosteal expansion that occurs during growth, it is one of the driving factors. I know the people at the USDA Human Nutrition Research Center in Grand Forks, North Dakota, are interested in the effects of trace minerals

167

on bone. Magnesium deficiency appears to affect trabecular bone at least in adults, but it doesn't seem to affect cortical bone. I am not sure on the mechanism, but perhaps it relates to the role of magnesium in ensuring adequate functioning of the parathyroid gland. Dr. Abrams, do you have any information on copper?

Dr. Abrams: There are considerable animal data related to copper deficiency, but there aren't any good human studies.

Dr. Specker: Very few pediatric studies have been done looking at calcium and vitamin D on bone, and those are the big nutrients in terms of pediatric bone research. There just aren't that many infant bone studies for the other micronutrients.

Dr. Castillo-Durán: Some countries even now use a high dose of vitamin D for the prevention of rickets. The effects for the prevention of rickets have been demonstrated, but I don't know about the safety of the high doses for the bone metabolism or the long-term effects on the bone metabolism. Do you have some information?

Dr. Specker: I don't think there is anything out there looking at the effects of Stoss therapy on bone. At least in later in childhood and adulthood it has been shown to be effective for the prevention of rickets and osteomalacia, especially in high-risk populations where you might have a problem with compliance.

Dr. Castillo-Durán: A study in our country some years ago compared those infants who were supplemented with daily doses and high doses, 2 or 3 times a day, and they demonstrated some effect in length, about 2 cm during the first years of life. Maybe it was related to the hypercalcemia and the effect on bone.

Dr. Specker: So the high-dose ones grew better?

Dr. Castillo-Durán: With the daily supplementation they grew better than the high dose of vitamin D supplementation.

Dr. Specker: So it is not a compliance issue.

Dr. Gebre-Medhin: If I were to start from the disease perspective and use rickets as an example, is it always possible to completely heal vitamin D deficiency rickets using only vitamin D? Is it also possible to treat vitamin D deficiency rickets at least in infants only using sunlight? What are the metabolic and bone consequences of these two statements?

Dr. Specker: You can effectively treat vitamin D deficiency rickets with vitamin D and without the minerals. By treating the vitamin D deficiency, you are correcting the mineral deficiencies because you increase 1,25-dihydroxy-vitamin D and absorb more calcium. In effect you are giving the infant more calcium. As far as sunshine is concerned, it is very effective treatment. In Scandinavia they use UV lights to prevent and treat rickets.

Dr. Batubara: I would like to ask you about attaining big bone mass in early adulthood for the prevention of osteoporosis. What is the optimal upper level calcium intake suggested, because as you know a higher calcium intake will interfere with the zinc absorption?

Dr. Specker: The new dietary reference intakes for North America are based on maximizing calcium retention, or at what level of calcium you no longer see additional retention by giving more, and that value around the time of peak bone mass is between 1,000 and 1,200 mg/day for both women and men.

Dr. Gibson: I just have a question in relation to a study that was carried out in New Zealand that you may know about: a multidisciplinary study on 1,000 infants who have been followed every 5 years up to 26 years of age [1]. Are you familiar with this study?

Dr. Specker: This last study I mentioned with the breast-fed and bottle-fed infants is from New Zealand? I am not sure if that is the study you are referring to.

Dr. Zlotkin: You showed data suggesting that there was some tracking at early infant nutrition on bone growth at age 8. There was a controversy about whether early breast-feeding had an impact on the bone mineral content at age 8. Is there any further tracking to an older age? Does it make any difference if we feed the infants in the first 2 years of life with regard to the two important outcomes which will be number of fractures and risk of osteoporosis or height growth for example? Does it matter if we feed the infants during the first 2 years?

Dr. Specker: When you say tracking, the data I showed at age 8 actually were opposite to what you would have expected if there was tracking. What I was showing was that those infants who had low mineral intake early in life should have had lower bone mass than those infants fed higher mineral, but at age 8 it had switched, so that the ones that had the low mineral early in life had high bone mass and vice versa. However, we have data showing that over 3 years during the toddler period there appears to be tracking. There are several studies done at different ages in childhood, so if you combine them all together you could speculate that in fact there is a point at which bone mass begins to track. What age that is, is not clear, but it is probably before puberty. Significant changes in bone occur during puberty. Those children with high values before puberty have high values after puberty. But no one has done a study looking over the entire pediatric age range. There are more mixed longitudinal studies and those tend to show that there is some tracking. In the adult literature, it has been found that the bone density made 11 years earlier predicts fracture risk just as well as the most recent bone density measurement. So we know that fracture risk is associated with bone density measurements up to 11 years earlier in adults. This has not been done in children. There also are studies, including some from New Zealand, that are case-control studies in which the bone density of children who fractured versus those who did not were compared [2, 3]. These studies find a lower bone density in the children with fractures versus those without fractures. In addition, those who fracture are then at a higher risk of fracturing later in childhood [4]. So early bone density is also thought to be a predictor of fracture risk in childhood, and once fractures occur then there is a higher risk of subsequent fractures. Therefore, there is immediate benefit of having a high bone density during childhood on a child's fracture risk, not necessarily just the prevention of osteoporosis later in life.

Dr. Zlotkin: Are you suggesting that early breast-feeding would decrease the risk of fracture based on that argument?

Dr. Specker: I am not willing to say that yet because I don't think there are enough studies showing the long-term impact of feeding during the neonatal period on bone mass later in childhood.

Dr. Pettifor: To follow up on Dr. Zlotkin's comments. I am left with the impression that you are suggesting that in fact a high calcium intake may not be beneficial in early life. Certainly from an exercise point of view you worry that calcium supplementation may not be appropriate. And yet in the food industry there is a push to increase calcium intake in this age group. Would you comment on that and speculate on whether one should be promoting high calcium?

Dr. Specker: It depends on what you mean by high calcium, but I think that it is very early to promote the feeding of high amounts of calcium early in life. I don't think the long-term effects on bone growth and size have really been determined. I think it would be premature.

Dr. Endres: I am delighted that you said for the treatment of rickets you would recommend the use of minerals; you didn't say calcium but you did mean calcium and phosphorus?

Dr. Specker: I was talking more biochemically. If you were to just treat with vitamin D then you would be correcting mineral deficiencies. You don't have to actually treat with calcium and phosphorus as well.

Dr. Endres: I think that calcium together with vitamin D would be enough, lets say 5,000 units/day over 3 or 4 weeks, but we never tried sunlight only because it is so easy over 3 or 4 weeks. One of the initial problems with vitamin D deficiency rickets is that nobody knows that. So we assume that in a first step, it is hypocalcemia, and then due to secondary hypothyroidism calcium is normalized and phosphorus decreases, and that is what we always find initially, i.e. hypophosphatemia. I think to prevent this tetany it is necessary, at least it is not harmful, to give calcium in addition to vitamin D. When we had more cases of rickets in Germany, we saw some children with tetany.

Dr. Specker: Venkataraman et al. [5] in Cincinnati found that treatment of vitamin D deficiency rickets with 400 IU vitamin D/day was sufficient to heal rickets. What I was trying to say about calcium is that if vitamin D is given to correct the vitamin D deficiency then 1,25-dihydroxyvitamin D increases and this will lead to an increase in intestinal calcium absorption, normalizing serum calcium concentrations, decreasing parathyroid hormone, and normalizing serum phosphorus. Initially, during early stages of vitamin D deficiency, 1,25-dihydroxyvitamin D concentrations are high, but then they drop. When you give vitamin D, 1,25-dihydroxyvitamin D will increase, intestinal absorption of calcium will increase and you have corrected the calcium deficiency.

Dr. Tolboom: I have a question on the fetal origin hypothesis of adult disease. What do you know of the fetal origin hypothesis in terms of bone disease or infections?

Dr. Specker: There was an abstract presented at the American Society for Bone and Mineral Research by Javaid et al. [6] from Southampton. They reported that maternal vitamin D status in late pregnancy was correlated with the child's whole body bone mineral content at the age of 9 years. It has not been published or peer-reviewed, only presented as an abstract.

Dr. Pettifor: I have a comment on the general data on the fetal origin of bone disease. The problem with the majority of studies is that they are influenced by the failure to adjust for bone size. So that actually if you adjust for bone size in children, later age groups in childhood and in adulthood, you adjust for differences in body stature which may be influenced by fetal environment. Then there is very little difference in bone mass if you are a low birth weight baby as opposed to a full size baby. I think most of the effects are seen on body size and therefore on bone mass, but once you adjusted for these there is very little evidence that there are major effects on bone density per se.

Dr. Abrams: I agree entirely. There have been several studies in preterm infants on bone mass up until early adolescence and they all show a decreased bone mass proportional to the decreased body size.

Dr. Specker: The abstract presented at the bone meeting had to do with maternal exposure to either vitamin D or calcium during pregnancy and long-term effects on the bone of the child, but I am not sure exactly what that was.

Dr. Gebre-Medhin: I am happy the issue of rickets and calcium and phosphorus came up again, that was my intention. The impression I have now is that you can effectively treat rickets on a pre-rickets diet by only providing vitamin D or sunshine, that is what we have had in Sweden, that is also the standard we have right now. Having said that, regarding bone and fractures and osteoporosis there is a heated debate concerning vitamin A along with increased calcium intake. You know the work by Melhus et al. [7] and the others. What is your comment on that?

Dr. Specker: There are quite a few studies. Melhus et al. [7] from Sweden originally reported this potentially adverse effect of vitamin A. Another study that supports these findings recently came from the Rancho Bernardo Study [8]. However, there are contradictory studies from Iceland [9]. There may be a possible vitamin A toxicity on bone at very high levels, at least in animal studies, but I am not sure about the human evidence because of these conflicting reports.

References

1 Silva PA, Stanton S: From Child to Adult. Auckland, Oxford University Press, 1996, pp 1–23.
2 Goulding A, Cannan R, Williams SM, et al: Bone mineral density in girls with forearm fractures. J Bone Miner Res 1998;13:143–148.
3 Goulding A, Jones IE, Taylor RW, et al: Bone mineral density and body composition in boys with distal forearm fractures: A dual energy X-ray absorptiometry study. J Pediatr 2001;139: 509–515.
4 Goulding A, Jones IE, Taylor RW, et al: More broken bones: A 4-year double cohort study of girls with and without distal forearm fractures. J Bone Miner Res 2000;15:2011–2018.
5 Venkataraman PS, Tsang RC, Buckley DD, et al: Elevation of serum 1,25-hydroxyvitamin D in response to physiologic doses of vitamin D in vitamin D-deficient infants. J Pediatr 1983;103: 416–419.
6 Javaid MK, Shore SR, Taylor P, et al: Maternal vitamin D status during late pregnancy and accrual of childhood bone mineral (abstract). J Bone Miner Res 2003;18:S13.
7 Melhus H, Michaelsson K, Kindmark A, et al: Excessive dietary intake of vitamin A is associated with reduced bone mineral density and increased risk for hip fracture. Ann Intern Med 1998;129: 770–778.
8 Promislow JH, Goodman-Gruen D, Slymen DJ, Barrett-Connor E: Retinol intake and bone mineral density in the elderly: The Rancho Bernardo Study. J Bone Miner Res 2002;17:1349–1358.
9 Sigurdsson G, Franzson L, Thorgeirsdottir H, Steingrimsdottir L: A lack of association between excessive dietary intake of vitamin A and bone mineral density in seventy-year-old Icelandic women; in Burckhardt P, Dawson-Hughes B, Heaney RP (eds): Nutritional Aspects of Osteoporosis. San Diego, Academic Press, 2001, pp 295–302.

Pettifor JM, Zlotkin S (eds): Micronutrient Deficiencies during the Weaning Period and the
First Years of Life. Nestlé Nutrition Workshop Series Pediatric Program, vol 54, pp 173–185,
Nestec Ltd., Vevey/S. Karger AG, Basel, © 2004.

Impact of Infections on Micronutrient Deficiencies in Developing Countries

Zulfiqar Ahmed Bhutta

Department of Paediatrics, Aga Khan University and Medical Center, Karachi, Pakistan

Introduction

Despite numerous advances and improvements in child health globally, malnutrition still remains a major problem [1, 2]. A large proportion of cases of malnutrition occur in South Asia [3], which also harbors almost three quarters of the global burden of low birth weight infants [4]. In other parts of the world high rates of HIV threaten to reverse all the gains made by child survival programs, with worsening malnutrition [5]. Such overt forms of malnutrition, however, do not reflect the true global burden of malnutrition, as a large proportion of the hidden burden of malnutrition is represented by widespread single and multiple micronutrient deficiencies.

The relationship between micronutrient deficiencies, such as vitamin A deficiency, and increased risk of childhood infections and mortality is well established [6]. Vitamin A supplementation is now recognized as an important public health intervention among young children in areas of endemic vitamin A deficiency. Other micronutrient deficiencies such as zinc and iron deficiency are also recognized to be widespread in developing countries and associated with increased risk of morbidity [7] and mortality [8].

A number of factors may influence micronutrient deficiencies in developing countries. These include poor body stores at birth as a consequence of maternal intrauterine malnutrition, dietary deficiencies and high intake of inhibitors of absorption such as phytates and increased losses from the body (fig. 1). To illustrate, in the case of iron deficiency, in addition to poor dietary intake and inhibitors of absorption [9], increased intestinal losses following parasitic infestation may also be an important cause of iron deficiency anemia [10]. Overall, although the effects of poor intake and increased micronutrient demands are well described, the potential effects of acute and chronic infections on the body's micronutrient status are less well appreciated. Even more

173

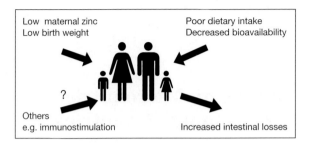

Low maternal zinc
Low birth weight

Poor dietary intake
Decreased bioavailability

?

Others
e.g. immunostimulation

Increased intestinal losses

Fig. 1. Pathogenesis of zinc deficiency. Determinants of body zinc status.

obscure is the potential effect of immunostimulation and intercurrent infections on the micronutrient distribution and homeostasis.

The potential bidirectional effect of micronutrient deficiencies on infections and immunity are increasingly being appreciated. The effect of micronutrient deficiencies on immunity and burden of infections in developing countries is well described. This review will, however, focus on the potential effect of infections on the homeostasis and body status of important micronutrients such as iron, zinc and vitamin A.

Biological Plausibility of the Effect of Infections on Micronutrient Deficiencies

A number of epidemiological studies support the close association of infections with micronutrient deficiencies. These include findings of lower serum concentrations of zinc with increasing burden and duration of diarrhea [7] as well as lower serum concentrations in patients with HIV infection [11]. Although children with hypovitaminosis A and low serum concentrations of vitamin A have higher rates of associated infections, the specific contribution of infection to vitamin A deficiency cannot be discounted. This relationship between low serum vitamin A and severity of disease has been observed with the increasing severity of HIV infection [12]. However, several infections are directly associated with an increased risk of micronutrient deficiency. These include diseases such as measles which have been directly implicated with unmasking as well as triggering vitamin A deficiency [13]. Therefore the association of relatively higher rates of micronutrient deficiencies with infectious diseases may be reflective of both an increased predisposition to infections in deficient populations as well as a direct effect of the infection itself on the micronutrient status indicators [14]. Low serum concentrations of micronutrients have frequently been described in subclinical infections. The levels also appear to be lowest where there are the highest levels of inflammatory

174

proteins. High serum concentrations of C-reactive protein and haptoglobin are known to be related to the density of malarial parasites in Tanzanian children [15], with correspondingly lower concentrations of plasma retinol. The levels of plasma retinol among apparently healthy children in Ghana were also found to be lowest in those with raised markers of acute inflammation [16]. The effects of infection on blood indicators of micronutrient status may be more marked in areas with widespread malnutrition. To illustrate, in an evaluation of the comparative effects of malnutrition and coexisting malaria on serum antioxidant levels in Nigeria, the reduction in plasma β-carotene concentrations was significant with malaria rather than malnutrition [17].

There may be a physiological reason or benefit for the observed effects of infection on micronutrient status and indicators. The reduction in circulating zinc may reduce available zinc for microbial metabolism during infection [18]. Recent evidence suggests that Zn^{2+} may also play a role in reducing cellular oxidative stress and thus the acute changes seen in the circulation may represent a physiological compartmental change by an intracellular shift in zinc [19]. These data thus provide evidence of a similar advantage to that achieved by reducing iron levels during the course of bacterial infection.

Impact of Infection on Indicators of Micronutrient Status

For many micronutrients it is unclear whether the best currently available indicators truly measure the current body status. The reasons for these are manifold. Firstly the alteration in the serum concentration of a particular micronutrient may not reflect the true body status but be an adaptive phenomenon. In other instances, the changes may be transient and related to the severity of coincidental infections.

In an evaluation of the relationship of concomitant infections with serum concentrations of zinc, copper and ferritin among Peruvian children, Brown et al. [20] concluded that the effect was variable and differed by nutrient, nutrition status of the population, and the severity of infections. Figure 2 indicates the mean serum zinc concentrations among a cohort of children under 36 months of age undergoing nutrition rehabilitation for persistent diarrhea in Karachi. No impact or reduction in plasma zinc was seen, except among those with the most severe infections, e.g. sepsis or pneumonia requiring systemic antibiotics. It has thus been suggested that this acute effect of coincidental infections on serum zinc levels may not be significant at a population level in developing countries and that serum concentrations of zinc can be used as a robust measure of population zinc status regardless of concomitant subclinical infections [21].

Reduced levels of circulating free iron as well as increased levels of iron-binding proteins are seen with infections [22] and may represent a physiological adaptation to reduce free iron availability to circulating pathogens. The

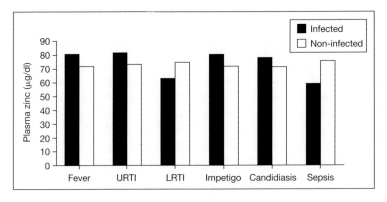

Fig. 2. Relationship of plasma zinc and coincidental infections. URTI = Upper respiratory tract infections; LRTI = lower respiratory tract infections.

effect of infections on serum ferritin, an important indicator of iron stores, is in the opposite direction and serum concentrations are elevated in the presence of infection [23]. Thus estimation of serum ferritin alone may lead to underestimation of the true prevalence of iron deficiency in subjects with high rates of coincidental infections and morbidity. However, this problem can be overcome if the ratio of the serum transferrin receptor and serum ferritin is assessed and the concentration of the serum-transferring receptor does not change during infection [24].

The most striking effects of infections on micronutrient status have been seen in volunteer human experiments assessing the serum levels following injection of low dose endotoxin. Gaetke et al. [25] studied the effect of endotoxin administration in 12 volunteers and demonstrated that serum cytokines went up and zinc concentrations decreased with the injections. However, no effect was seen on serum albumin or albumin-zinc binding.

There is some evidence at a cellular level of a reduction in liver retinol-binding protein (RBP) synthesis in animals injected with endotoxin [26]. RBP, if not bound efficiently to transthyretin (TTR), could also move to the extravascular space or be lost in the urine [27] following endotoxin challenge. It has also been suggested that it may be possible to use the RBP/TTR ratio as a measure of vitamin A status in the presence of acute inflammation [24]. These findings indicate that inflammation-induced hyporetinemia does not necessarily imply a loss of vitamin A, but rather represents a redistribution of tissue vitamin A brought about by a reduced hepatic synthesis of RBP.

The aforementioned acute changes in serum concentrations of zinc and iron may not accurately reflect the changes in the body status of these micronutrients, and there is thus considerable interest in exploring other measures. Earlier studies employed intravenously administered radioactive isotopes such as ^{65}Zn to study a multi-compartment model of zinc kinetics [28].

These techniques have now been largely supplanted by stable isotope studies. Stable isotopes of zinc namely ^{68}Zn and ^{67}Zn have been used to study zinc homeostasis in a six-compartment model [29]. Although some information is available to indicate the high turnover rates of acute phase proteins during infection [30], to date no zinc kinetic studies have evaluated whole body and compartment changes in zinc metabolism during infections using stable isotopes.

Pathogenesis and Mechanisms of Micronutrient Deficiency with Coexisting Infections

There is little information on the short-term compartment changes in micronutrients such as iron, zinc and vitamin A. However, other mechanisms underlying net body losses and homeostasis are well described. It is possible to elucidate the mechanism of alteration in micronutrient status and consequent deficiency from other direct studies and observations.

The gut has a special role in the pathogenesis and severity of micronutrient deficiencies.

The association of helminthic infections, especially hook worms, with iron deficiency in young children is well established and largely relates to direct intestinal losses [31]. Although the association between diarrheal disease-control programs and malnutrition or growth rates has been questioned, in many parts of the world there is a close relationship between the two. In particular prolonged and recurrent episodes of diarrhea, frequently in association with HIV infection, are a frequent cause of morbidity and micronutrient deficiency. In recent years, the association of increased micronutrient losses such as those of zinc and copper with acute diarrhea has been well recognized [32]. These findings may explain the high rates of subclinical zinc deficiency among children with frequent and recurrent bouts of diarrhea, and may be particularly marked among children with persistent diarrhea.

Figure 3 indicates data from sequential metabolic and trace element balance studies among 20 children with persistent diarrhea who underwent inpatient nutritional rehabilitation in Karachi. These findings indicate significant intestinal losses of zinc during diarrhea, which frequently exceed the dietary intake leading to a net negative balance during the diarrheal episode. These trends reversed with recovery from diarrhea and nutritional rehabilitation over a 14-day period. These data support the continued use of zinc supplements during the nutritional rehabilitation.

In addition, it is also recognized that children with shigellosis can lose a significant amount of vitamin A in the urine, thus further aggravating preexisting subclinical vitamin A deficiency [33]. As already illustrated, the risk of micronutrient deficiency in infancy and early childhood can be compounded several fold by the presence of low body stores from birth as in low birth

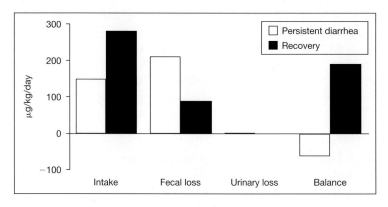

Fig. 3. Metabolic balance of zinc in children (n = 20) with persistent diarrhea and after recovery.

Table 1. Suggested regimen for micronutrient supplementation in infectious illnesses during infancy and childhood

Disorder	Recommended micronutrient	Dose	Duration
Acute diarrhea	Zinc	10 mg/day	7–10 days following diarrhea
Persistent diarrhea and malnutrition	Zinc	10–20 mg/day	14–30 days
	Vitamin A	50,000–100,000 units	Once only
Pneumonia	Zinc	10 mg/day	10–14 days
Pneumonia in malnourished children	Vitamin A	50,000–100,000 units	Once only
Measles	Vitamin A	200,000 units daily	2 days

weight infants, and further aggravated by poor breast-feeding and complementary feeding practices [34].

Conclusions and Implications

The aforementioned data indicate that although coincidental infections may lead to transient alterations in serum concentrations of micronutrients, the physiological basis and significance of these changes are unclear. However, available information from large scale surveys indicate that these transient alterations may not be significant at a population level and thus serum or plasma estimation of micronutrients can be used as an adequate measure of micronutrient status in such populations.

On the other hand the important contribution of some infections to aggravation of micronutrient deficiencies in at-risk populations cannot be ignored. Increased losses of micronutrients such as vitamin A and zinc during infectious illnesses such as diarrhea are important contributors to micronutrient deficiencies. This may be particularly marked with prolonged diarrhea and dysentery and lead to clinically significant deficits and overt micronutrient deficiency.

Given that the epidemiological association between micronutrient deficiencies, such as zinc and diarrhea, is well established, supplementation strategies are logical in endemic areas. The growing body of evidence on the key role of zinc supplementation in accelerating recovery from diarrheal illnesses in developing countries supports its use in public health strategies in endemic areas. The association of measles with overt and subclinical vitamin A deficiency is also recognized, and administration of vitamin A to all such malnourished and at-risk children forms a corner stone of such management strategies. Table 1 summarizes some of the suggested regimens for supplementation with key micronutrients during specific childhood infectious illnesses, in which a contributory relationship of the disorder to precipitating or unmasking the micronutrient deficiencies is recognized.

References

1 Black RE, Morris SE, Bryce J: Where and why are 10 million children dying every year? Lancet 2003;361:2226–2234.
2 Measham AR, Chatterjee M: Wasting Away: The Crisis of Malnutrition in India. Washington, World Bank, 1999.
3 de Onis M, Frongillo EA, Blossner M: Is malnutrition declining? An analysis of changes in levels of child malnutrition since 1980. Bull World Health Organ 2000;78:1222–1233.
4 Sachdev HPS: Low birth weight in South Asia; in Gillespie S (ed): Malnutrition in South Asia: A Regional Profile. Kathmandu, UNICEF Regional Office for South Asia, 1997.
5 Ainsworth M, Waranya T: Breaking the silence: Setting realistic priorities for AIDS control in less-developed countries. Lancet 2000;356:55–60.
6 Beaton GH, Martorell R, Aronson KJ, et al: Effectiveness of Vitamin A Supplementation in the Control of Young Child Morbidity and Mortality in Developing Countries. ACC/SCN Nutrition Policy Discussion Paper No. 13, 1993, pp 1–120.
7 Black RE: Micronutrient deficiency – An underlying cause of morbidity and mortality. Bull World Health Organ 2003;2:79–81.
8 World Health Report: Reducing Risks, Promoting Healthy Life. Geneva, World Health Organization, 2002.
9 Hunt JR: Moving towards a plant-based diet: Are iron and zinc at risk? Nutr Rev 2002;60: 127–134.
10 Dossa RAM, Ategbo EAD, Koning FLHA, et al: Impact of iron supplementation and deworming on growth performance in preschool Beninese children. Eur J Clin Nutr 2001;55: 223–228.
11 Bahskaram P: Micronutrient malnutrition, infection and immunity: An overview. Nutr Rev 2002;60:S40–S45.
12 Tang AM, Graham NM, Semba RD, Saah AJ: Association between serum vitamin A and E levels and HIV-1 disease progression. AIDS 1997;11:613–620.

13 D'Souza RM, D'Souza R: Vitamin A for the treatment of children with measles – A systematic review. J Trop Pediatr 2002;48:323–327.
14 Filteau SM: Vitamin A and the acute-phase response. Nutrition 1999;15:326–328.
15 Hurt N, Smith T, Tanner M, et al: Evaluation of C-reactive protein and haptoglobin as malaria episode markers in an area of high transmission in Africa. Trans R Soc Trop Med Hyg 1994;88: 182–186.
16 Filteau SM, Morris SS, Raynes JG, et al: Vitamin A supplementation, morbidity, and serum acute-phase proteins in young Ghanaian children. Am J Clin Nutr 1995;62:434–438.
17 Adelekan DA, Adeodu OO, Thurnham DJ: Comparative effects of malaria and malnutrition on plasma concentrations of antioxidant micronutrients in children. Ann Trop Pediatr 1997;17: 223–227.
18 Haraguchi Y, Sakurai H, Hussain S, et al: Inhibition of HIV-1 infection by zinc group metal compounds. Antiviral Res 1999;43:123–133.
19 Sakaguchi S, Iizuka Y, Furusawa S, et al: Role of Zn(2+) in oxidative stress caused by endotoxin challenge. Eur J Pharmacol 2002;451:309–316.
20 Brown KH, Lanata CF, Yuen ML, et al: Potential magnitude of the misclassification of a population's trace element status due to infection: Example from a survey of young Peruvian children. Am J Clin Nutr 1993;58:549–554.
21 Brown KH: Effect of infections on plasma zinc concentration and implications for zinc status assessment in low-income countries. Am J Clin Nutr 1998;68:425S–429S.
22 Weinberg ED: The role of iron in protozoan and fungal infectious diseases. J Eukaryot Microbiol 1999;46:231–238.
23 Friis H, Gomo E, Koestel P, et al: HIV and other predictors of serum folate, serum ferritin, and hemoglobin in pregnancy: A cross-sectional study in Zimbabwe. Am J Clin Nutr 2001;73: 1066–1073.
24 Beesley R, Filteau S, Tomkins A, et al: Impact of acute malaria on plasma concentrations of transferrin receptors. Trans R Soc Trop Med Hyg 2000;94:295–298.
25 Gaetke LM, McClain CJ, Talwalkar RT, et al: Effects of endotoxin on zinc metabolism in human volunteers. Am J Physiol 1997;272:E952–E956.
26 Langley SC, Seakins M, Grimble RF, Jackson AA: The acute phase response of adult rats is altered by in utero exposure to maternal low protein diets. J Nutr 1994;124:1588–1596.
27 Willumsen JF, Simmank K, Filteau SM, et al: Toxic damage to the respiratory epithelium induces acute phase changes in vitamin A metabolism without depleting retinol stores of South African children. J Nutr 1997;127:1339–1343.
28 Wastney ME, Aamodt RL, Rumble WF, Henkin RI: Kinetic analysis of zinc metabolism and its regulation in normal humans. Am J Physiol 1986;251:R398–R408.
29 King JC, Shames DM, Lowe NM, et al: Effect of acute zinc depletion in men on zinc homeostasis and plasma zinc kinetics. Am J Clin Nutr 2001;74:116–124.
30 Jahoor F, Gazzard B, Phillips G, et al: The acute-phase protein response to human immunodeficiency virus infection in human subjects. Am J Physiol 1999;276:E1092–E1098.
31 Crompton DW, Nesheim MC: Nutritional impact of intestinal helminthiasis during the human life cycle. Annu Rev Nutr. 2002;22:35–59.
32 Castillo-Duran C, Vial P, Uauy R: Trace mineral balance during acute diarrhea in infants. J Pediatr 1988;113:452–457.
33 Mitra AK, Alvarez JO, Guay-Woodford L, et al: Urinary retinol excretion and kidney function in children with shigellosis. Am J Clin Nutr 1998;68:1095–1103.
34 Bhutta ZA: Iron and zinc intake from complementary foods: Some issues from Pakistan. Pediatrics 2000;106:1295–1297.

Discussion

Dr. Abrams: When we look at zinc the problem is that unless you are severely zinc deficient you don't tend to drop your serum zinc very much and so that the stable isotope in the kinetic studies pick up more subtle changes than the serum zinc does. So all these studies tend to underestimate or can potentially underestimate the role of mild deficiencies. The problem is that it is not easy to make stable isotope kinetics, and attempts to do so have not been terribly successful. So I think some isolated groups that may be relatively small are needed. But one can look at all sorts of different markers, always different things, with complete kinetic studies in mild deficiency states, and that is the kind of gap that hasn't been done at this point.

Dr. Bhutta: I couldn't agree more. The important issue, the challenge that I made is really to take the science where it matters. I believe that with some of this stable isotope work we at least have the tools to study populations in representative groups in depth, where there is the reality, the real-life concomitant burden of infections and morbidity which are such an important part of the equation. So I would very much like to see that work being done. Unfortunately according to what I have read in the literature, much of this is induced by necessity and it is also not in association with populations that are largely the focus of public health intervention programs. So we don't quite know what the relationship of all body zinc status measurements in developing countries is with other simpler markers that may be available.

Dr. Hurrell: You mentioned the influence of infection on the loss of micronutrients, how to redistribute them, but you didn't mention absorption. Is there any influence of infection on micronutrient absorption?

Dr. Bhutta: From a few studies that have been done there are data available on vitamin A in terms of the association of diarrhea with a reduced uptake. There are a lot of data available on the iron which I have not touched upon in terms of reduced absorption of iron with chronic enteropathy, and the difficulty in that literature is how do you dissociate that with chronic anemia of infections. There is very little work on bioavailability as well as absorption in children with persistent diarrhea aside from our own work. I think there are probably only 3 groups which have looked at zinc balance studies in diarrhea, one is Castillo-Durán et al. [1] in Chile. We have done studies on this and I think there has been some preliminary work at the International Centre for Diarrheal Disease Research, Bangladesh (ICDDRB), but it has not been able to sort out whether or not there is reduced absorption in a situation with persistent diarrhea and enteropathy and it is probably implicit that children with enteropathy and reduced mucosal surface area would have induced absorption. So to summarize I think your point is valid, I am just not aware of studies which have looked at that very specifically in terms of either mechanisms of absorption or net fluxes.

Dr. Castillo-Durán: Can you comment on the potential use of zinc in oral rehydration solutions (ORS) as a potential new tool for the treatment of diarrhea?

Dr. Bhutta: I think there are two issues with zinc. First of all I think the public health community needs to unravel the zinc story and to really decide if we are looking at zinc deficiency in isolation or is zinc deficiency in most instances out of the multiple micronutrient deficiency scenario? If the latter is the case then I think we really need to look at combined approaches of micronutrient supplementation. Currently the thinking on zinc supplementation during diarrhea and prevention is also to look at a delivery system of zinc which may be in the form of either dispersible zinc tablets or a large scale zinc supplementation trial such as the one that has been started in Bangladesh. There isn't a whole lot of support for using zinc in ORS because you need to use such a large amount of it, and also the evidence is that oral rehydration therapy with ORS intake goes down so rapidly as the diarrhea recovers that you would not be able to replete a deficient state unless you were able to continue ORS intake for several days unnecessarily. So I think the tendency is really to use a different vehicle like a tablet, or to look at additional approaches such as supplementation or fortification.

Dr. Zlotkin: Thank you for your really clear talk on the impact of infection on micronutrient status. As you spoke I realized that perhaps our strategy or focus on the strategy of providing micronutrients is naïve because as you quite clearly said the effect of infection on micronutrient status is impacted in a number of ways: there can be stool loss; anorexia can be associated with infection and therefore not as much is eaten; there can be a number of impacting factors which affect micronutrient status. In our sessions we really are talking about a strategy for a nutritional approach looking at ways to prevent infections, for example, immunization might be a way to improve micronutrient status: access to clean water; access to ORS; access to health care providers, and perhaps antibiotics. Although they are not directly related to micronutrient status they are certainly very directly related to the general strategy that one has to think about. What you have done is to emphasize that we have to be broad in our thinking, we cannot only approach this as nutritionists but have to think of the infection in the whole scenario.

Dr. Bhutta: I couldn't agree more. In paper 2 of the Bellagio series [2] where we looked at the impact of interventions on reducing child mortality, this is precisely the point that was made that nutrition strategies need to be intertwined with additional strategies to reduce the burden of diarrhea, the burden of respiratory infections, the burden of measles. I think unless you reduce and eliminate measles in developing countries you are going to be chasing the vitamin A requirement for the next 20 years. So I couldn't agree more; we should be looking at integrated strategies where there are additional measures to pure nutrition strategies.

Dr. Gebre-Medhin: The most striking message that I take to heart is the very strong association between deficiency and protein energy malnutrition. As you very well know more than anybody, the average child between 1 and 5 years has something like 7 infections per year. In most instances these infections have a viral character where C-reactive protein (CRP) is not of very much use. Could you comment on other indicators or infections other than CRP which is a very non-robust thing. The second comment is that if you look at Swedish children and their vitamin A status, at any given time there would be something like 15 or 20% who could be looked upon as being vitamin A deficient, but if they are followed up they bounce back again every month. The infection goes away, they bounce back in their status, which shows the very strong impact of this low-grade infection that is possible to correct. I would like to have your views on that.

Dr. Bhutta: I think the second point you made is indeed very important because I personally do not know the answer to it. But on the basis of what we see in the field, I believe that immunostimulation, as a response to chronic low-grade infections in these children, some of which are viral, some of which are bacterial and produce a state of chronic inflammation, is a real entity. In the slide I showed the kind of environment that many of these children are living in in developing countries with recurrent burdens of diarrhea, and therefore the impact of these short-term and also sustained bouts of infection on full body status micronutrients is very poorly recognized. We know from work done years ago what happens in terms of recurrent infections and stunting. I think if you could extrapolate, expand on what happens to micronutrient status in a child with recurrent infections and a continuous background of infection, you would see something quite analogous to what we see in asthma and inflammation, a state of continuous inflammation in some of them. Now whether or not we will be able to reverse that with micronutrient interventions singly or in combination, I personally don't think it is possible. I think there need to be additional measures to reduce the burden of infections themselves. Coming back to your first question as to what can be done in viral infections when CRP does not seem to be elevated. There has been a lot of work with other indicators as you know, and currently Thurnham et al. [3] are looking at whether or not some kind of adjustment for vitamin A can be developed using markers. The indicators that have been developed are alpha 1-antichymotrypsin

(ACP) and α_1-glycoprotein (AGP), you can take your pick and they all behave almost the same. CRP seems to be better in certain hands, and ACP and AGP in others. None of them are exceptional. CRP is simple to do, certainly ACP and AGP are beyond the reach of most laboratories in developing countries. So to answer your question I think there is a lot of work to be done in this area to develop better indicators for an acute phase response than we currently have. I believe CRP is probably the one that has been studied most.

Dr. Tolboom: I have two questions. One on the methodology to measure morbidity. You showed a slide in which a recent cough was associated with a decline in vitamin A; but a cough itself doesn't do that. Have you got an answer to that; is that a problem of methodology?

Dr. Bhutta: Very good question and clearly. When a survey is going to be done at the national level in a population, the community health workers and physicians need to be trained before hand using a tool. In the morbidity complex that I showed, standard definitions were used. For recent morbidity from acute respiratory infections we used indicators that the parents would be able to relate back in terms of recall. This was a 2-week recall period and clearly simple things were used such as 'did your child have a cough'. So what I said was that recent cough was really the only measure that we have from that 2-week recall period, and it does not represent pneumonia.

Dr. Tolboom: Then there was a point about chronic infestations, particularly parasitic diseases. Do you think there is some relationship between, for example, giardiasis that is quite common in most developing countries in 20–25% of schoolchildren, and micronutrient status?

Dr. Bhutta: Again an excellent question and the answer to that is I have looked at the literature in preparation for this as to what is known about helminthiasis in general and micronutrient status. Absolutely nothing has been prospectively studied and done on zinc status in giardiasis or helminthiasis, there is some work available from the National Institute of Nutrition on helminthiasis and vitamin A absorption which indicates that perhaps a high helminth load may be associated with vitamin A deficiency. Obviously there is a whole body of literature on helminthiasis and iron status and again, to illustrate, the most recent publication in that area is 13 years old. So it is not a focus of attention and fertile ground for much greater work.

Dr. Ribeiro: Congratulations on your presentation. Based on your clear summary of the correlation of zinc losses in diarrheal disease, are you convinced that there is a broad place for zinc supplementation during the acute phase of diarrhea and during persistent diarrhea treatment?

Dr. Bhutta: We are part of the International Zinc Nutrition Consultive Group Steering Committee. Clearly in public health sectors there is now growing recognition of the need for zinc interventions. Now whether that takes the shape and form of intervening in any specific diarrheal syndromes has really not been resolved. Most of us are of the opinion that you tend to see zinc deficiency in relation with diarrhea in settings where there is a preexisting background of zinc deficiency. So ideally we should be in the highest category which is really infancy and children who have had hyper-diarrhea, with a view to preventive strategies to replete body zinc and therefore treat all diarrheal episodes with some form of zinc. It is logical because to try and sort out in public health settings which episode will get zinc and which episode will not is very difficult. Again the logic is that if you repeatedly treat episodes of diarrhea in public health settings with perhaps 2-week courses of zinc, then you may be able to improve status over time. Actually the most exciting data on this have come from the ICDDRB and Black's work [4] in which zinc supplementation was given through community health workers for diarrheal episodes and they were able to show a difference in mortality. But more importantly they were able to show a reduction in antibiotic prescribing at a community level. So when you are giving zinc there may be additional benefits beyond an impact on diarrhea, there may be benefits on nutrition, and certainly if you can reduce antimicrobial prescribing by physicians for diarrhea that may have a huge impact on antimicrobial resistance. So as they say, watch this space, because I hope we will have consensus on what might be the best strategies within a year.

Dr. Gibson: I just wanted to make a comment in response to Dr. Zlotkin's view about a more holistic approach, and just a comment about a program that has been undertaken by World Vision Canada [5] in which they have a very comprehensive micronutrient health program that has been running in Tanzania, Zambia and Malawi. In their comprehensive micronutrient health program which included immunization, fortification, supplementation and health education, they have certainly shown some very impressive results in terms of reducing stunting and reducing anemia and improving infant mortality.

Mr. Parvanta: Thank you very much for that stimulating presentation. I just have a question on the issue of the Pakistan survey. In most population surveys the way the sample sizes are calculated are determined based on the expected prevalence of the deficiency one is looking for and so on. Given what you said about the impact of infections on prevalence estimates, in most surveys nobody accounts really for that in estimating the sample size. Do you have any suggestions on what type of an estimate one could make on the expected prevalence of infections and so on, assuming you even had CRP or AGP or something of that sort.

Dr. Bhutta: That is an excellent question and I wish we had been at this state when we were designing the survey. By the way the survey of a population of 140 million is on a preschool cohort of 6,000 children, so even that was a logistic challenge. It is not provincially representative, so most national surveys have to compromise the ideal with the pragmatic. Now if I was to review this whole thing again, and I wish I had believed that by just accepting that there would be a 20% prevalence of subclinical infections, which is more or less what we found, not subclinical but real infections, we would have adjusted the sample size for that. So in developing countries when looking at high burdens of morbidity, some of those data may not be interpretable on the basis of coexisting infections. Until we get a robust measure using these measures you need to adjust for that. So maybe the 20% adjustment is what I would recommend, at least in the South Asian context. I can't speak for HIV prevalent populations.

Mr. Parvanta: So with the adjustment you are also saying that you would obviously have to have some indicators of infection status afterwards?

Dr. Bhutta: Yes, which we do.

Dr. Lönnerdal: I would like to come back to one of the questions brought up and I think you were fairly cautious in your response. One of the things you missed earlier was when I talked about iron supplementation. I think that in any developing country there would be a significant proportion of infants who will have iron deficiency and anemia and will certainly benefit from iron. But what we have seen is that, in those who actually do have a satisfactory iron status, there could actually be a negative effect, and therefore the cost-benefit or the whole reason of what you should do becomes a little bit more murky. I would like to take this a little bit further and talk about the set of experiments we did in infant rhesus monkeys. We used this model because we can be a little bit more aggressive about what we can do in this setting than in human infants. We used infant formula and fed them for 4 months: one group was fed regular formula; another formula containing probiotics, and a third group was fed formula with extra zinc. We induced enteropathogenic *Escherichia coli* infection in these infant monkeys, which of course we cannot do in human populations. The outcome was that the probiotics group had a reduced severity and duration of the *E. coli* infection.

184

What we also found was that the group with probiotics and zinc had a significantly worse outcome when it came to diarrhea than the control group. What we retrospectively found was that of course the zinc status of these infants was satisfactory when they were infected. So if they received extra zinc when they had an infection the outcome was actually worse; possibly the extra zinc stimulated bacterial growth or whatever. But again a little bit of caution, in any given population we may have 40 or 50% of the infants that are zinc-deficient and still have some 50–60% that perhaps are zinc-adequate. The question is if you aggressively treat with zinc in order to reduce the severity of diarrhea, then what happens with the group that actually is satisfactory from the beginning?

Dr. Bhutta: Very important question and I think therefore as zinc intervention trials become more skilled, it is very important that we get precise answers to the question, what happens to zinc-replete or zinc-sufficient infants when there is a large zinc supplementation trial. There is a zinc mortality study that is coming to closure very soon and we will have the data from those large-scale studies. So far in the work that we and others have done on zinc supplementation in large-scale population settings, we have not seen evidence of either biochemical zinc sufficiency or levels which may reach toxic levels. So we have not seen it, but that is not to say that it may or may not exist. Your question on probiotics is a very interesting one. I would like to refer you back to one of the earliest publications on zinc and diarrhea that we did [6], and one of the interesting things that we found in infants with persistent diarrhea supplemented with zinc was that when their breath hydrogen excretion was measured, the pattern was very high. We don't understand why this is, but it was like the bacterial overgrowth that you saw and a pattern which was similar to bacterial overgrowth. The conjecture at that time was that zinc is doing something in the gut that we need to be aware of. Having said that I think one of the most exiting opportunities that we have now is to look at probiotics and prebiotics in susceptible populations, both as a means of reducing the burden of diarrhea and potentially improving micronutrient absorption through the gut, and status thereof. So I think some of the studies really need to be done in terms of addressing micronutrient status in populations with diarrhea.

References

1 Castillo-Duran C, Vial P, Uauy R: Oral copper supplementation: Effect on copper and zinc balance during acute gastroenteritis in infants. Am J Clin Nutr 1990;51:1088–1092.
2 Jones G, Steketee RW, Black RE, et al, Bellagio Child Survival Study Group: How many child deaths can we prevent this year? Lancet 2003;362:65–71.
3 Thurnham DI, McCabe GP, Northrop-Clewes CA, Nestel P: Effects of subclinical infection on plasma retinol concentrations and assessment of prevalence of vitamin A deficiency: meta-analysis. Lancet 2003;362:2052–2058.
4 Black RE: Zinc deficiency, infectious disease and mortality in the developing world. J Nutr 2003;133(suppl 1):1485S–1489S.
5 World Vision Canada: MICA Phase I Results 1995–2001. Mississauga, World Vision Canada, 2002.
6 Bhutta ZA, Nizami SQ, Isani Z: Zinc Supplementation in malnourished children with persistent diarrhea in Pakistan. Pediatrics 1999;103:e42.

Pettifor JM, Zlotkin S (eds): Micronutrient Deficiencies during the Weaning Period and the
First Years of Life. Nestlé Nutrition Workshop Series Pediatric Program, vol 54, pp 187–202,
Nestec Ltd., Vevey/S. Karger AG, Basel, © 2004.

The Economic Impact
of Micronutrient Deficiencies

Susan Horton

Munk Centre for International Studies, University of Toronto, Toronto, Ont., Canada

Micronutrient deficiencies have significant adverse consequences on key aspects of body functioning, such as on immune systems and hence resistance to infection, on hearing, cognition, endurance and peak work capacity. The impacts are particularly significant at vulnerable times (pregnancy, the perinatal period, infancy, and likely in old age). Micronutrient deficiencies therefore have important effects on the global burden of disease, with important outcomes on morbidity and mortality. They also have direct economic effects on work productivity and, via morbidity and premature mortality, on work output, as well as more indirect ones on the costs of health system usage, via cognition on the success of the education system, on the incentives to save and invest in children.

Although the human costs alone (burden of disease) justify interventions to alleviate micronutrient malnutrition, efforts have also been made to quantify the economic costs. Information on the burden of disease attributable to micronutrient deficiencies can help to persuade Ministers of Health to devote additional resources within the health budget to micronutrients. But information on the economic consequences of deficiencies may help to persuade Ministers of Finance to allot more resources to health, and away from other competing economic priorities.

Hence, advocacy for increased investment in micronutrient interventions has followed two different approaches. One has been the approach preferred by the World Health Organization, namely to estimate the cost-effectiveness of micronutrient interventions – the currently preferred metric being cost per disability-adjusted life-year (DALY) saved. The other approach has been to estimate economic costs of micronutrient deficiencies as a first step towards undertaking a cost-benefit analysis of micronutrient interventions, an approach that development banks have been willing to take. The approaches are complementary but cannot readily be combined in a single metric. Saving lives of small children (or preventing stillbirths) has enormous human benefits, but these typically do not show up as large economic benefits. Likewise, some micronutrients may have large effects on cognition or productivity, but relatively modest benefits in terms of saving lives. In some cases, the approaches may overlap: some micronutrient interventions may improve health as well as avert important costs to the health care system.

In this article we focus on the economic benefits. The World Health Organization (WHO) [1] has already done important work on the relative cost-effectiveness of micronutrient supplementation/fortification for vitamin A, iodine and iron. (The WHO website has more extensive discussion on their website, as part of the CHOICE project – CHOosing Interventions that are Cost-Effective.) The literature discussed in here does indeed suggest that micronutrient interventions are highly worthwhile investments, and also a fruitful area for public-private partnership [2].

In this short survey, we first examine in more detail the mechanisms through which micronutrient deficiencies can have economic impacts. We then use some specific micronutrients as examples to give estimates of the magnitude of the economic effects. The four mechanisms elaborated upon in the next section are the effects of micronutrients on productivity (generally of adults, in market work), on cognition, on morbidity, and on mortality, and we trace possible economic impacts through each route. In the following sections we survey numerical estimates for three specific nutrients, namely folate, iodine and iron. Again, this is not exhaustive. This survey does not go as far as comparing the economic costs of micronutrient malnutrition, with the economic costs of micronutrient interventions (cost-benefit) [for explicit cost-benefit, see for example, 3, 4]. The final section provides some policy suggestions and recommendations for future work.

Selected Mechanisms by Which Micronutrient Deficiency Can Adversely Affect Economic Outcomes

Here some of the key effects on productivity, cognition, morbidity and mortality, and their corresponding economic impacts are catalogued in turn. While this is not necessarily an exhaustive list, it represents some of the major mechanisms, beginning with those with the strongest empirical documentation of impact.

Productivity

Some micronutrients have well-documented effects on adult productivity. A large number of laboratory and field studies document the adverse effects of anemia on performance in laboratory tests and in the field [for summaries see, 3, 5]. Intervention studies, for example providing iron convincingly demonstrate that these productivity effects can be reduced/reversed by reducing the level of deficiency. Biological studies provide the underpinning mechanisms for the underlying causes (reduced maximal work capacity; reduced endurance). The largest body of work exists for iron, but other micronutrient deficiencies such as zinc and iodine may directly affect productivity. The zinc results are more speculative, but productivity is known to be associated in some occupations with height, and zinc has effects on growth and stature.

Cognition

There is evidence that some micronutrients have effects on cognitive outcomes, both from studies correlating cognitive performance and deficiency, and from studies of interventions which find performance improvements. The most intriguing studies are those which follow up nutritional interventions over the long run, for example the INCAP supplementation studies in Guatemala, where participants received supplements both of energy and micronutrients [6]. There are relatively few such longitudinal studies, but they have the potential to find the broadest range of impacts. These studies of effect are supported by biological studies of the mechanisms. Evidence of cognitive outcomes exists for iron, iodine, and vitamin B_{12}, and is also hypothesized for zinc.

Morbidity

Some micronutrients are associated with impaired immune function and hence increased morbidity. Morbidity is most evident at vulnerable stages of life, for example in young children. There may also be effects in the elderly, but few such studies exist in developing countries. Morbidity in infants and children involves costs, such as costs of health care (visits to health practitioners, purchase of medicine) and costs of taking care of sick children and transporting them to hospital. These costs are hard to document in developing countries. Several micronutrient deficiencies are also associated with increased risk of premature birth (iodine, iron, folate for example). In developing countries the primary outcome may be increased neonatal mortality and stillbirth, whereas in developed countries with more developed health systems there are increased health care costs for the care of premature babies. Some deficiencies may lead to birth outcomes with implications for expensive long-term care, e.g. folate deficiencies which lead to neural tube defects.

Mortality

In the extreme, micronutrient deficiencies can lead to increased mortality. This has been documented for iron deficiency in both maternal mortality as well as perinatal mortality; for iodine deficiency in stillbirths and perinatal mortality, and for vitamin A in infant and child mortality. The WHO [1] attributes 0.8 million deaths worldwide to iron deficiency, 1.5% of the annual total,

0.8 million to vitamin A, 1.4% of the annual total, and 0.8 million to zinc deficiency, 1.4% of the annual total. One area not much examined is the effect of micronutrient deficiency in the elderly, where increased mortality may also plausibly be observed. One could make the case that calcium deficiency (via increased bone loss and falls) contributes to mortality in elderly women.

It is difficult to quantify the economic impact of stillbirths and deaths of infants and young children. The direct economic effect of these deaths in developing countries is likely more modest than for example the death of working-age adults from cardiovascular disease and stroke. The economic effect of the death of mothers in childbirth may be hard to demonstrate in countries where the assumption is that the man will simply take another wife, although the human costs are considerable. There are for example studies documenting the increased mortality rate for other children, if the mother dies.

However, there may be other important, but more subtle, effects. In societies with elevated infant and child mortality rates, there may be adverse effects on investments in children, affecting learning and education and hence long-run productivity. Savings depend on life expectancy since one important motive for saving is provision for one's old age, hence shorter life expectancy may reduce savings, with impacts on economic growth. Individuals who are malnourished are less likely to play an active role in the community, possibly impacting social capital. All these effects are speculative and difficult to quantify.

The next three sections in turn examine the economic impacts of three nutrients, namely folate, iodine and iron (in alphabetical order). Readers will notice that vitamin A, one of the 'big three' micronutrients in recent policy, is not included. This does not imply that there are no economic consequences of vitamin A deficiency, rather that its major effects show up in health outcomes, and its effects on morbidity and mortality are the primary rationale for intervention. There are economic consequences of other micronutrient deficiencies which are not covered in this brief survey (the effects of zinc, calcium, and vitamin B_{12} have all been mentioned above).

Economic Impact of Folate Deficiency

A number of recent studies have modeled the economic and health impacts of folate deficiency. One key area is in plasma homocysteine and the incidence of coronary heart disease, as well as stroke and peripheral vascular disease [7]. Another is in peri-conceptional supplementation and the prevention of birth defects, especially neural tube defects (spina bifida being an extreme case) [8], as cleft lip/palate, conotruncal (heart) defects, and limb defects.

Studies of birth defects suggest that based on recall data, there was a 30% reduction in the risk of heart defects and a 36% reduction in the risk of limb

Table 1. Estimated costs associated with birth defects, potentially avertable with periconceptional supplementation with folic acid (in USD for 1992)

Condition	Cost/case USD	Medical costs USD (millions)	Total costs USD (millions)	Possibly avertable medical costs USD (millions)	Possibly avertable total costs USD (millions)
(1)	(2)	(3)	(4)	(5)	(6)
Spina bifida	294,000	205	489	102.5	244.5
Cleft lip/palate	101,000	97	696	63	466
Tetralogy of Fallot	262,000	185	360	56	108
Truncus arteriosus	505,000	108	209	32	63
Single ventricle	344,000	62	172	19	52
Upper limb reduction	99,000	11	170	4	61
Lower limb reduction	199,000	17	167	6	60

Columns 1–4 are based on data from the California Birth Defects Monitoring Program [9]; columns 5 and 6 were calculated by the present author assuming the following relative risk reduction with periconceptional folic acid supplementation: 50% (spina bifida); 65% (oral clefts); 30% (heart defects including tetralogy of Fallot, truncus arteriosus and single ventricle), and 36% (upper and lower limb reduction defects). See references in text for sources for relative risk data.

defects if mothers had taken folic acid-containing multivitamins during the month before conception or the first 2 months of pregnancy [9]. In families at high risk of oral clefts because of a parent or previous child with the condition, there was a 65% reduction in risk in an intervention study if women received multivitamins and high-dose folic acid beginning 2 months before conception [9, 10]. The risk reduction for spina bifida with folic acid supplementation from at least 4 weeks before until at least 8 weeks after conception is 50% [8].

There are approximately USD 8 billion lifetime costs associated with birth defects related to births in a single year in the US. USD 2 billion of these are direct medical costs, and USD 6 billion are other direct costs such as special education and lost productivity due to premature death and occupational limitations; costs of caregiving are not included [9]. Table 1 (summarized from the California Birth Defects Monitoring Program [9], with additional calculations by the author) shows that, by applying the risk reductions associated with folic acid supplementation, about one quarter of these could potentially be averted by peri-conceptional supplementation of folic acid (about USD 1 billion total costs, including about USD 0.25 million in direct medical costs).

This type of data has contributed to the implementation of flour fortification with folic acid in the US and efforts to encourage supplementation for pregnant women as well as women seeking to become pregnant.

There are additionally billions of dollars in annual medical costs that are potentially avertable with folic acid supplementation in the area of cardiovascular disease [for cost-effectiveness analysis and some data on medical costs see, 7]. It seems likely that more economic work will be done in this area to encourage other developed countries to adopt folic acid fortification and supplementation programs, in some cases linked to efforts to deal with deficiencies in vitamin B_{12}.

Economic Impact of Iodine Deficiency

Iodine is an excellent example of a case where data on the size of the economic costs of deficiency were used effectively to help mobilize support for international action to reduce deficiency. Iodine's role in thyroid hormones and hence regulation of metabolic activities of all cells throughout the life cycle means that severe deficiency can lead to lower metabolic rates, growth retardation and brain damage. The success of international efforts to intervene are summarized in the WHO's Third Nutrition Report [11]. Based on Clugston et al. [12] and Bleichrodt and Born [13], it can be estimated that there is an average 10.27% productivity loss per birth to a mother with goiter: 3.4% of such births are cretins with an assumed zero market productivity in adult life; 10.2% are severely mentally impaired with 25% lower productivity, and the remainder are 5% less productive than normal, using the estimate from Bleichrodt and Born [13] that IQ is 13.5 points lower.

This can be used to generate a crude estimate of economic losses by region, utilizing data on the prevalence of goiter from the WHO [14]. The dates of the goiter data are not specified but are likely from the mid 1990s. When these are combined with data on the gross domestic product (GDP) and per capita GDP by WHO regions (calculated by the author from data from the World Bank [15]), and assuming (to be conservative) that all the goiter is concentrated in the areas of poorer health and hence lower GDP within each region (i.e. that none exists in the 'A' regions categorized by health), table 2 provides estimates of economic losses by region. The estimates suggest that worldwide economic losses around 1994 (before salt iodization began to be rapidly expanded) could have exceeded USD 36 billion annually, exceeding USD 6 billion in each of three regions, namely the Americas (Latin America and the Caribbean), lower income Europe (Eastern Europe particularly Turkey, former Soviet Union), and Western Pacific (particularly China, parts of Southeast Asia). The losses were proportionately largest in the Eastern Mediterranean region where soils are particularly deficient and the prevalence of goiter was the highest.

Table 2. Estimates of worldwide economic losses potentially attributable to iodine deficiency prior to widespread salt fortification (mid 1990s)

Region	Population with goiter		Per capita GDP USD 1998 excluding healthiest regions (A)	Estimated losses due to iodine deficiency	
	n (millions)	%		% GDP excluding healthiest regions	USD (billions) 1998
Africa	73	11.4	632	0.5	1.9
Americas	41	5.0	4,240	0.2	7.1
Eastern Mediterranean	91	18.9	1,583	1.8	5.9
Europe	98	11.2	2,424	0.5	9.8
Southeast Asia	206	13.4	489	0.5	4.1
West Pacific	124	8.0	1,335	0.3	6.8
Total	633	10.5	n/a	n/a	35.7

Notes: the number and percent with goiter from the WHO [14], date not specified, but likely around 1994 prior to widespread salt iodization in developing countries; per capita GDP from the World Bank [15] and is a (population) weighted average for all countries excluding the A countries in each region (WHO category: the healthiest countries), i.e. excludes the developed countries. Hence Americas excludes the US and Canada; Europe excludes Western Europe; West Pacific excludes Japan, Australia and New Zealand, etc. The assumption is that economic losses attributable to iodine deficiency are virtually zero in the developed countries, to be conservative.

Since widespread salt iodization has occurred, the predicted economic losses will decline dramatically. In the future, new methods to calculate losses will need to be developed, using urinary iodine as a measure of iodine status and relating functional impairments of children to the urinary iodine status of pregnant women (goiter rates only respond to improved iodine status with a long lag, and become a much less useful indicator).

Economic Impact of Iron Deficiency

Much work has been done on the economic impact of iron deficiency (although the success of interventions to reduce iron deficiency has proven more elusive). We summarize here the main effects directly on adult productivity, indirectly via cognitive development in childhood, and some illustrative dollar estimates for selected countries, based on Horton and Ross [3].

The effects of iron supplementation on adult productivity have been convincingly demonstrated both in the field and in the laboratory. There are some limitations, for example the studies demonstrate impacts *within* narrowly defined occupations where productivity can be readily measured, and omit more subtle effects (such as in white collar occupations where productivity is hard to measure, or effects causing workers to choose less demanding and lower productivity occupations, or even to drop out of the labor force entirely).

Two frequently cited studies give estimates of the order of magnitude of the productivity impact.

The first study of male rubber plantation workers in Indonesia [16] showed that iron supplementation of anemic workers (undertaken in a placebo-controlled, double-blind trial) was associated with a 17% increase in the weight of latex collected. This suggests that large increases in productivity can be associated with iron supplementation in very heavy manual labor, where maximal work capacity is a factor. The second study, [17] of female textile factory workers found that iron supplementation (again in a placebo-controlled double-blind trial) was associated with a 5% increase in productivity. This study suggests that even in occupations involving light manual labor, there are effects of iron deficiency on productivity likely via endurance. Although the productivity effects are more modest than in heavy manual labor, they occur over a broader range of occupations.

The effects of iron supplementation on cognition are somewhat speculative since there are as yet no long-term studies of interventions, although the INCAP studies may capture the effects of iron supplementation as well as supplementation of calories [6]. Our earlier work [3] relies on a series of inferences. We surveyed 11 studies of interventions for children below 2 years of age, which found evidence of effects on motor skills as well as mental skills, which tend to be more significant when children are initially anemic and when the intervention has a longer duration. The effects on motor skills are of more interest, since these are correlated with mental tests on older children (whereas mental skills below the age of 2 years do not correlate well with mental tests on older children). In 4 supplementation studies in developing countries on children over 2 years old, 3 studies found improvements on cognitive tests. The one with a quantitative measure of effect [18] found this to be about 0.5 SD, similar to the difference between anemic and non-anemic children in observational studies. Suppose there is some attenuation of effect over time (the intercorrelation between IQ scores of children ages 6–8 years, with those of the same children age 17 years, is about 0.62–0.65 [19]. Finally, 5 studies we surveyed for developing countries suggested that a 1 SD increase in cognitive achievement, was associated with an 8% increase in adult wages. Accordingly, a plausible estimate is that iron interventions in children in childhood could result in a 2.5% productivity impact in the labor market (8% $\times$ 0.5 $\times$ 0.65). This is conservative, since it does not include the

Table 3. Economic losses expected due to iron deficiency, as % GDP and in absolute USD for 1994

Country	Loss	
	USD (millions) 1994	% GDP
Tanzania	24	0.59
Bangladesh	451	1.74
Mali	21	0.84
India	4,294	1.47
Nicaragua	11	0.81
Pakistan	501	0.92
Honduras	16	0.33
Egypt	180	0.42
Bolivia	29	0.54

Source: updated calculations based on Horton and Ross [3].

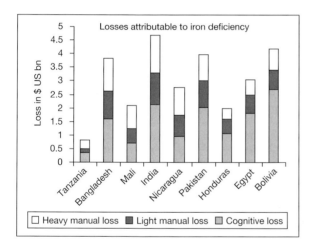

Fig. 1. Per capita loss due to iron deficiency.

well-documented effects of improved cognitive performance on higher schooling, and of schooling on wages (and hence implied productivity).

When these effects (17% impact on heavy manual labor, 4% impact on light manual labor, and 2.5% effect on other labor) are combined, along with information about the level of anemia in men and women, women's share of the labor force, and the relative importance of heavy manual and light manual labor in total work, one can make estimates as to the US dollar value of economic losses associated with insufficient iron intake.

Figure 1 presents these estimates in USD per capita for 9 countries, showing the contribution of losses in different kinds of work. Table 3 provides similar information as to the absolute dollar value of losses and the loss as percent of the GDP for the same countries. A couple of things stand out. Broadly speaking, the share of the loss associated with cognitive effects increases with the level of development (figure 1 and table 3 are arranged in order of ascending GDP per capita). Losses tend to go up absolutely with the level of development (the exception is that the level of anemia is much higher in the South Asian countries showing correspondingly higher losses). Losses as a percentage of the GDP tend to be highest in the poorest countries, particularly the South Asian poor countries which have the highest levels of anemia. Table 2 also points out the fact that the annual losses in South Asia exceed USD 5 billion. The losses in sub-Saharan Africa would also be substantial.

Policy Implications, and Areas for Future Research

This brief survey shows that the economic costs of micronutrient deficiency are substantial, and provide a compelling rationale (in addition to the health consequences) for intervention. The results need to be interpreted cautiously. The economic costs estimated here are generally costs existing in cross-section at the current point in time and accumulated due to past deficiencies (deficiencies in utero or during childhood, with the exception of the immediate effects of iron on adult productivity). Hence programs of intervention will not have dramatic effects instantaneously, but will take time to show economic gains. One way to see this is to undertake a formal cost-benefit of interventions, appropriately discounting future gains, and using an 'incidence methodology'.

The three micronutrients examined here are of interest, being at different stages in the policy lifecycle. The adverse effects of iodine deficiency were recognized and quantified during the 1980s, and led to a policy thrust to iodize salt broadly throughout the developing world in the 1990s. Although the productivity effects of iron were well known in the 1980s, the technical issues to reduce deficiency had not been solved. Quantifying the economic costs in the late 1990s has underpinned current ongoing efforts for widespread iron fortification. Finally, the economic impact of folate deficiency has only been more recently calculated: countries with existing fortification are very few (the US has fortification, but Netherlands which has calculated the costs, has not yet opted to fortify), but it is likely that efforts to fortify and supplement will become more widespread.

Some of the nutrients not covered in detail in this survey are at too early a stage in the policy lifecycle to include. It is likely that there are economic impacts of zinc deficiency, but the relative lack of studies of impact and the difficulties in measuring zinc status mean that little progress has been made. The economic effects of vitamin B_{12} deficiency are likewise understudied.

Some useful areas for future research would include: the effects of micronutrient deficiency in the elderly; those micronutrients for which the evidence base is not as strong (such as zinc, vitamin B_{12}), and micronutrients for which policy implementation has as yet occurred in only a few countries (folic acid).

References

1 World Health Organization: The World Health Report 2002. Geneva, WHO, 2002.
2 Asian Development Bank (with Micronutrient Initiative and International Life Sciences Institute): Manila Forum 2000: Strategies to Fortify Essential Foods in Asia and the Pacific. Manila, Asian Development Bank Nutrition and Development Series, 2000, vol 2.
3 Horton S, Ross J: The economics of iron deficiency. Food Policy 2003;28:51–75.
4 International Food Policy Research Institute: Effects of Diet in Improving Iron Status of Women: What Role for Food-Based Interventions? Gender and Intrahousehold Aspects of Food Policy Project Brief No 4. Washington, IFPRI, 2000.
5 Haas JD, Brownlie T: Iron deficiency and reduced work capacity: A critical review of the research to determine a causal relationship. J Nutr 2001;131:676S–688S.
6 Pollitt E, Gorman K, Engle P, et al: Nutrition in early life and the fulfillment of intellectual potential. J Nutr 1995;125:1111S–1118S.
7 Tice JA, Ross E, Coxson PG, et al: Cost-effectiveness of vitamin therapy to lower plasma homocysteine levels for the prevention of coronary heart disease. JAMA 2001;286:936–943.
8 Postma MJ, Londeman J, Veenstra M, et al: Cost-effectiveness of periconceptional supplementation of folic acid. Pharmacy World of Science 2002;24:8–11.
9 California Birth Defects Monitoring Program website: http://www.cbdmp.org; accessed August 20, 2003.
10 Tolarova M, Harris J: Reduced recurrence of orofacial clefts after periconceptional supplementation with high-dose folic acid and multivitamins. Teratology 1995;51:71–78.
11 World Health Organization: The Third World Nutrition Report. Geneva, WHO, 1997.
12 Clugston GA, Dulberg EM, Pandav CS, Tiden RL: Iodine deficiency disorders in South East Asia; in Hetzel BS, Dunn JT, Stanbury JB (eds): The Prevention and Control of Iodine Deficiency Disorders. New York, Elsevier, 1987.
13 Bleichrodt N, Born MP: A meta-analysis of research on iodine and its relationship to cognitive development; in Stanbury J (ed): The Damaged Brain of Iodine Deficiency: Neuromotor, Cognitive, Behavioural and Educative Aspects. Elmsford, Cognizant Communication, 1994.
14 World Health Organization: Guidelines on Food Fortification with Micronutrients for the Control of Micronutrient Malnutrition. Geneva, WHO, 2003.
15 World Bank: World Data Indicators. Available from http://www.worldbank.org/data/dataquery.html, accessed August 30, 2003.
16 Basta S, Karyadi D, Scrimshaw NS: Iron deficiency anemia and the productivity of adult males in Indonesia. Am J Clin Nutr 1979;32:916–925.
17 Li R, Chen X, Yan H, et al: Functional consequences of iron supplementation in iron-deficient female cottonmill workers in Beijing. Am J Clin Nutr 1994;59:908–913.
18 Seshadri S, Gopaldas T: Impact of iron supplementation on cognitive functions in preschool and school-age children: The Indian experience. Am J Clin Nutr 1989;50:675–686.
19 Jensen AR: Bias in Mental Testing. New York, Free Press, 1980.

Discussion

Dr. Endres: I think physicians don't very much like to compare cost versus treatment, but if we have to convince policy makers then it must be done. Only in one small case did you mention how much we save if we spend money, for example, to fortify flour with folate or salt with iodine. I could imagine that in countries where unemployment is very high, policy makers don't pay much attention to these benefits because they believe there are enough people to compensate for the loss of productivity due to illness. Do you have any figures proving that a non-reaction by policy makers has happened? In the past 20 years we have seen how difficult it is to add iodine to salt in many countries. For example in Germany it was extremely difficult to convince people, and it is the same and still true for folate fortification of flour in some countries.

Dr. Horton: I think you are absolutely right. It is very difficult to do a case-control study because you either fortify for the whole country or you don't. And if you fortify you don't have case controls; you don't have groups that are not receiving the flour. It is much less good quality evidence than nutritionists would like to work with. Many times also you are working with the counterfactual of what would have happened if we didn't do this. I think now we will begin to see problems if countries like New Zealand and Switzerland start to slip back and get iodine deficiency because they let up on the effort on salt. But unfortunately, because we are doing this counterfactually it involves modeling and it involves making assumptions. You also made a very good point about unemployment. People won't care so much about adult productivity if unemployment is high, and how I would counter that is to say that cognitive effects are really important. No developing country can argue that they have an excess of cognitive skill. Clearly to succeed in the world economy, education and cognition are increasingly important, and I think this is a really important area for more work.

Dr. Tolboom: I have a question about the mortality you mentioned in adults which is clearly a great loss economically. But I would like to have your ideas as a professional on infant and child mortality. As doctors we do our best and try to save life, but if I were an economist I would perhaps say, so what? So I would like to have your ideas on that one.

Dr. Horton: That is why I carefully avoided doing any estimates on the cost-benefit of vitamin A. As an economist I am very uncomfortable with attaching low values to lives of children and infants, but unfortunately that is what convention and economic assumptions will do. So I think to some extent you have to use both techniques. The global burden of a disease is one calculation, as the economic loss is another, and for certain nutrients the economic losses matter more than for others. For iodine the economic case is much more important than the global burden of disease, but it is the reverse for vitamin A. So in my own work I have always refused to make that trade off.

Dr. Bhutta: Thank you for these very interesting economic arguments. I just want to support the need for them in countries where health budgets are very low and where not enough priority and attention have been paid to health and nutrition issues. It is very important that we further develop and expand on these economic arguments if policy makers, who are driven a lot by economic arguments, are asked to increase their investment in this very critical area of human development.

Dr. Gebre-Medhin: I very much enjoyed listening to you and I think this is a very important component of our deliberations. Dr. Tolboom partly took up my question and the issue of calculating the impact on mortality. Many years ago, when I worked as a pediatrician in Ethiopia, we tried to calculate the impact of death in families from a cultural perspective. Every family is culturally bound to perform in a certain way and this may go over a period of several years, having to invite the community, not working for periods of time, coming back again and celebrating the death of children, for example. We came up with horrendous figures on loss of work and productivity because of this cultural impact. Have you done any work on that? Working in Sweden we are now worried about initiating a folate-supplementation program in Sweden because side supplementation may lead to an increase in twin births, and the calculations for Sweden seem to point in the direction that the benefits are balanced off. I would like to hear your comments on that.

Dr. Horton: On the first question, on the cost of mortality, let me give you one example. I was in Pakistan doing work on the high level of maternal anemia and maternal mortality rates, which were shockingly high. But then my collaborator, who is a nutritionist from Pakistan, asked me the 'so what?' question. He said 'so what, these people will just take another wife'. So it was hard in that context to attach a value to it. There are studies showing that the death of the mother has significant effects on death of other small children in the household, so that there are social consequences that are perhaps hard to capture economically. As to your second question about the down side, sometimes in addition to benefits from the intervention there are down sides as well, and the same is true for the fluorination of water that has been strongly resisted in some countries because people perceive a negative effect of adding substances to food you can't avoid consuming. As an economist I would just take the cold-hearted approach that you calculate the value of the benefits and those of the additional costs, but one thing you have to take into account is that different people will bear the benefits and the costs, and that is a very hard value judgment to make.

Dr. Semba: You talked about applying these analyses to older adults, and there is this idea with the compression of morbidity hypothesis that you would keep older adults healthier longer. We can compress all their morbidity and all the cost of the health care into a very short period of their life. I am just wondering if these types of analyses have been applied to something like vitamin D deficiency and hip fracture in older adults?

Dr. Horton: Probably there are people here who would know more about this than I do. Since I primarily work in developing countries I haven't surveyed the literature on older adults; it has been less relevant for developing countries. But clearly with the increase in life expectancy in countries like China, I think there would be increased interest in this for developing countries as well, and I think we should encourage much more work on this. In the developed countries older adults have effects on the economy, not primarily through their work output because often they are retired, but through huge costs to the health system from health effects such as fractures.

Dr. Pettifor: I wish to discuss the issue of child mortality and, as Dr. Tolboom brought up, that mortality has very little cost on productivity. In fact it may have a benefit as one is removing a child from the family and the cost of feeding that child. So a much bigger problem is in fact morbidity rather than mortality during childhood. Have you studied that?

Dr. Horton: It tends to be very specific to the country. I mentioned birth defects. These have huge costs in the US but I would expect much lower costs in developing countries. I think even if you did the work very carefully, and often we are hampered by the lack of data from doing it, the costs for morbidity in children still would not bear up against the costs of morbidity in adults, even though for families they may be quite significant. Sometimes a severe illness in a child could be the thing that pushes a family into poverty, so I think we shouldn't neglect that.

Mr. Parvanta: I guess you are really a very good economist because you certainly have learned the value of nutrition or micronutrients. In the United States, for example, there has been a very successful nutrition program for women and children, the Women, Infants, Children (WIC) program has lasted now for about 30 years. A number of evaluations have been done, and as I recall the last time I looked some years ago, they came out with an estimate that for every dollar spent on the program there was a savings of USD 3–4 on future health care cost. I am wondering whether you have used this kind of information in some of the calculations you have made?

Dr. Horton: Yes, I am familiar with them. For example vitamin A in WIC products, there have been studies associating this with less otitis media and ear infections, and showing that there are net economic savings. 20 years ago I also did work on the food stamp program in the US, and you know the economic benefits associated with that.

The Economic Impact of Micronutrient Deficiencies

Yes, definitely you can make an economic case associated with these kinds of social and health interventions in developed countries; in the Head Start program (an education intervention), people have done the cost-benefit of that. These studies tend to be better than for the developed countries because we have more data, we have more panel studies, we can control for things better, we have much better cost data for the health system.

Mr. Parvanta: I am not an economist and certainly I have a lot of trouble saving money. But the question I have is the issue of cost, if you could perhaps help me understand this a little better. Often when I am speaking with colleagues and governments and public agencies, development agencies, when we talk about cost it almost seems as though we are approaching them with the perception that the government has to pay, to cover the cost, or the development agency has to cover the cost. Yet in a lot of these programs, especially the fortification of salt or flour, the idea is essentially that the cost will be passed on to the consumer. Are those costs the same kinds of costs? I guess in terms of fund money it is, but can you give us an idea of how we might use that to help convince certain governments or public agencies how to deal or how to think about those costs?

Dr. Horton: I should mention that economists don't have the monopoly on doing savings; I also do not balance my check book very well. But the 'who pays?' perspective is really important and if you read a cost-benefit study it often tells you from whose perspective it has been written. Sometimes for the US, the study is done from the point of view of the government as payer or the health system, and then the government makes the decision. If it is going to save the government money then it will implement the project. But economists would advocate that you should take a more general perspective and you should be concerned about social costs. The social costs may not even be monetary costs, sometimes there are resources which appear to be free because there are no charges but that doesn't mean that there is no social cost. For example, suppose you make a nutrition intervention that takes a lot of the mother's time. Many mothers are not working in developing countries or in developed countries, or they are not working in the market and not being paid. Does that mean we can freely use their time in a project at zero cost? No, of course not, there are opportunity costs, there are costs of the things that they are not doing. A part of the methodology of doing cost-benefit studies appropriately is to think of the payer perspective, and also attaching true economic societal costs to resources.

Dr. Lozoff: I am curious, when you present this kind of economic analysis, what sort of attacks do you get? What criticisms come up?

Dr. Horton: Perhaps I have been lucky, I have had good experiences. I remember being in Vietnam where UNICEF has been trying to convince the government to do investment planning and the government was really more interested in economics, trying to get the economy to grow, and perhaps let the social consequences take care of themselves. The minute they started hearing rates of return on iron investments, it had an effect on the Minister of Finance, the financial people's discussions. There are a couple of organizations, the Micronutrient Initiative and the Food and Agriculture Association of the UN have been developing tools in which you can plug into economic models' data for your own country, and come out with the results for the economic costs of iron deficiency in your own country, and the rates of return. From what I understand these are quite convincing for policy makers. But on the other hand people do raise doubts about the assumptions, for example the issue that many people are unemployed. Actually you could quite validly criticize the results, the assumptions I have made on the cognitive effects of iron saying we don't have longitudinal data to support that, you are making a big assumption. That plus the general dislike of economists' ideas about assumption, the idea that you should be able to put a value on human life is very distasteful to many people, so not everyone is convinced.

Dr. Zlotkin: One of the problems I think with iron is that as you describe the costs, you list four costs in the area of productivity, cognitive cost, morbidity cost and mortality cost. But unlike the example for vitamin A deficiency or iodine deficiency where for vitamin A you have something that population people can understand, they understand blind, what it means to be blind, and with iodine deficiency people understand what it means to have a big lump in their throat. What you are doing in terms of the economic advocacy is really important but part of our overall problem is finding the right hook for physicians to advocate their governments to do something about anemia, teachers to advocate their ministry of education to do something about anemia, and the economic ministry to do something because I think the argument you make whether it is owed by 1 or 2 degrees is a very powerful argument. Most of us would say that if we were to invest USD 2 and get a return of USD 10 or 20 everyone in this room would do it. So the question is why haven't we done it? I think one of the reasons we haven't done it is that we do need popular support for this type of advocacy and we lack this blindness when we are talking about anemia. So I think what you are doing is extremely important and the information you provide is important, but I really do think it is up to all of us in the room to be the advocates for this particular health issue.

Dr. Horton: I think you are right and zinc is an even more extreme example. It is difficult to measure zinc status, we don't have good estimates of prevalence of zinc deficiency and it is going to be even harder with zinc than with iron.

Mr. Parvanta: I would like to follow up on Dr. Zlotkin's comment as far as the delivery of the message or the hook that you mentioned. Dr. Galar told me about the work he tried to do in Egypt. When he made appointments with the Minister of Education of Egypt to explain the issue of anemia and how the children were sick and anemic and not feeling well, and to talk about iron deficiency anemia. He said that the minister was very kind and gracious but told him to go and see the Minister of Health. He had two visits like this. On the third visit, he became wiser and did not talk about iron deficiency to the Minister of Health; he said nothing about anemia, he talked about the cognitive and education skills of the students and the fact that they were not learning as well at school. This time, on the third visit, the minister not only listened but he actually got out from behind his desk, came around, put his arms around Dr. Galan's shoulders and asked him to sit on the couch and talk about iron deficiency once again. So the type of message that we give is very important. One final observation I made in China. As I understand, and I suppose our colleagues from China can verify this, micronutrients and nutrition interventions are components of the national development plans, the economic plans of the country, and part of the reason why that came about, as I understand from the stories I was told by colleagues there, is that there was a meeting in 2000 in Manila on fortification and micronutrients actually had a lot to do with it. The meeting was sponsored by the Asian Development Bank and so the report of the meeting was put together in English and was sent to the various countries. The copy that went to China went routinely to the Ministry of Economy to be translated. It was sent to the group that handles the economy or finance, and so the economists could actually read this entire document in order to translate it into Chinese. As a result they actually paid attention to essentially every sentence and that is when they became aware: 'Oh, we didn't realize that nutrition had so much to do with economic development', and that lead to the next steps. So it is a coincidence that the report went there. What we have to do is give this type of information to the right source with the right hook.

Dr. Semba: I understand why you are avoiding the cost of the child or infant dying. I think it has much broader implications for society. There was a book published years ago by Scheper-Hughes [1] who is an anthropologist working in Bahia who wrote about the high mortality rates, and how it just was accepted. A child dies and the mother has another child, and I think when it gets to a point where society comes to accept this, then we have all failed.

The Economic Impact of Micronutrient Deficiencies

Dr. Sablan: The real issue with food fortification is that the economic burden has actually shifted to the industry. In our country we have a food fortification program which has actually been shown to be more cost-effective than actual supplementation, and the Ministry of Health agrees that it is a good program and it will actually address a lot of vitamin and mineral deficiencies. As an economist, is it not a little hard to convince the industry that they will actually be carrying the cost of fortification? In the long run they will probably look at the long-term effects and realize that it is probably very good to fortify and will improve the economy. But what would be your answer to their question on the short-term so that they will fortify?

Dr. Horton: I think there are several things that you can do. Firstly industries may bear the costs of the initial investment but typically they will pass the costs on to the consumer, the recurrent cost of the fortificant. So in those cases it is really important to do social marketing. It is really important to make the consumers aware that what they are consuming is a better quality product, that they should be willing to pay these few cents additional cost because of the benefits that will accrue to them and their children, and that may be something where assistance is required for social marketing. So that is one thing that is really important. Another thing that is really important is legislation. There have been some attempts in small African countries to go for fortification of sugar, for example, but if you are acting in isolation without all the countries surrounding also acting in this legislation you run into problems of cheaper unfortified supplies coming in. So this is not a problem in big countries like the Philippines or India, but in Africa it indicates that it is going to be more difficult to fortify because we will have to get regional groups of countries to act in concert.

Reference

1   Scheper-Hugher N: Death without Weeping: The Violence of Everyday Life in Brazil. Berkeley, U California Press, 1992.

Pettifor JM, Zlotkin S (eds): Micronutrient Deficiencies during the Weaning Period and the
First Years of Life. Nestlé Nutrition Workshop Series Pediatric Program, vol 54, pp 203–211,
Nestec Ltd., Vevey/S. Karger AG, Basel, © 2004.

Practical Considerations for Improving Micronutrient Status in the First Two Years of Life

Ibrahim Parvanta and Jacky Knowles

International Micronutrient Malnutrition Prevention and Control Program,
Division of Nutrition and Physical Activity, Centers for Disease Control and Prevention,
Atlanta, Ga., USA

Introduction

Six- to 24-month-old children are at especially high risk for micronutrient deficiencies due to their rapid rate of growth and their ability to consume only small amounts of food at any one time. Continued breast-feeding during this age provides significant nutritional and health benefits for the children. However, after 6 months of age, breast milk alone will not meet the infant's needs for some key minerals, such as iron and zinc. Thus, additional dietary sources of these nutrients are needed, and it has been estimated that adequate complementary foods for infants older than 6 months should provide 75–100% of daily zinc and iron requirements [1]. However, even if iron- and zinc-rich foods such as meats were readily available, it would require unrealistically high daily intakes of these foods to achieve the recommended intakes of iron and zinc during the second half year of life [1]. In most developing countries, where complementary foods are mainly based on cereal products of low vitamin and mineral density, iron and zinc intakes are insufficient for optimum development of children less than 24 months old [2, 3].

Public health authorities now agree that infants should be exclusively breast-fed until 6 months of age, followed by the introduction of micronutrient-rich complementary foods [4, 5]. International guidance also clearly specifies that the widespread use of fortified complementary foods and/or universal micronutrient supplementation is essential to prevent micronutrient deficiencies in infants and young children [1, 4, 6].

Innovative strategies to make fortified complementary foods and micronutrient supplements widely available and accessible in non-industrialized

203

countries are urgently needed. Yet, except for mostly donor-supported vitamin A capsule distribution, few developing countries have effective programs to prevent deficiencies of other micronutrients in preschool children. This is partly due to a lack of understanding among public and private sector decision makers regarding the detrimental impact of micronutrient deficiencies on the physical development and mental and learning capacity of populations and, consequently, on the socioeconomic development of their communities and nations. Additional constraints to the development of programs to prevent micronutrient deficiencies in infants and young children, especially related to fortification of complementary foods, include: a perceived threat to breast-feeding; concerns about lack of clean water and sanitation needed to safely prepare complementary foods; hesitation about the role of multinational baby food companies, and the high cost of commercially produced fortified complementary foods, making them inaccessible to a large proportion of the population.

Recent developments of new micronutrient delivery products such as Sprinkles [7], Foodlets [8], and Spreads [9], offer new opportunities for sustainable elimination or reduction of micronutrient deficiencies in young children through the principle of in-home fortification of traditional complementary foods [10].

Practical Considerations

Evaluations of iron and folic acid supplementation programs for pregnant women in developing countries have found that the typical strategy of delivering supplements through the health system is ineffective on a large scale. Some key reasons for this include: poor public health sector logistics and incentives that result in unreliable supplies and distribution of tablets; poor or nonexistent program communication and community promotion of supplements; inadequate patient counseling and lack of information by health care providers, and lack of choice of supplements through the health system [11].

Preventive micronutrient supplementation efforts are also hindered in developing countries because in many societies, micronutrient supplements are synonymous with 'medications' and 'cures' [11, 12]. In many developing countries, the classification of micronutrient preparations as pharmaceuticals, with access to them only by prescription and through medical centers or pharmacies, further add to the perception of supplements as curative medical interventions. Thus, consumers in these countries do not perceive supplements as components of, or adjuncts to, good nutrition. Instead, the population is often hesitant to use the products on a regular basis and for extended periods of time because of the fear of 'over medication' [11, 12]. Furthermore, the limited and high-priced varieties of fortified complementary foods in developing country markets also have a connotation as 'special' foods with 'medicinal' properties which should be consumed by children when they are ill.

In contrast, in developed countries such as the US, there is widespread availability and use of affordable and competing brands of fortified complementary foods and pediatric micronutrient supplements through the commercial sector. Thus, the average consumer perceives and utilizes fortified complementary foods as the 'normal' diet for infants and young children, and can access many varieties of micronutrient supplement preparations in the market without medical prescription.

The Women, Infants and Children's Supplemental Nutrition Program (WIC) has been implemented in the United States since the 1970s and is designed to provide nutrition screening and counseling services, as well as nutritious foods, to low-income children <5 years old and pregnant women [13]. It is quite likely that one important reason for the success of this 30-year-old national maternal and child nutrition program is that beneficiaries purchase specific authorized foods from the commercial market using special program coupons or credit mechanisms. Enabling WIC Program participants to access the nutrient-rich foods through the existing market eliminated the need for the government to create an independent and costly logistics network to deliver food products to program participants through government clinics. Anecdotal information also suggest that the promotion of specific types of micronutrient fortified foods helped to encourage the private sector to increase the number of commercially fortified products that meet WIC Program requirements, including lower priced generic ones (fig. 1). Thus, over time, WIC Program recipients have had more fortified food options to choose from and, perhaps even more importantly, the remainder of the US population not receiving WIC Program services have also benefited from the availability of competitively priced fortified foods on the grocery store shelves.

Examples of effective market-based public health intervention programs in developing countries include local production and commercial distribution of oral rehydration solutions, and more recently, retail level distribution of safe water storage vessels and chlorine-based disinfectant solutions [14, 15]. It is highly likely that lessons from these programs could be adapted to improve the distribution and coverage of micronutrient supplements, in-home fortificants, and centrally produced fortified complementary foods in developing countries. Furthermore, with continued success and expansion of safe-water programs [14, 15], it might be possible to combine this effective disease prevention measure with efficacious fortified water strategies to prevent iron and perhaps other micronutrient deficiencies, as have been reported in Brazil [16, 17].

Considerations for Future Program Development

It would be safe to say that, although treatment of micronutrient deficiencies requires intervention by the health sector, the sustainable widespread prevention of these deficiencies cannot be achieved through interventions

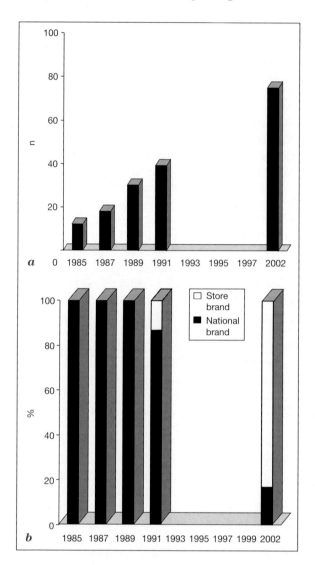

Fig. 1. The increase, over time, in the number of breakfast cereal products (**a**) and percent of store vs. national brand breakfast cereals (**b**) authorized by the Women, Infants and Children Supplemental Nutrition Program (WIC) in the state of Maine, USA, 1985–2002. Source: Personal communication from Mr. Ron Bansmer, Director, Maine WIC Program.

delivered by public health agencies alone. The long term improvement of micronutrient status of young children requires that appropriate, low-cost, fortified complementary foods and micronutrient supplements are available through the commercial market and other community-based delivery channels, and that their production and use become the norm among industry and consumers.

It is important for the health sector to acknowledge the essential role of private industry in the production, marketing and distribution of high-quality micronutrient-rich foods and supplements for various consumer segments in society. This supportive role of the health sector is essential to ensure public acceptance of the products. By 'sharing the burden' of micronutrient deficiency interventions with the private sector, public health agencies could channel limited resources to target the most vulnerable populations with limited access to markets, and to better monitor the process and impact of micronutrient intervention programs.

It is also essential to recognize that, if a particular strategy is not applicable to one part of the world or may not reach the most vulnerable or most remote populations within countries, the implementation of that strategy may still benefit populations in other parts of the world or of a nation; i.e. no single intervention will cover all populations or is 100% effective. For example, children under 24 months old in both rural and urban areas of developing countries are often iron deficient. With adequate marketing and promotion, it may be possible to distribute appropriately priced fortified complementary foods, in-home fortificants, and/or micronutrient supplements through the market sector in urban and peri-urban communities using various pricing schemes, while the most underprivileged could be served through improved government or nonprofit sector distribution networks.

Retail level delivery of micronutrient-rich products will likely also lead to more regular use of such products. For example, the high compliance with pre-pregnancy and early prenatal folic acid supplementation program in China is in part attributed to the sale of the supplements to program beneficiaries. The sale of the supplements provides monetary incentives for those responsible for ensuring high coverage of the program, and improves compliance by overcoming the population's perception that a freely distributed product is not beneficial or is of poor quality (Li Zhu, Beijing University, personal commun.).

Finally, appropriate partnerships between the public, private, and civic sectors are essential for implementation of sustainable public health interventions, including prevention of micronutrient deficiencies. For example, the tremendous achievement in increasing the proportion of households in the world using iodized salt from less than 20 to almost 70% during the 1990s [18], was only realized once public health authorities acknowledged that the salt industry 'held the key' to success, and together with Kiwanis International, a civic organization, initiated an active engagement with salt producers. In 2000, the partnership led to the salt industry publicly acknowledging its role in salt iodization and a collaborative international coalition of public, private, and civic organizations was formed to support national efforts for sustained elimination of iodine deficiency [19]. Another example of public and private sector partnership to improve public health can be found in the development of an effective water purification system which was the result of collaboration between the US Centers for Disease Control and Prevention (CDC) and the Proctor and Gamble Health Sciences Institute. This collaboration has further led Proctor and Gamble Health Sciences Institute, the CDC, the International Council of Nurses, and other organizations to establish an International Network to Promote Safe Household Water Treatment and Storage in developing countries [20].

Conclusion

Successful and sustainable prevention of micronutrient deficiencies will require public, private, and civic sector commitment to collaborate, based on the resources and expertise of each group. No single sector, intervention method, or product can reach all of the target populations. Multiple intervention strategies are needed which involve multiple sectors of society, multiple forms of fortified foods, multiple types of micronutrient supplements, and especially, a combination of market- and community-based access points, as well as government sector distribution networks, to make nutrient-rich foods and supplements accessible and acceptable by consumers in developing countries.

References

1 World Health Organization: Complementary Feeding of Young Children in Developing Countries: A Review of Current Scientific Knowledge. Geneva, WHO, 1998.
2 Gibson RS, Ferguson EL, Lehrfeld J: Complementary foods for infants in developing countries: Their nutrient adequacy and improvement. Eur J Clin Nutr 1998;52:764–770.
3 Gibson RS, Hotz C: The adequacy of micronutrients in complementary foods. Pediatrics 2000; 106:1298–1299.
4 Pan American Health Organization/World Health Organization: Guiding Principles for Complementary Feeding of the Breastfed Child. Washington, PAHO/Geneva, WHO, 2003.
5 World Health Organization: The Optimal Duration of Exclusive Breastfeeding: A Systematic Review. Geneva, WHO, 2001, WHO/NHD/01.08;WHO/FCH/CAH/01.23.
6 Stoltzfus R, Dreyfuss ML: Guidelines for the Use of Iron Supplements to Prevent and Treat Iron Deficiency Anemia. Washington, ILSI Press, 1998.
7 Zlotkin S, Antwi KY, Schauer C, Yeung D: Use of microencapsulated iron (II) fumarate sprinkles to prevent recurrence of anemia in infants and young children at high risk. Bull WHO 2003;81:108–114.
8 Gross R (ed): Micronutrient Supplementation throughout the Life Cycle. Report of a Workshop Held by the Ministry of Health Brazil and UNICEF, Rio de Janeiro, 1996. Rio de Janiero, UNICEF, 2000.
9 Briend A: Possible use of spreads as a FOODlet for improving the diets of infants and young children. Food Nutr Bull 2002;23:239–243.
10 Nestel P, Breind A, de Benoist B, et al: Complementary food supplements to achieve micronutrient adequacy for infants and young children. J Pediatr Gastroenterol Nutr 2003;36:316–328.
11 Galloway R, McGuire J: Determinants of compliance with iron supplementation: Supplies, side effects, or psychology? Soc Sci Med 1994;39:381–390.
12 Parvanta I, Galuska D, Simpson ME: Gaza Nutrition Survey: October 1998. Report Prepared for the United Nations Relief and Works Agency and Centers for Disease Control and Prevention, September 15, 1999.

13 Burich MC, Murray JR: Study of WIC Participant and Program Characteristics 1990, Final Report. Alexandria, United States Department of Agriculture, Food and Nutrition Service, Office of Analysis and Evaluation, 1992.
14 http://www.psi.org/our_programs/products/water_chlorination.html
15 http://www.cdc.gov/safewater/default.htm
16 Dutra-de-Oliveira JE, Ferreira JB, Vasconcellos VP, Marchini JS: Drinking water as an iron carrier to control anemia in preschool children in a day-care center. J Am Coll Nutr 1994;13: 198–202.
17 Dutra-de-Oliveira JE, Scheid MMA, Desai ID, Marchini JS: Iron fortification of domestic drinking water to prevent anemia among low socioeconomic families in Brazil. Int J Food Sci Nutr 1996;46:213–219.
18 http://www.iodinepartnership.org
19 van der Haar F, de Long J, Haxton D, Mannar MGV: Salt 2000: Marking and Sustaining Global Progress in Universal Salt Iodization. IDD Newslett 2000;16:33–37.
20 Proctor and Gamble Health Sciences Institute: Promising New Technology Proven Effective in Purifying Water for the Developing World. Press release, 19 June 2003.

Discussion

Dr. Semba: You talked about one last potential solution being the introduction of fortified complementary foods after 6 months, and I would like to give you two scenarios. For example, in Indonesia the most common complementary food is rice, rice porridge, and in Malawi it is corn porridge, and both of these are locally produced and not centrally distributed. So how would you fortify these?

Mr. Parvanta: In some countries centrally produced fortified foods may not be the option. In those situations, there are other strategies that could be used. These include in-home fortification, using micronutrient Sprinkles which will be discussed later by Dr. Zlotkin, and micronutrient supplementation. However, fortification of complementary foods is possible in some parts of the world. Thus, we at the CDC, are collaborating with UNICEF to support complementary food fortification efforts in South and Central America and Eastern Europe and the former Soviet Union regions because centrally produced complementary foods are used by relatively large population segments. The main point is that where it is possible, production and utilization of fortified complementary foods must be promoted.

Dr. Bhutta: I agree with a lot of what you have said. As a member of the WHO expert panel on breast-feeding I would like to clarify a few things. One, there was extensive discussion within the group on micronutrient supplementation, not just after 6 months but even within the first 6 months. I believe within the recommendations there are recommendations for high-risk groups such as small-for-date infants, and there was clear recognition even though it may not appear for reasons of parsimony in that paragraph that you alluded to. The challenge therefore is how this can be done in developing countries where commercial or centrally processed complementary foods only represent at best about a third of the entire repertoire of complementary foods in households. There is a mix of strategies that needs to be adopted which at one end really needs to look at what the market will provide in terms of complementary foods, and at the other end looks at alternative strategies such as fortification of staples. Just to conclude, I strongly endorse moving forward by bringing the industry into this entire debate. Pakistan, where I come from, has had a central food fortification program with regard to vitamin A for over 40 years in terms of vegetable oil fortification. Yet in four decades it has not been possible to expand it to include additional micronutrients or additional vehicles, and this is partly because at the public health level the importance of this for children in general has not been recognized.

Mr. Parvanta: Thank you for this point. Let me just add that developing countries vary, just as developed countries vary. Thus, we should consider opportunities by country, or perhaps by region. In those countries where fortification of complementary foods is a potential option, their governments and relevant industries should be encouraged and supported to make such fortification happen. We should note that in countries where food fortification programs are in place, often the food producers are not informed of their important contributions to public health. For example, a few months ago at a meeting of flour millers, a miller from El Salvador pointed out that their industry had not been informed if fortification of flour with iron and folic acid had had any impact on the health of the population of El Salvador. Thus, the public health sector should make a special effort to inform food industry partners about the impact of fortification programs and acknowledge their contribution accordingly.

Dr. Bloem: I have two comments for you. It is very interesting when you say we have to give people more choices, but poverty means that there is a lack of choice. It is almost like poor people denying that they have no choices, but giving them more choices is almost a contradiction. The other issue you talked about is industry, and I think it is a little bit dangerous to talk about industry because industry is quite different in different places. In China of course you see an incredibly increased food industry, but because of globalization the food industry is no longer working in isolation.

For example a big industry in Indonesia was bought by Heinz, and that happens in many places, supermarkets are growing, all these global companies are actually influencing many different countries, and you have small countries like Bangladesh where there is hardly any industry and where in fact people still eat what they produce to a certain extent. So it is more complicated than just saying let's involve industries. We have to be more specific when we talk about industry.

Mr. Parvanta: Obviously, the situation varies from country to country, and one has to address each situation accordingly. For example, in India about 20–25% of wheat flour consumed is milled by large scale mills while the remaining 75–80% of flour is by the small milling sector. Given India's large population, the public health benefits of fortifying industrially produced flour would affect tens of millions of people in that country. So, why not move ahead with such efforts?

Dr. Vasquez-Garibay: You were talking about infants and mentioned the rapid growth rate and low gastric capacity as a limitation for receiving a high nutrient density diet. I didn't understand what you were trying to say with that because perhaps that high density diet might mean adipose proliferation and obesity, that is the problem now in Mexico. The second point is that the most vulnerable people in Mexico, something like 26 million people, cannot afford to buy fortified foods.

Mr. Parvanta: Let me take the second issue first. Yes, there are people in every country that cannot purchase fortified commercial foods. However, there are also large segments of the population who can purchase such foods and would benefit accordingly. Furthermore, there is a range of incomes among the poor, and they make purchasing choices. For example, I pointed out in my presentation the poor purchase cigarettes which are relatively expensive. Thus, they choose how to spend their limited resources. We, public health and the food industry, need to inform and encourage them to choose to purchase healthier fortified foods instead. With regard to the point about low gastric capacity, fortification of complementary foods would provide a richer diet with regard to micronutrient content without increasing the caloric content of infants' diets.

Dr. Tolboom: You shared some very stimulating ideas with us and you showed an interesting slide on the recommendation of exclusive breast-feeding. You are quite happy with that but I am still quite worried. I recall an earlier Nestlé Nutrition Workshop. Series [1], in which we looked at the time of introduction of complementary foods. If you look at Malawi or Zambia you see that children get complementary foods at the age of 2 or 3 months. So I think that the breast-feeding expert committee's use of terms such as 'you should', 'exclusive', 'continue for 6 months' etc. do not adequately address what actually happens in the field. With your clear intuition for client perspective, I would like you to elaborate a little bit on that.

Mr. Parvanta: I feel exactly as you do that the reality of infant feeding practices in most populations is far different than the expert guidelines on type and length of breast-feeding. By our just focusing public health programs to implement the breast-feeding guidelines and ignoring actual consumer practices, we severely jeopardize infant health and development. While good breast-feeding practices should be promoted, there is an urgent need to improve the vitamin and mineral content of complementary foods, no matter how early such foods are offered to infants. For example, in the late 1960's a very small proportion of infants in the United States were breastfed. To improve nutritional status of infants, starting in the early 1970's, use of fortified breast milk substitutes were encouraged by health and nutrition programs, while breast-feeding was also promoted. Over time, breast-feeding rates have improved, but non-breast-fed infants have also been protected from micronutrient deficiencies because of widespread availability of fortified formulas and other baby foods.

Reference

1   Ballabriga A, Rey J (eds): Weaning: Why, What, and When. Nestlé Nutrition Workshop Series. New York, Raven Press, 1987, vol 10.

Pettifor JM, Zlotkin S (eds): Micronutrient Deficiencies during the Weaning Period and the First Years of Life. Nestlé Nutrition Workshop Series Pediatric Program, vol 54, pp 213–232, Nestec Ltd., Vevey/S. Karger AG, Basel, © 2004.

Specific Strategies to Address Micronutrient Deficiencies in the Young Child: Targeted Fortification

Lynnette M. Neufeld[a] and Usha Ramakrishnan[b]

[a]Division of Nutritional Epidemiology, National Institute of Public Health, Cuernavaca, Morelos, Mexico, and
[b]Department of International Health, Rollins School of Public Health, Emory University, Atlanta, Ga., USA

Introduction

Micronutrient deficiency during early childhood may be related to a series of factors including inadequate stores accumulated during the fetal period, low intake from maternal breast milk, early abandonment of breast-feeding, increased losses due to infections and inadequate micronutrient intake from complementary foods (foods taken in addition to breast milk from ~6 months until the child eats from the family diet, ~24 months). Current guidelines recognize that, while in most settings full breast-feeding is adequate to meet nutrient requirements for the first 6 months of life, the appropriateness of complementary feeding practices from 6 to 24 months is a major concern in many developing countries [1], especially micronutrient density (micronutrient content/100 kcal) and frequency of feeding due to small gastric capacity.

Assuming an average breast-milk intake, almost all iron and zinc, 5–30% of vitamin A, and 50–80% of thiamin, riboflavin and calcium must be supplied by complementary foods [2]. Very little or no vitamin B_6, B_{12} and folate are needed from complementary foods because of their higher concentration in breast milk. In settings where women do not breast-feed for extended periods, breast milk intake is low or breast-feeding women are deficient in these vitamins, the proportion provided by complementary foods should increase.

213

Micronutrients Most Likely to Be Inadequate in Complementary Foods

The density of many micronutrients, including zinc, iron, calcium, vitamin A, and vitamin B_{12} is low in foods of plant origin, typically used as the basis of complementary feeding in developing countries [2]. Dietary factors that inhibit absorption of some nutrients (phytates, polyphenols and dietary fiber) tend to be high [3] particularly in maize and legumes and although these foods also contain moderately high levels of trace elements such as iron and zinc, they are poorly absorbed.

Analysis of typical diets of breast-fed infants (6–24 months) indicate that several foods consumed by 6- to 11-month-old infants in Peru and Mexico have iron densities that could meet infant requirements, but only if 2–3 times more of the food was consumed than that reported for any child [2]. Zinc and calcium densities were adequate for children aged 18–24 months when animal source foods were included. Gibson et al. [3] found that very few complementary foods from Africa and Asia could meet the iron, zinc, calcium and riboflavin needs of infants 9–11 months of age. Vitamin A density may also be inadequate especially if breast milk retinol intake is low due to maternal deficiency or low breast milk intake. Recent studies have shown that the bioavailability of vitamin A from plant-based foods is much lower (~50%) than earlier estimates [4], and that in the absence of any preformed retinol, young children would have to consume about 4–5 times the current amount of plant-based foods such as spinach to meet their requirements [5].

Similar analyses of dietary intake data from Bangladesh, Ghana, Guatemala, Peru and the USA [6] using the updated nutrient requirements [7–11] indicate that iron, zinc and calcium densities remain low in almost all foods for children <12 months of age, despite the lower energy requirements. Calcium and iron densities were inadequate for children aged 12–23 months. Although the results were inconsistent for other micronutrients (riboflavin, vitamin B_6, niacin, thiamine, folate and zinc), they are most likely limiting in the diets of infants <2 years of age and it was concluded that more research is needed to establish appropriate nutrient densities for complementary foods.

Rationale for the Use of Targeted Fortification to Improve Micronutrient Status of Small Children

It is clear that the density of zinc, iron, calcium and possibly other micronutrients in unfortified foods from developed and developing countries is insufficient to meet the needs of infants and small children. Improved micronutrient density may be feasible through daily consumption of poultry, meat, fish or eggs and vitamin A-rich fruits and vegetables [1]. In many populations, however, economic and other constraints limit the inclusion of sufficient animal-source food to breech this gap [2]. Other mechanisms (fermentation, germination, ascorbic acid) can improve the availability of iron and zinc from plant-based foods, but are likely insufficient to meet the needs of infants [3]. Micronutrient supplement distribution can be very efficacious in improving micronutrient status especially when high-risk groups are targeted [12]. It has been challenging, however to implement supplementation programs due to technical and logistical problems, including interactions between nutrients in multinutrient syrups, safety, frequency of consumption (at least weekly for nutrients such as iron, zinc and water soluble vitamins), compliance, reliance on health systems for distribution, and sustainability [13].

The increased use of processed foods facilitates fortification as an effective strategy to improve micronutrient intakes of populations. Universal fortification of staples and condiments, however, is unlikely to improve micronutrient intakes of small children due to the small amount of these foods consumed. Commercial complementary foods have been available and used extensively in many developed countries since the 1950s. Consistent with nutrition knowledge at that time, emphasis was placed on adequate protein intake [6]. Fortified complementary foods (FCFs) now provide an important alternative to meet the micronutrient needs of young children [14]. As urbanization and women's participation in the work force increase, commercial complementary foods provide a convenient and timesaving alternative to home preparation and reduce the risk for microbial contamination [6].

Barriers to the Use of Fortified Foods in Developed and Developing Countries

There are a number of barriers to the widespread production and use of FCFs, particularly among the rural poor in developing countries. Because this is where the highest prevalence of micronutrient deficiencies exists, fortified foods have had little impact on the prevalence of child malnutrition to date [6].

Barriers on the Production Side

The amount of micronutrients needed from FCFs depends on total requirements and intake from breast milk and other sources. A large range in consumption of complementary foods can be expected, depending on child age and intake from other sources [6] and it may be difficult for manufacturers to estimate appropriate levels of fortification when target populations are heterogeneous. Lutter [15] recommends that the level of fortification be set to meet the needs of the largest possible proportion of non- or minimally breast-fed infants over the range of target ages. Typical breast milk intake, portion size, bioavailability, micronutrient interactions and inhibitors of absorption naturally occurring in the food vehicle should be taken into consideration in determining the level of fortificant. Nutrient bioavailability studies of fortified foods have been conducted in older children and adults [16–18] and in FCFs with different iron fortificants in the presence of enhancers (ascorbic acid) and inhibitors (phytates and milk) of iron absorption [19]. Unfortunately, there is a paucity of information on the bioavailability of other nutrients and the role of interactions when more than one nutrient is added to complementary food.

Quality control of food fortification, including fortification to the specified level and control of microbial contamination must be monitored; although this may be logistically difficult if foods are prepared by many disperse manufacturers. Where livelihood depends on small-scale agriculture, locally produced crops should be used in the production of FCFs to avoid undermining local markets [6].

The potential role of industry in the production of safe, affordable and high-quality FCFs is great, both as a partner in the production of FCFs for national programs and for sale in the market. A number of barriers must be overcome before industry is likely to make the investment needed for FCF production. Raw material costs can only be reduced to a certain degree, after which packaging and marketing expenses must decrease [20]. The demand for FCFs in developing countries is very low, especially among high-risk groups and a large investment would be necessary to create demand and brand loyalty in this setting [15]. Finally, many producers shy away from foods for small infants for fear of consumer boycott [20, 21] or even liability due to concerns of contamination from inadequate hygienic practices during food preparation that could be attributed to the product itself [20]. Public sector and advocacy groups must work with industry to reduce perceived risks related to FCF production and increase the market for high-quality, low-cost FCFs.

Reaching the Most Needy

In developing countries, FCFs have traditionally been expensive and available only to the wealthier, urban population. Recently FCFs have been included as part of national poverty alleviation programs in various Latin American countries, including Mexico, Peru, Guatemala, Columbia, Costa Rica and Chile (Neufeld and Hotz, unpublished document prepared for Global Forum, 2003). One such program, *Oportunidades* (previously *Progresa*) has been operating in Mexico since 1997 and has been evaluated by the National Institute of Public Health (INSP), Mexico, since its inauguration. A description of this program was published as part of a previous Nestlé Nutrition Workshop [22].

Creating a demand for FCFs among poor families with little disposable income may be a major barrier, particularly among rural dwellers, less accustomed to the use of commercial foods. Although some national programs distribute FCFs to poor families, they reach a small portion of those who could benefit [15], and unless steps are taken, may ultimately create dependency [6]. Furthermore, the nutritional quality of the products distributed through national programs has not always been adequate [15].

Education and social marketing may help create consumer demand for FCFs [15] and provide an opportunity to educate the population about appropriate feeding practices and promote breast-feeding [6]. Unlike breast-feeding, clear policy support and advocacy have been lacking for specific recommendations related to complementary feeding [21]. An abundance of research exists on issues related to complementary feeding including nutrient composition, consistency, hygiene, control of microbial contamination and feeding environment (e.g. responsive feeding practices) but the implementation of this information into action has been inadequate [21].

Fortification and Micronutrient Status of Infants and Young Children: Experiences from Universal and Targeted Food Fortification

Many examples of the effectiveness of untargeted fortification to improve the micronutrient status of older children and adults have been published. The iron status of children improved after universal fortification of rice (Philippines) and flour (Venezuela) [23]. Several studies have also evaluated the efficacy of fortified foods targeted to school-age children (drinks, cookies, candies) with positive effects on iron [24–28], vitamin A [24–26], and zinc status [24]. In Morocco, the iron and iodine status of children improved with the use of salt fortified with microencapsulated iron and iodine [29].

Recent studies suggest that fortified foods may contribute 10–20% of micronutrient intakes in older children and adults from developed countries. Fortified foods were shown to contribute ~80% vitamin B_6, 40–50% vitamins C, B_2, E and niacin, 10–20% iron, vitamin A and folate, and 5% calcium intakes in German children (2–15 years) [30]. Fortified ready to eat cereals and fruit juices are significant sources of iron and vitamin C, respectively, among US children (2–18 years) [31]. Berner et al. [32] concluded that fortification substantially increased micronutrient intakes in all age/sex groups in the US, especially young children, based on nationally representative dietary intake data. However, micronutrient intakes from fortified foods among children <2 years of age are not well documented.

Although essential to improve the micronutrient status of older children and adults, these strategies are unlikely to have substantial impact on the micronutrient status of children <2 years of age. Micronutrient density is insufficient to meet requirements during complementary feeding and the small quantities that can be consumed due to limited gastric capacity will not compensate for lower nutrient density.

217

Developed Country Experiences in Targeted Fortification

Breast milk substitutes and complementary foods have been fortified, especially with iron, since the 1970s in many developed countries and the observed decline in rates of anemia and iron deficiency has been attributed to this [33]. The best evidence comes from the United States where the prevalence of anemia declined among low income young children between 1974 and 1985 [34, 35], corresponding to the introduction of iron-fortified formula and complementary foods in the national Women, Infants and Children program.

An important lesson from developed countries is the active role of the private sector in the development and marketing of FCFs. A wealth of experience exists in the selection of appropriate fortificant, acceptability of the final product, etc. For example, many efficacy trials [36–38] have compared the impact of different iron fortificants on young child iron status and the advantages and disadvantages are well documented [39]. The challenge is to share this knowledge and make it relevant to developing country settings where it is most needed.

Developing Country Experiences in Targeted Fortification

While evidence exists that FCFs may improve outcomes such as child growth and morbidity [2, 22], less is known about their impact on micronutrient status in developing country settings. The results of published efficacy trials [40–44] are mixed and methodological details (table 1) show that there is considerable variability in study design, micronutrients and food vehicles used.

Most studies showed positive effects of complementary foods fortified with iron on iron status. In China [44], no drop in hemoglobin concentration was observed in the fortified food group ($-0.8 \pm 0.1\,\mathrm{g/l}$) while it declined significantly in the control group ($-7.9 \pm 1.2\,\mathrm{g/l}$). Similarly, a significant drop in ferritin and hemoglobin concentration was observed in infants receiving unfortified porridge or porridge with fish powder in Ghana, while no drop occurred among those receiving fortified porridge [43]. At 12 months of age, 11% of infants receiving the fortified porridge had low serum ferritin compared to 50% in all other groups. In South Africa [42], a smaller drop in serum iron but not hemoglobin concentration was observed in the fortified food group. In Chile [41], infants receiving iron fortified rice cereal had a higher hemoglobin concentration and a lower prevalence of anemia at 8, 12 and 15 months of age than infants receiving unfortified cereal.

FCFs provided protection against a drop in serum retinol in South Africa [42] and Ghana [43]. In Ghana, the prevalence of vitamin A deficiency (retinol $<0.7\,\mu\mathrm{mol/l}$) was 10.4% in the fortified group and 27.0–34.3% in the other groups. There was no change in serum zinc in South Africa, China or Ghana and no data were reported for Chile. In one older study [40], riboflavin status was adequate in the fortified food group at 9 months of age while riboflavin status worsened in the group not receiving the fortified food.

Therefore, there is some evidence that FCFs may help prevent micronutrient deficiencies under ideal circumstances. However, few program effectiveness trials have been conducted. Considering that national programs in different parts of the world provide FCFs, it is essential to determine whether FCFs provide benefits for infant micronutrient status over and above other program components (e.g. economic transfers).

Case Study of a Fortified Complementary Food in Mexico

The nation-wide poverty alleviation program, *Oportunidades* was implemented in 1997 in rural areas and expanded to urban areas in 2001. A fortified, milk-based complementary food, 'Nutrisano' is distributed to all participating low-income families with children 4–23 months of age and underweight children 2–4 years of age. Considering the enormous investment involved in the production and distribution of Nutrisano, a series of studies were conducted to determine the efficacy to improve micronutrient status, iron bioavailability and stability and acceptability of various iron fortificants.

Efficacy to Improve Infant Micronutrient Status
The efficacy of Nutrisano to improve iron, zinc and vitamin A status was assessed using supplementation with multiple micronutrient syrup as positive control [45]. This was used instead of placebo due to the high prevalence of micronutrient deficiency and provides the opportunity to compare two strategies currently implemented in Mexico. The micronutrient content and percent recommended intake are presented in table 2. Infants 4–12 months of age were randomly assigned to receive Nutrisano or syrup daily. After 4 months, the ferritin concentration dropped significantly in the Nutrisano group (-12.4 ng/dl) while no change was observed in the syrup group ($+0.87$ ng/dl). The prevalence of iron deficiency (ferritin <12.0 ng/dl) was significantly lower in the syrup group (12.5 vs. 37.5% Nutrisano). There was no difference between groups in hemoglobin concentration or anemia prevalence. Micronutrient syrup, but not Nutrisano provided protection against a drop in iron stores during the weaning period and further research was carried out to determine why. Laboratory results for serum zinc and retinol will be available shortly.

Bioavailability, Stability and Acceptability of
Different Forms of Iron in Nutrisano
Following the efficacy trial, the bioavailability of ferrous sulfate (FS), ferrous fumarate (FF), or reduced iron + sodium EDTA (Fe-EDTA) in Nutrisano was assessed in children 2–4 years of age using stable isotope procedures [46]. Nutrisano labeled with [58]Fe was consumed after fasting and a reference dose of [57]Fe dissolved in grape juice with 50 mg ascorbic acid was administered the following day. Incorporation of iron into erythrocytes was

Table 1. Efficacy trials of the impact of fortified complementary foods on infant micronutrient status in developing countries

Country	Fortificant	Age at initial feeding in months	Food vehicle	Duration and details of supplementation	Micronutrient status outcomes measured
South Africa	MM[1]	6	Complementary food	12 months Randomized to fortified or unfortified food	Hemoglobin, serum iron, zinc, retinol
Chile (n = 515)	Elemental iron 55 mg/100 g dry cereal (no information-mentioned for other micronutrients)	4	Rice cereal (Gerber) 30 g/day	Randomized to fortified or unfortified cereal Stratified by breast or formula fed and by iron fortification within the formula group Daily feeding with encouragement to 15 months Ascorbic acid present in iron-fortified formula	Hemoglobin, prevalence of iron deficiency anemia (low Hb + 2 values low for mean corpuscular volume, serum ferritin, transferrin saturation)
Ghana (n = 190)	1 MM (electrolytic iron, zinc oxide) 2 Dried anchovy powder	6	Traditional maize porridge or improved porridge (Weanimix)	Randomized to traditional porridge plain or with fish powder, Weanimix plain, with fish powder or multiple micronutrients Daily feeding to 12 months	Hemoglobin, hematocrit, plasma retinol, zinc, TIBC, erythrocyte riboflavin

China (n = 226)	10 micronutrients (ferric ammonium citrate 10%, zinc gluconate 5%, retinol acetate 375% of RDA)	6–13	Rusk	Randomized to fortified or unfortified rusk by village. Daily feeding for 3 months. Direct monitoring of consumption	Hemoglobin, erythrocyte porphyrin, plasma vitamin A and erythrocyte glutathione reductase activity (riboflavin)
Gambia (n = 178)	Riboflavin in fortified wheat flour (1.4 µg/g fresh weight of supplement)	3–12	Locally prepared with wheat, soya, skim milk, ground nut oil, sugar	Supplemented 3–12 months of age with or without mother receiving supplement during pregnancy and lactation or nothing. Assignment by community	Erythrocyte glutathione reductase activity (riboflavin)

[1]MM = Multiple micronutrients, stated as quantity similar to recommended dietary allowance (RDA).

Table 2. Nutrient content of a fortified food (Nutrisano) and a micronutrient syrup, distributed in different national poverty alleviation programs in Mexico

Nutrient	Nutrisano		Syrup	
	content[1]	% new DRI[2]	content	% new DRI
Energy, kcal	194	23	0	–
Protein, g	5.8	–	0	–
Total fat, g	6.6	–	0	–
Total carbohydrates, g	27.9	–	0	–
Sodium, mg	24.5	–	0	–
Vitamin A, μg	40.0	8	0	–
Vitamin E, mg	6.0	–	0	–
Vitamin C, mg	40.0	80	60.0	120
Vitamin B$_{12}$, μg	0.7	140	1.1	220
Folic acid, μg	50.0	63	95.0	119
Zinc (zinc sulfate), mg	10.0	333	20.0	666
Iron[3], mg	10.0	91	20.0	182
Riboflavin, mg	0	–	1.2	300
Thiamin, mg	0	–	1.1	367

[1]Content in one daily portion (44 g of dry mix Nutrisano; 20 drops, syrup).
[2]Selected micronutrients, US dietary recommended intakes (DRI) for 9–11 months of age [7–10] and energy based on WHO/UNICEF recommendations for total energy 9–11 months of age [2].
[3]Reduced iron in Nutrisano; ferrous sulfate in syrup.

assessed 15 days after administration. Iron absorption from Nutrisano with FS was 7.9%, 2.4% from FF, and 1.4% from Fe-EDTA. Considering 1 mg/day requirement, daily iron absorbed from Nutrisano fortified with FS would provide 144% of the requirement, and 50% if fortified with FF. Iron absorption from Nutrisano fortified with Fe-EDTA would be negligible.

Government authorities requested a recommendation for changing the iron fortificant in Nutrisano and further testing was conducted (Morales J, unpublished data). The taste, color, viscosity and microbial content of Nutrisano with each fortificant were assessed immediately after production and after 6-month storage. Expert judges were able to identify a slightly metallic taste in the food fortified with FS. Approximately 10–20 min after addition of water, color changes and jellification occurred in Nutrisano fortified with FS but not FF or Fe-EDTA. All samples were within acceptable limits for microbiological tests.

Acceptability and intake of Nutrisano with 3 fortificants was evaluated in blind testing among infants 4–23 months of age [47]. All forms received a rating of 4 on a 5-point Likart scale from the infants' mothers. Infants >12 months of age consumed more Nutrisano fortified with FF (28 g), than FS (23 g) or Fe-EDTA (24 g).

Based on this series of studies, researchers at the Instituto Nacional de Salud Publica recommended that the fortificant be changed from reduced iron to ferrous fumarate. This recommendation is now being implemented. Ongoing program evaluations should provide results for the effectiveness of Nutrisano to improve micronutrient and other outcomes.

Conclusions

Micronutrient intakes of children <2 years of age are inadequate in many parts of the world and specific interventions must be undertaken to improve micronutrient status and avoid deleterious consequences for child survival, growth and development. FCFs play an important role in maintaining adequate micronutrient status of small children in developed countries and are likely to play an increasing role in developing countries in the near future.

The inclusion of FCFs in national programs has great potential to improve micronutrient intakes in vulnerable groups. Nonetheless, additional marketing and promotion strategies to improve the use of FCFs is necessary as programs are unlikely to reach all those who could benefit from FCFs and may not be economically sustainable for some countries. Clear documentation of the cost-effectiveness of programs distributing FCFs through close monitoring and evaluation may provide the motivation necessary to expand the use of FCFs in programs, where feasible. Interchange between government policy-makers and researchers, such as the case in Mexico for the design and improvement of Nutrisano, are essential to ensure that state-of-the-art knowledge in the field is incorporated into program planning. Cooperation with industry should be increased by reducing real and perceived risk associated with investment in FCF production and by increasing consumer demand though education and social marketing. Communication of the effectiveness of FCFs for preventing micronutrient deficiencies and their negative consequences in a manner meaningful to rural populations with limited resources may increase demand for the products.

To make appropriate decisions about food vehicle and level of fortification in each population setting, manufacturers will require information regarding the range of nutrient intakes in the population (from breast milk and other complementary foods), the likely range of consumption of the fortified food, cultural traditions and taboos of foods appropriate for young children, prevalence and severity of micronutrient deficiency in the population and capacity of the population to purchase complementary foods. At least part of this information may exist for some developing countries. The impetus to motivate industry to get more involved in the production of FCFs lies with public and advocacy organizations. Ideally, these same bodies should then work with industry to ensure a product that responds to needs of the target population.

Recommended Research Areas

Experience in both developed and developing countries has resulted in a wealth of information on micronutrient needs, appropriate densities, bioavailability of different fortificants, interaction between nutrients, and enhancers and inhibitors of absorption. The food industry, especially manufacturers of infant foods also have considerable experience but this information is typically proprietary in nature and often not available in a manner that would benefit disadvantaged populations. Without doubt, better cooperation and trust between industry and public health/policy sectors with appropriate technology transfer (north–south) would help both increase demand and supply for low-cost FCFs. In this scenario, developing countries would evaluate FCFs in their own context, with appropriate assistance. This type of research is essential to reduce barriers related to the production of low-cost, acceptable and high-quality FCFs.

Many of the previously identified research needs [22] have not yet been adequately addressed and maintain relevancy. In addition:

(1) Appropriate nutrient densities based on type of diet including breast-feeding, amount and frequency of food consumed and foods typically consumed needs to be clarified.

(2) Bioavailability of micronutrients, particularly iron and zinc in various food vehicles needs to be established and guidelines should be produced for the use of specific fortificants, depending on food vehicle characteristics.

(3) Formative research at the population level must be conducted to understand how to appropriately present, promote and market FCFs, particularly in rural areas of developing countries.

(4) The effectiveness of programs distributing FCFs to improve child micronutrient status and incremental improvement over and above other program benefits needs to be assessed, as does cost-effectiveness. Clear solutions to ensure sustainability when programs are effective must be found.

(5) On-going process evaluation is essential to understand why programs distributing FCFs work or do not work, and provide feedback for their improvement.

(6) The relative contribution of FCFs to improving micronutrient status compared to other interventions in varying contexts should be evaluated.

References

1 Pan American Health Organization/World Health Organization: Guiding Principles for Complementary Feeding of the Breastfed Child. Washington, PAHO/Geneva, WHO, 2001.
2 World Health Organization/UNICEF: Complementary Feeding of Young Children in Developing Countries: A Review of Current Scientific Knowledge (who/nut/98.1). Geneva, WHO, 1998.
3 Gibson RS, Ferguson EL, Lehrfeld J: Complementary foods for infant feeding in developing countries: Their nutrient adequacy and improvement. Eur J Clin Nutr 1998;52:64–770.

4 West CE, Eilander A, van Lieshout M: Consequences of revised estimates of carotenoid bioefficacy for dietary control of vitamin A deficiency in developing countries. J Nutr 2002; 132(suppl):2920S–2926S.
5 Miller M, Humphrey J, Johnson E, et al: Why do children become vitamin A deficient? J Nutr 2002;132(suppl):2867S–2880S.
6 Dewey KG, Brown KH: Update on technical issues concerning complementary feeding of young children in developing countries and implications for intervention programs. Food Nutr Bull 2003;24:5–28.
7 Institute of Medicine: Dietary Reference Intakes for Calcium, Phosphorus, Magnesium, Vitamin D and Fluoride. Washington, National Academy Press, 1997.
8 Institute of Medicine: Dietary Reference Intakes for Thiamine, Riboflavin, Niacin, Vitamin B_6, Folate, Vitamin B_{12}, Pantothenic Acid, Biotin, and Choline. Washington, National Academy Press, 1998.
9 Institute of Medicine: Dietary Reference Intakes for Vitamin C, Vitamin E, Selenium, and Carotenoids. Washington, National Academy Press, 2000.
10 Institute of Medicine: Dietary Reference Intakes for Vitamin A, Vitamin K, Arsenic, Boron, Chromium, Copper, Iodine, Iron, Manganese, Molybdenum, Nickel, Silicon, Vanadium, and Zinc. Washington, National Academy Press, 2001.
11 Joint Food and Agriculture Organization/World Health Organization Expert Consultation: Vitamin and Mineral Requirements in Human Nutrition. Geneva, WHO, 2002.
12 Allen LH: Iron supplements: Scientific issues concerning efficacy and implications for research and programs. J Nutr 2002;132(suppl):813S–819S.
13 Mora JO: Iron supplementation: Overcoming technical and practical barriers. J Nutr 2002;132(suppl):853S–855S.
14 World Health Organization/UNICEF: Global Strategy for Infant and Young Child Feeding 2002. Document A55/15. Geneva, WHO, 2002.
15 Lutter CK: Macrolevel approaches to improve the availability of complementary foods. Food Nutr Bull 2003;24:83–103.
16 Mendoza C, Viteri FE, Lönnerdal B, et al: Absorption of iron from unmodified maize and genetically altered, low-phytate maize fortified with ferrous sulfate or sodium iron EDTA. Am J Clin Nutr 2001;73:80–85.
17 López de Romaña D, Lönnerdal B, Brown KH: Absorption of zinc from wheat products fortified with iron and either zinc sulfate or zinc oxide. Am J Clin Nutr 2003;78:279–283.
18 Herman S, Griffin IJ, Suwarti S, et al: Cofortification of iron-fortified flour with zinc sulfate, but not zinc oxide, decreases iron absorption in Indonesian children. Am J Clin Nutr 2002;76: 813–817.
19 Walter T, Olivares M, Pizarro F, Hertrampf E: Fortification; in Ramakrishnan U (ed): Nutritional Anemias. Boca Raton, CRC Press, 2001, pp 153–184.
20 Setiadi A: Manufacturing Complementary Foods in Indonesia: Current Constraints and Future Opportunities. Conference on Food Fortification in Asia, Manila, 2000.
21 Piwoz EG, Huffman SL, Quinn VJ: Promotion and advocacy for improved complementary feeding: Can we apply the lessons learned from breastfeeding? Food Nutr Bull 2003;24:29–43.
22 Rivera-Dommarco JA, Lutter C: The potential role of processed complementary food in Latin America; in Martorell R, Haschke F (eds): Nutrition and Growth. Nestlé Nutrition Workshop Series Pediatric Program. Philadelphia, Lippincott Williams & Wilkins, 2001, vol 47, pp 281–304.
23 Mannar V, Boy GE: Iron fortification: Country level experiences and lessons learned. J Nutr 2002;132:856S–858S.
24 Abrams SA, Muchi A, Hilmers DC, et al: A multinutrient-fortified beverage enhances the nutritional status of children in Botswana. J Nutr 2003;133:1834–1840.
25 Ash DM, Tatala SR, Frongillo EA, et al: Randomized efficacy trial of a micronutrient-fortified beverage in primary school children in Tanzania. Am J Clin Nutr 2003;77:891–898.
26 van Stuijvenberg ME, Kvalsvig JD, Faber M, et al: Effect of iron-, iodine-, and β-carotene fortified biscuits on the micronutrient status of primary school children: A randomized controlled trial. Am J Clin Nutr 1999;69:497–503.
27 Giorgini E, Fisberg M, de Paula RA, et al: The use of sweet rolls fortified with iron bis-glycinate chelate in prevention of iron deficiency anemia in preschool children. Arch Latinoam Nutr 2001;51:48–53.
28 Sari M, Bloem MW, de Pee S: Effect of iron-fortified candies on the iron status of children aged 4–6 y in East Jakarta, Indonesia. Am J Clin Nutr 2001;73:1034–1039.

29 Zimmermann MB, Zeder C, Chaouki N, et al: Dual fortification of salt with iodine and micro-encapsulated iron: A randomized, double-blind, controlled trial in Moroccan schoolchildren. Am J Clin Nutr 2003;77:425–432.
30 Sichert-Hellert W, Kersting M, Manz F: Changes in time-trends of nutrient intake from fortified and non-fortified food in German children and adolescents – 15 year results of the DONALD study. Dortmund Nutritional and Anthropometric Longitudinally Designed Study. Eur J Nutr 2001;40:49–55.
31 Subar AF, Krebs-Smith SM, Cook A, Kahle LL: Dietary sources of nutrients among US children, 1989–1991. Pediatrics. 1998;102:913–923.
32 Berner LA, Clydesdale FM, Douglass JS: Fortification contributed greatly to vitamin and mineral intakes in the United States, 1989–1991. J Nutr 2001;131:2177–2183.
33 Ramakrishnan U, Yip R: Experiences and challenges in industrialized countries: Control of iron deficiency in industrialized countries. J Nutr 2002;132:820S–824S.
34 Leads from the MMWR: Declining anemia prevalence among children enrolled in public nutrition and health programs. Selected states, 1975–1985. JAMA 1986;256:2165.
35 Yip R, Walsh KM, Goldfarb MG, Binkin NJ: Declining prevalence of anemia in childhood in a middle-class setting: A pediatric success story? Pediatrics 1987;80:330–331.
36 Haschke F, Male C: Iron nutritional status during early childhood. The importance of weaning foods to combat iron deficiency; in Haltberg L, Asp NG (eds): Iron Nutrition in Health and Disease. London, Libbey, 1996, pp 325–329.
37 Haschke F, Pietschnig B, Vanura H, et al: Iron intake and iron nutritional status of infants fed iron-fortified beikost with meat. Am J Clin Nutr 1988;47:108–112.
38 Stekel A, Olivares M, Pizarro F, et al: Absorption of fortification iron from milk formulas in infants. Am J Clin Nutr 1986;43:917–922.
39 Hurrell RF: Fortification: Overcoming technical and practical barriers. J Nutr 2002;132:806S–812S.
40 Bates CJ, Prentice AM, Paul AA, et al: Riboflavin status in infants born in rural Gambia, and the effect of a weaning food supplement. Trans R Soc Trop Med Hyg 1982;76:253–258.
41 Walter T, Dallman PR, Pizarro F, et al: Effectiveness of iron-fortified infant cereal in prevention of iron deficiency anemia. Pediatrics 1993;91:976–982.
42 Oelofse A, van Raaij JM, Benade AJ, et al: The effect of a micronutrient-fortified complementary food on micronutrient status, growth and development of 6- to 12-month old disadvantaged urban South African infants. Int J Food Sci Nutr 2003;54:399–407.
43 Lartey A, Manu A, Brown KH, et al: A randomized, community-based trial of the effects of improved, centrally processed complementary foods on growth and micronutrient status of Ghanaian infants from 6 to 12 mo of age. Am J Clin Nutr 1999;70:391–404.
44 Liu DS, Bates CJ, Yin TA, et al: Nutritional efficacy of a fortified weaning rusk in a rural area near Beijing. Am J Clin Nutr 1993;57:506–511.
45 Neufeld LM, Rivera JA, Villalpando S, Shamah Levy T: Changes in iron status after 4 mos supplementation with a micronutrient syrup or a fortified complementary food. FASEB J 2003; LB375.
46 Pérez-Expósito AB, Villalpando S, Abrams A, et al: Evaluación de la biodisponibilidad de hierro en el suplemento infantil distribuido por el programa Progresa utilizando isótopos estables (Evaluation of the bioavailability of iron in the infant food supplement distributed in the program, Progresa, using stable isotopes). X Congr Invest en Salud Pública, Libro de Resúmenes, 2003, TL087:155.
47 Flores ME, Safdie M, Sotres D, Rivera J: Evaluation of acceptability and intake by women and children of nutritional supplements fortified with three forms of iron. FASEB J 2003;LB371.

Discussion

Dr. Hurrell: I enjoyed your presentation very much. I have several comments on the iron fortification trials that you did. I was wondering what the composition of the complementary food was? You said it was just milk-based. Were the iron absorption studies in adults or were they in infants? The absorption of ferrous sulfate was about 3 times that of fumarate and in most of the adult studies they have been the same.

So if it was an infant study I was wondering why the absorption of fumarate was less than sulfate? Perhaps you could comment on that. Just one other point, and that is that it was not iron EDTA which was studied, but reduced iron plus EDTA which is not actually iron EDTA. So the results which you gave were not from iron EDTA but from elemental iron.

Dr. Neufeld: Yes, it is elemental iron with EDTA. The iron bioavailability studies were conducted in infants. I am not the person to answer the question about the difference between ferrous fumarate and ferrous sulfate. In our group it is Salvador Villalpando who does the isotope bioavailability studies, so I really wouldn't know.

Dr. Abrams: What about the data compared with what was found in Bangladesh?

Dr. Hurrell: I think that is part of the important finding that iron absorption from fumarate is less in infants than we would have expected. The present study agrees exactly with what we reported in Bangladesh where fumarate was found to have 25% the absorption of ferrous sulfate. Most of the guidelines for infant feeding recommend the use of fumarate based on adult studies which show that it is also absorbed as ferrous sulfate. I think that is quite an important finding.

Dr. Abrams: I would also point out that there are methodological problems in assessing the bioavailability of reduced iron because the isotope methods would probably overestimate the absorption. So I would consider 1.4% to be an upper limit of what was truly absorbed because the fumarate is certainly much more accurate than sulfate, and there are huge differences that you found previously. I am glad it has been found, but I think it needs to be discussed as the real impact on how we fortify foods.

Dr. Hurrell: The lower absorption of ferrous fumarate in infants may be due to gastric acid secretion. It may be that infants have less gastric acid than do adults, and perhaps this was one of the reasons why ferrous fumarate is less well dissolved in their gastric juices.

Dr. Tolboom: There is not much difference between the gastric acid secretion in infants compared to older children and adults, only in the very young, about the first weeks perhaps, so thereafter it is the same.

Dr. Barclay: Coming back to the absorption of ferrous fumarate versus ferrous sulfate versus iron EDTA: were these studies done as acute absorption studies or were the children consuming these products for a certain period of time beforehand for adaptation?

Dr. Neufeld: Yes, they were given an adaptation diet. So they were adapted and then given the different forms.

Dr. Zlotkin: The two strategies that have worked in terms of targeted fortification in the Western environment, one of which you emphasized and the other you didn't. It may be because you are unwilling to use the F word in a Nestlé meeting. But I do want to emphasize that two strategies for targeted fortification that have worked extremely well in the West are the targeted fortification of commercial infant foods and the targeted fortification of infant formulas, that is the F word I was referring to. It is worthwhile mentioning that, although everyone in this meeting would of course agree that the primary feeding methodology for infants everywhere in the world should be exclusive breast-feeding for 6 months followed by the appropriate introduction of fortified complementary foods, there are situations in which formula is going to be used in infants who cannot be breast-fed. One of the targeted fortification studies that we should emphasize is that if formula is to be used it should be a fortified formula because there is no doubt and good epidemiologic evidence that fortified formulas do work to prevent at least iron deficiency and probably most micronutrient deficiencies. So the two strategies where there is good proof of efficacy and effectiveness are the commercial formulas and the commercial cereals. A further point I would like to make, and maybe you could respond to this, is that I am not sure that it is necessary for us to reinvent the wheel in each and every country around the world. We do have multinationals who have the capacity to produce fortified cereal products at a relatively low cost, and although it may be possible that national companies can produce the cereal at lower cost, this may be at the expense of quality control. So I do think that one of the strategies that we should think about is ways to make the multinationals continue to distribute their highly fortified cereal products at a very reasonable cost even if that means strategies to subsidize the cost for those who can't pay for it.

Dr. Neufeld: I was hoping that somebody from Nestlé would discuss that because I agree with you. There are many fortified foods but they are not distributed at low cost. They are distributed at exorbitantly high cost for poor families in developing countries. So I don't know the answer to why that hasn't been done already, if we are already assuming that this is a need.

Dr. Guesry: We have been collaborating with the Minister of Health of Chile for more than 20 years in producing first infant formulas and milk fortified with iron and all the trace minerals. So this does exist. I don't know of any infant formula which is not fortified. There are norms and all the industry respects these norms. So discussing the existence or not of fortified infant formula is a bit esoteric to me.

Dr. Zlotkin: If I could just comment. In Canada and the US a percentage of formula is not fortified with iron.

Dr. Neufeld: That is true. In Mexico too there are many formulas not fortified with iron available on the market. You can get formula not fortified with iron if you want to.

Dr. Amancio: What do you think of these rules adopted for fortification?

Dr. Neufeld: I am not that familiar with the food industry development of these products. As we showed, the bioavailability of iron in this milk-based formula is dependent on the form of iron, and all of those estimates were made based on this milk-based formula.

Dr. Armancio: It is also the amount of calcium, as calcium decreases iron bioavailability.

Dr. Neufeld: Right, but I think that would be the major issue. If I understand the industry correctly, the level of iron that is put into the product needs to be set in order to have the amount of available iron. So in this product it has been set considering bioavailability, and what we are trying to deliver to the infants.

Dr. Lozoff: In the last several presentations people have been talking about the need to consider local beliefs and customs about food. I want to mention an analysis we did quite a number of years ago, using the Human Relations Area Files. There was a standard anthropologic sample of 186 pre-industrial societies representing all of the world cultures and communities. In that sample one third of the world societies introduced solid foods before 1 month, one third introduced between 1 and 6 months, and only one third introduced after 6 months. So in the context of our customs and beliefs, there may be room for discussion about the length of exclusive breast-feeding. These anthropologic data are there directly in front of us [1].

Dr. Neufeld: We find similar results in Mexico. Exclusive breast-feeding goes down dramatically at 1 month of age and is almost nonexistent by 3 or 4 months. They are called prevaritas, you give little bits, you give little tastes of food to children, but that happens from very early age. That is one, and second in terms of the importance of this more qualitative research, in terms of the development of a product. What we have found since the implementation of this program is that even though the program suggests that this product is consumed as a pabulum, as a sort of a thicker product, most women give it as a drink. It is the most common means of giving this food to the children. So what we are now working on is trying to decide whether that is all right in terms of the micronutrients that we want the child to consume and, if it isn't, we might have to change the concentration of the product as opposed to trying to convince these people to give the food in a form that they are not accustomed to use. This is one of the areas where local work needs to be done because cans of some kind of commercial product that sells all over the world wouldn't necessarily be consumed at the level that we would want in certain groups of the population.

Dr. Abrams: The low iron formula in the United States is less than 4.5–5 mg/l. So there are only two formulas that I am currently aware of in which the content of iron is 4 mg/l, which is truly low iron. Canada may have some lower ones. In the iron–calcium interaction, a long story we talked about before, there is no evidence whatsoever that complementary foods are a long-term problem.

Mr. Parvanta: Just one question. If I understood you correctly the pabulum is distributed by the government sector to a low income population. What products of similar nutrient quality or nutrient content are there for those populations that are just above that poverty level cutoff but may have just about the same high risk, and are there some products available for them?

Dr. Neufeld: I don't know if you are supposed to say this at Nestlé meetings but it is Gerber. On the Mexican market Gerber infant cereals and Gerber foods are available, but pretty much only the urban upper and middle classes would consider purchasing those because they are expensive; in terms of the general income, very expensive. This pabulum is actually produced by the government. The government has an organization called Liquanza. It is the milk, the government's milk production. So the product itself, the pabulum, and the milk that is the product for women, is produced by the government for this program. They are not for sale on the open market. They are exclusively distributed as part of this program. Now there has been debate about whether they should be, about whether they should put this product on the market, but it hasn't been done.

Dr. Mogrovego: I work at Nestlé in Ecuador and I would like to make some comments. First of all in my country nearly half of the population has iron deficiency. So the government implemented a policy directed to fortifying flour with iron, and also Nestlé mixed formulas and cereals with iron for children, and now we are introducing some complementary foods.

Dr. Neufeld: Distribution as part of a program or for sale?

Dr. Mogrovego: Only for sale, this was introduced 2 weeks ago. We also have communication and education programs for the consumers. We are beginning part of the education program that the government does not do. We are doing something that the government does not do, like working together to build a collaboration with local municipalities in the city. We have to work together: government, industry and policy makers.

Dr. Barclay: I would like to come back to the statement by Dr. Amancio about the relationship between calcium and iron absorption. It really would be doing a great disservice to children to deprive them of iron-fortified milk under the misconception that calcium has a significantly negative impact on iron nutrition. This has already been discussed in detail during this workshop; in the acute short-term studies, sharply increasing calcium intake has a negative effect on iron absorption, but in the long-term the effect is not there. In long-term studies looking at calcium intake versus iron status, there is only a very small negative correlation between calcium intake and iron status. I would even go further by saying that this is even more reason to have some iron in milk products if indeed calcium does have a slightly negative effect on iron absorption.

Dr. Neufeld: Actually in his presentation Dr. Castillo-Durán mentioned that Chile has been fortifying milk with iron and other micronutrients for many years with a positive impact on iron status in the country. Mexico has recently also started fortifying the milk that is redistributed as part of a program to older children; that milk is now fortified with iron and other micronutrients. We are currently evaluating that program too, so in a few years we will be able to say whether we find an impact on iron status.

Mr. Parvanta: Going back to the issue of consumer choice and the statistics. What was mentioned first about the issue of when and the age of the child at which certain micronutrients may be introduced. The reaction to that may be different, very young infants have a different risk versus the older infants. Given the reality of the world, people introduce different products at a much younger age, complementary foods at a very much younger age, what are your thoughts about that? I am not talking about formulas but the other products, about fortification of other products with nutrients, and which nutrients you might want to consider making sure that those foods have some kind of fortification.

Dr. Neufeld: First of all, although this is the reality I think we do need to do interventions to try to encourage exclusive breast-feeding according to the WHO recommendations. Because it is happening that doesn't mean we should not try to encourage people and improve those debates on breast-feeding. That being said, in Mexico a lot of what is given at very early ages isn't necessarily given for food reasons. For example teas are given, sweetened teas are given but they are considered medicinal, they are considered purgatives, and are given for many different reasons. So there are very traditional cultural beliefs and we might not want to influence those, we might not change them. But I don't know if we should be saying if you are going to give sugared tea why don't you give sugared fortified tea? I have to think about that a lot more before I could comment on that. It is the mothers who introduce the foods early by eating the tortillas and letting the child suck on a little bit. So the contribution at those very early ages is really minor, and I don't think we want to give the message that here is a good product, therefore give it early, because it is going to completely contradict our breast-feeding messages.

Dr. Gebre-Medhin: Thank you for an excellent presentation. You are doing remarkable and very important work and we wish you good luck. I would like to reinforce what Dr. Zlotkin and Dr. Guesry have said, and that is I don't think we can get away from the importance, imperative importance of the necessity of breast milk substitutes, commercially produced and enriched. Sweden is a remarkable example of a situation where the prevalence of breast-feeding was very low in the 1940s. It continued that way until the mid 1970s and during this time, in addition to socioeconomic development, it was possible to virtually eradicate all forms of deficiency and malnutrition, and that is no doubt due to the remarkable cooperation between health workers, pediatricians, nutritionists and the industry. I think it is very important to underline these things. As Dr. Guesry has said, it is very important to remember that these products are very carefully regulated, so the question of these products being additionally supplemented or fortified is not relevant at all. Now Sweden has decided to go over to exclusive breast-feeding and extended breast-feeding until the age of 6 months, and they do it extremely well. It is also important for us that wherever breast-feeding is low the solution is not the production of commercially produced formula, rather investing in breast-feeding, more breast-feeding. The problem that we have in Sweden is that we don't know whether we should give complementary feeding at 4 or 6 months as the WHO is recommending. We have no data for that. We need to do more research work on that. So I think the issue is cooperation around this, between different nations, and the production of complementary feedings that are enriched or fortified according to standard procedures, we have to work on that. In addition to that in areas where breast-feeding is not prevalent, our first emphasis, our first advocacy should be to elevate that part and complement it with production of industrially produced products and complementation.

Dr. Lozoff: Why would the government decide to go with ferrous fumarate based on those infant absorption data you had? There was a 4-gram difference in intake, but the absorption was much better.

Dr. Neufeld: It was much more a matter of cost and the characteristics of the supplement because there were physical changes in the product, in the pabulum, the formation of small red and green spots, and if I see green spots I do not give that food to my 1.5-year-old son. So there was that consideration and also ferrous sulfate is considerably more expensive than ferrous fumarate.

Dr. Vasquez-Garibay: The majority of formulas in Mexico, I would say almost all, have between 8 and 12 mg iron/l. The problem as I see it is how to decide to complement the infants between 6 and 12 months of age and to separate them from the 12- to 24-month-olds, because many, the majority, of the infants in rural areas are in fact receiving breast milk as opposite to the urban areas of Mexico. So the problem sometimes with this policy from Mexico is how to decide to give this kind of fortified food to the population which is most vulnerable to malnutrition and iron deficiency.

Dr. Neufeld: This program, Oportunidades, which probably has close to 2 million households in Mexico, including rural areas, was started in rural areas in 1997 but has now expanded to small and large urban areas. The only areas that are not included are the very large metropolitan areas such as Mexico City. As part of the health education and health services, the program itself strongly promotes breast-feeding in the first months of life, very strongly. The messages to improve breast-feeding are very strong. That is something we haven't monitored yet, but we are doing ongoing evaluations and we are always asking about exclusive breast-feeding and what else is given and for how many months. So eventually we will be able to monitor whether there are changes in the population, improvements in the prevalence of breast-feeding. The program was implemented when the WHO recommendations were still 4–6 months, so the program was reexamined a little bit according to that recommendation, providing the supplements as of 4 months of age. They are given universally to all children between 4 and 24 months of age, with the assumption that over 2 years of age the children gradually become more accustomed to the family diet and by 3 years they should be fully accustomed. But certainly there is strong encouragement to improve breast-feeding.

Dr. Bhutta: There are two issues that I would like to highlight. One is that in developing countries there is also the converse of continued exclusive breast-feeding well beyond 6 months of age, which is a real phenomenon at least in the part of the world where I come from. It is not insubstantial, we see it in something closed to 20–30% of the rural populations that we see. So I think the message in terms of appropriate complementary feeding at the right time is critical. I also think there is a need to emphasize that breast-feeding alone is not really the panacea in terms of micronutrient deficiency. In perhaps the most vulnerable part of infancy, micronutrient deficiency doesn't just magically develop at 6 months of age. In parts of the world we have low birth weight, it is a real phenomenon and these infants are significantly micronutrient deficient by 2–3 months of age, if not earlier, and there is the real challenge in terms of what strategies one needs. So I think one needs to throw micronutrient supplementation strategies into the equation for the mothers during pregnancy, and in lactation which may influence breast milk content, and also the real challenge of developing vehicles for giving micronutrients to young infants who are at risk of deficiency such as low birth weight infants well under 6 months of age. I don't think anybody in public health programs has got an answer to that yet.

Dr. Neufeld: I agree completely. I didn't stress it here at all because I was really speaking about complementary feeding but this program does provide the same type of products. It is a beverage to pregnant and lactating women, it is actually a fortified milk drink, with exactly that reason to improve infant stores at birth and to improve maternal micronutrient content of milk.

Dr. Barclay: In reply to your challenge to the food industry to produce lower-cost fortified infant cereals, if we wish to offer products that consumers will want to use, they have to be of a highest nutritional and organoleptic quality. I don't think this can be done cheaply. High-quality products require modern factories, quality ingredients, modern processing techniques, quality control, etc., and so they are going to come at a cost. The other solution that you describe, which has indeed been shown to be effective, is the WIC program whereby high-quality products are made available to those that need them.

Dr. Neufeld: Even if you lower packaging costs?

Dr. Guesry: We have done this. About 25 years ago we started a program called PPP, popularly positioned product. We looked at the raw material, the production cost, the packaging, and the distribution, In Nigeria for example, a soy maize product was launched which was very successful for this reason, and in the Philippines, Indonesia, and so forth. So this could be done, but only to a certain extent because we don't want to compromise on safety and quality.

Reference

1 Lozoff B: Birth and 'bonding' in non-industrial societies. Dev Med Child Neurol 1983;25:595–600.

Pettifor JM, Zlotkin S (eds): Micronutrient Deficiencies during the Weaning Period and the
First Years of Life. Nestlé Nutrition Workshop Series Pediatric Program, vol 54, pp 233–248,
Nestec Ltd., Vevey/S. Karger AG, Basel, © 2004.

Specific Strategies to Address Micronutrient Deficiencies in the Young Child: Supplementation and Home Fortification

Stanley Zlotkin and Mélody Tondeur

Departments of Paediatrics, Nutritional Sciences, and
Centre for International Health, University of Toronto;
Division of Gastroenterology and Nutrition and the Research Institute,
Hospital for Sick Children, Toronto, Ont., Canada

Iron deficiency results from an imbalance between iron uptake, iron utilization and iron loss [1]. It can arise from several risk factors, alone or in combination, such as premature birth or intrauterine growth retardation, early cord clamping, inappropriate use of cow's milk, prolonged exclusive breast-feeding and malabsorption [2, 3]. However, the most important risk factors predisposing infants to iron deficiency and associated anemia include: low intake and low bioavailability of the dietary iron, and the presence of infection and blood loss [4].

During the first 2 years of life, infants require relatively large amounts of iron due to their high growth rate. On average, during the 1st year of life, the birth weight and blood volume of the full-term, normal birth weight infant will triple [5]. By 4–6 months of age, the abundant iron stores present at birth are usually exhausted and thus the full-term, normal birth weight infant can no longer depend on breast milk alone to meet iron requirements [6–8]. It is then recommended to introduce iron-rich complementary foods to meet the infant's iron needs [9]. The selection of weaning foods determines in large part whether an infant will be at risk of developing iron deficiency and associated anemia [6]. Complementary foods that have a low iron content of low bioavailability will increase the risk of iron deficiency.

Strategies to Treat and Prevent Iron Deficiency in Infants

There are three nutrition intervention strategies that can be used to prevent iron deficiency anemia in infants. These include: dietary diversification/ modification; targeted iron fortification of infant foods, and iron supplementation [10, 11]. This article will primarily focus on the latter approach that can also be used to treat iron deficiency anemia [12].

Dietary Diversification/Modification

Dietary diversification/modification is an approach that aims at increasing the availability, access and utilization of foods with a high quantity and high bioavailability of micronutrients [10]. It is the most desirable and sustainable method of preventing micronutrient deficiencies [9]. It can improve and maintain not only iron status, but also nutritional status in general [9]. It involves changes in food production practices, food selection patterns and traditional methods for preparing and processing traditional foods with relatively low technological requirements [10, 13].

In most developing countries, complementary foods are usually prepared as thin gruels made from cereals or starchy roots and tubers high in phytic acid, a major inhibitor of non-heme iron absorption [8, 14, 15]. There are several methods that exist to increase iron intake or enhance the bioavailability of iron in these types of complementary foods. First, strategies such as soaking, fermentation and germination can be used to increase the bioavailability of non-heme iron and other minerals in cereal-based complementary foods by reducing the content of phytic acid [8, 16]. All three methods based at the household level induce some enzymatic and/or non-enzymatic hydrolysis of phytic acid [8]. Second, the bioavailability of non-heme iron in the complementary foods can also be improved by promoting the intake of enhancers of non-heme iron absorption such as ascorbic acid [8, 15, 16]. This can be achieved by consuming fruit juices with the meal or adding fruits and vegetables to the complementary foods. Finally, animal foods such as meat, poultry and fish, and small whole fish bones, all known to enhance non-heme iron absorption, can be added to complementary foods to increase iron intake and bioavailability [6, 8, 15]. However, consumption of such foods is rare in most developing countries due to economic, cultural and religious constraints [10, 16]. In addition, if such foods are available in a household, the adult males of the family will most likely benefit from it over the children because of cultural beliefs [17]. In contrast, in most developed countries, there is a high consumption of animal foods, especially meat, which partly explains why infants have better iron status in these countries [18].

Gibson et al. [8] studied the nutrient content of typical complementary foods used throughout the developing world and concluded that, even if the strategies outlined above are used to improve iron intake and bioavailability, they may not be sufficient to overcome the deficits in iron. The authors proposed fortification of plant-based complementary foods as a solution [8].

Targeted Iron Fortification of Foods

Fortification is defined by the Codex Alimentarius as the addition of one or more essential nutrients to a food, whether or not it is normally contained in the food [19]. Fortification of foods with micronutrients is an effective strategy to increase micronutrient intake of a population [19]. It can be passively targeted to some or all population groups and thus does not necessitate any cooperation from the individuals who benefit from it [16]. An industrial infrastructure is required, and the fortified food needs to be well accepted by the targeted population group and affordable [16].

Iron fortification of complementary foods has been demonstrated to be efficacious and effective in preventing iron deficiency in infants [20, 21]. The reduction in the prevalence of iron deficiency anemia in infants in most industrialized countries during the latter half of the 20th century can be attributed in part to the introduction of iron-fortified complementary foods in the 1960s and 1970s [18, 22]. The success of iron fortification of complementary foods has been limited to developed countries primarily because of the reliance on processed foods by all income groups of the population [12, 23]. In most developing countries, access to industrially processed complementary foods is very limited if not impossible due to the high cost of these foods [9, 14, 15, 18, 24]. This partly explains why infants in the developing world are more affected by iron deficiency and its anemia as compared to infants in developed countries.

Davidsson [15] proposed that new approaches be explored such as fortifying complementary foods at the household level. Such an approach can be achieved through the use of Sprinkles, which will be outlined below.

Iron Supplementation

In clinical practice, once a patient is diagnosed with iron deficiency anemia, treatment with medicinal iron is prescribed accordingly. However, in large-scale public health programs, it is financially and logistically impossible to screen the entire population at risk of developing iron deficiency anemia, especially in developing countries [16]. Therefore, the most cost-effective approach is to give iron supplements to the entire population group at risk [16]. One of the advantages of iron supplementation is that it produces rapid improvements in iron status [16]. The INACG/WHO/UNICEF (1998) recommend providing iron supplementation to all children between 6 and 24 months of age if the prevalence of anemia in this age group is at least 40% or more. Similarly, where the prevalence of anemia in the same age group is lower than 40% but the diet does not include or is limited in iron-fortified complementary foods, it is recommended to provide iron supplements to all infants between 6 and 12 months of age [9, 20]. This type of intervention is aimed at reversing the anemia in anemic individuals and preventing it from developing in the non-anemic individuals [16]. Infants are a challenging group to give iron supplements as they do not have the ability to swallow pills [16]. Two interventions targeting infants will be outlined below, and the advantages and drawbacks of each will be considered.

Iron Drops or Syrup

For the past 150 years or more, oral ferrous sulfate has been the main source of iron for the treatment of iron deficiency anemia [25]. When a proper dose of iron is ingested for a sufficient duration, this intervention has been shown to be efficacious in treating iron deficiency anemia [11]. Oral ferrous sulfate remains the standard against which the efficacy of other forms of iron treatment is compared [17]. For infants and young children, ferrous sulfate in the form of drops or syrup can be used for the treatment and prevention of iron deficiency anemia [16], and the recommended daily dosage for large-scale public health programs is 12.5 mg of iron for normal birth weight babies between 6 and 24 months of age [20]. However, to date, there has been no successful large-scale effectiveness trial with this form of iron therapy [14, 18, 26]. In 1994, an effectiveness trial in Romania involving about 2,000 infants showed a smaller improvement in hemoglobin concentrations than expected with the administration of ferrous sulfate drops once daily for a minimum of 3 months [27]. Low parental compliance in administrating the drops to their infants was suggested to be one of the reasons for the limited reduction in anemia prevalence. Indeed, compliance to long-term ingestion of oral iron drops is known to be poor [14, 16]. Low compliance has been attributed to several factors and these include: the gastrointestinal side effects when the dose of iron is high; the unpleasant and strong metallic taste of the drops which can also stain a child's teeth if not wiped off immediately, and the complicated dispensing instructions, especially for illiterate individuals as the caregiver is required to measure a decimal volume from a dropper [17, 28, 29]. There are also technical disadvantages associated with the use of a liquid iron preparation such as short shelf life and expensive transportation costs due to the weight of the bottles in which the liquid is stored [14, 16]. Another disadvantage of the iron drops is the potential for overdose if a child ingests the entire contents of a bottle [17, 26].

Due to the limitations associated with the use of liquid iron supplements for the treatment and prevention of iron deficiency anemia in infants and young children, a group of UNICEF consultants who met in 1996 encouraged the development of new methods for the delivery of micronutrients, including iron, to infants and young children [14].

Home Fortification

Responding to the UNICEF directive, Zlotkin [11] and his research team at the Hospital for Sick Children developed a new form of iron supplementation in powder form, Sprinkles, containing microencapsulated ferrous fumarate. More recently, instead of being referred to as an iron supplement, Sprinkles have been called a home fortificant [3, 28] or a complementary food supplement [24]. The iron in Sprinkles is encapsulated with a soya-based hydrogenated lipid to prevent any interaction with the food thereby avoiding any changes in color, taste or texture [30]. It is packaged in single-dose sachets which need to be sprinkled once daily onto infants' weaning food immediately before feeding [30]. Each sachet also contains a filler, maltodextrin, in order to add volume to the micronutrients so that they can be easily handled [24]. In vitro dissolution studies were initially performed to ensure the lipid encapsulation would dissolve in the low pH medium of the stomach, thereby leaving the iron available for absorption [11].

Sprinkles have several advantages: (i) other essential micronutrients such as vitamins A, C and D, folic acid, iodine or zinc can be added to the sachets; (ii) the sachets are lightweight and thus are simple to store, transport and distribute; (iii) the sachets are easy to produce, have a relatively low production cost (USD 0.02–0.03, depending on the volume produced) and are easy to use since one does not have to be literate to learn how to use them, and (iv) the potential for overdose is unlikely [26, 28, 30]. In addition, the use of Sprinkles does not require any change in food practices [24] and can help promote the transition from exclusive breast-feeding to complementary foods at 6 months of age. Moreover, Sprinkles can provide the daily dose of micronutrients to each child regardless of the quantity of complementary food that is fed [24]. A drawback is the waste disposal challenge that it poses due to the single-dose sachets [24]. However, packaging is necessary to protect the product from light, air and moisture for a long shelf life [24] and to avoid any potential overdose. The HJ Heinz Company has been assisting in the packaging and distribution of Sprinkles from various manufacturing facilities around the world, and has been producing Sprinkles on a 'cost-recovery' basis for research and humanitarian distribution purposes.

Between 1999 and 2000, two large clinical trials were conducted in rural Ghana to test the efficacy of Sprinkles in treating anemia in infants. The first study was a large randomized controlled trial involving approximately 560 anemic infants aged 6–18 months. The study demonstrated that Sprinkles were as efficacious as the ferrous sulfate drops in treating anemia after 2 months of therapy (table 1) [30]. In both groups, the mean recovery rate was about 60% and there were minimal side effects. In another trial involving about 300 infants 6–18 months of age, between 63 and 75% of the subjects were successfully treated after receiving Sprinkles for a 2-month period [31]. Treatment failure was attributed to several potential factors causing anemia

Table 1. Mean hemoglobin and percent anemic by treatment group at baseline and after 2 months of treatment (mean ± SD)

	Sprinkles (n = 246)	Drops (n = 247)
Baseline		
Hemoglobin, g/l	87 ± 8[a]	87 ± 9
Anemic, %	100[b]	100
Final		
Hemoglobin, g/l	102 ± 16[c]	100 ± 17
Anemic, %	42.3	43.7

[a]Values at baseline (p = 0.63) and final visit (p = 0.23) were similar in both groups.

[b]Values are percent anemic where anemia is defined as hemoglobin values of <100 g/l.

[c]Mean hemoglobin values significantly increased from baseline to the final visit in both groups (p < 0.001).

other than iron deficiency such as: malaria, parasitic infections, *Helicobacter pylori*, gastroenteritis, respiratory infections, or subclinical vitamin A deficiency [30]. To test the safety of Sprinkles, a study in China evaluated hemoglobin and serum ferritin levels in mainly non-anemic preschool children. Of the 285 children who received Sprinkles for 3 months (either 5-days/week or once/week) none had elevated ferritin levels (>400 µg/l) at the end of the trial, thus demonstrating the safety of the intervention [32]. Small trials in northern Canada and Bolivia also demonstrated that Sprinkles were efficacious in treating and preventing anemia when added to complementary foods at the household level (unpublished data).

The acceptability of Sprinkles by both the caregivers and their infants was evaluated in both Ghana and China [28]. It was shown that caregivers found the sachets easy to use and more acceptable than the iron drops. Children did not object to ingesting the foods to which Sprinkles were added because it did not change the taste of the food. In addition, Sprinkles were not associated with any major side effects other than changes in the color of the child's stool which is known to occur with any iron therapy.

The effectiveness of Sprinkles in non-study settings remains to be fully tested [26]. However, a large distribution program in Mongolia sponsored by World Vision Mongolia is currently under way. In this program, the sachets contain iron and vitamin D (with ascorbic acid, folate and zinc) since iron deficiency anemia and vitamin D deficiency rickets are the two most prevalent nutritional problems in young children in Mongolia. Although post-intervention biological outcome indicators (hemoglobin and clinical signs of rickets) have yet to be collected, Sprinkles have been successfully distributed

Table 2. Percent iron absorption from Sprinkles (%)[a,b]

Iron dose[c]	Hb group[d]	
	anemic (Hb <100 g/l)	non-anemic (Hb ≥100 g/l)
30 mg	8.7 (3.5–17.8; n = 19)	4.6 (1.1–12.3; n = 21)
45 mg	7.0 (2.9–13.0; n = 19)	4.5 (1.7–10.6; n = 19)

[a]Values are geometric means, with ranges and number of subjects in parentheses.
[b]Calculated with the use of oral (^{57}Fe) and intravenous (^{58}Fe) stable iron isotopes.
[c]There was no significant main effect for iron dose (p = 0.35).
[d]Significant main effect for Hb group, p < 0.0001.

to about 11,200 infants and young children over a 12-month period with 74% adherence to the intervention [33].

To determine iron absorption from Sprinkles in infants 6–18 months of age, we recently conducted bioavailability studies in Ghana (unpublished data). Results from these studies will help to determine the most appropriate dose of iron to add to a Sprinkles sachet that would be safe and effective in treating and preventing iron deficiency and associated anemia in infants. In our first bioavailability study, a dual stable isotope method was used to determine the amount of iron absorbed from two different doses of iron from Sprinkles provided to both anemic and non-anemic infants. Results indicated that the iron from Sprinkles, when added to a maize-based complementary food, was relatively well absorbed by both anemic and non-anemic infants (table 2). Data also demonstrated that anemic infants absorbed significantly more iron from Sprinkles as compared to non-anemic infants. From a 30-mg dose of iron, with an average iron absorption of about 9%, net absorbed iron was 2.6 mg/day in the anemic infants. In contrast, non-anemic infants had a mean percent absorption of about 5% and thus net absorbed iron was 1.4 mg/day. Therefore, it was concluded that administration of Sprinkles in a maize-based complementary food given to infants would result in significant iron absorption. To further determine the most appropriate dose of iron to add to a Sprinkles sachet, we recently conducted a dose-response randomized controlled trial using three iron doses from Sprinkles (12.5, 20 and 30 mg/day) compared to one dose of ferrous sulfate drops (15 mg/day) provided to infants 6–18 months of age (unpublished data). All infants were anemic at baseline. At the end of the 2-month intervention, the prevalence of anemia in all groups dropped to 45%, with no difference among the groups. Therefore, it was concluded that the three doses of iron from Sprinkles tested were as efficacious as ferrous sulfate drops in treating anemia in infants.

We are currently conducting a randomized controlled trial to determine the optimal intervention time for the treatment of iron deficiency anemia and maintenance of an anemia-free state in 'at risk' infants. One of our earlier studies demonstrated that, when infants are provided with a large dose of iron (80 mg/day) from Sprinkles, the positive effect on anemia status and iron stores may last for as long as 18 months after the intervention [34]. Our current study is designed to determine the long-term impact of Sprinkles on anemia status at a smaller iron dose (12.5 mg/day) when provided to infants for 2, 3 or 4 months.

Based on our clinical trials conducted to date in Ghana, China, northern Canada and Bolivia, and our bioavailability and dose-response studies conducted in Ghana, we have determined that doses of iron from Sprinkles ranging from 12.5 to 20 mg/day are efficacious for the treatment of iron deficiency anemia in infants. We can also conclude that Sprinkles are well accepted by caregivers, with few side effects. Based on our current distribution program in Mongolia, we have demonstrated so far that wide-scale distribution via nongovernmental organizations is feasible.

The etiology of iron deficiency anemia is complex and multifactorial. It can result from a combination of limited iron reserves at birth, blood loss due to infections, and an inadequate source of iron-rich foods. Moreover, it occurs mostly in the poorest countries. The challenge of overcoming this complex social-biological amalgam is daunting. Although international activities, such as the GAIN initiative, are dealing with a part of the problem (i.e. fortification of staple foods), this strategy may not significantly benefit young children (who do not eat enough fortified staple foods). It is somewhat ironic that iron deficiency anemia is a serious public health problem with a potentially simple solution. As researchers, we must think (and act) 'out of the box' to redefine a framework for safe, sustainable, integrated and effective approaches to meet iron needs of 'at risk' infants and children including new systems to deliver iron and other essential problematic nutrients. We must continue to work towards convincing policy-makers and educating the public about the importance of the problem and must improve our abilities to do so. It is essential to form partnerships to address the problem and to use sustainable distribution systems once the right form and type of iron are determined. It is our belief that Sprinkles may be one of the ways of addressing this urgent and preventable problem.

References

1 Yip R: The challenge of improving iron nutrition: Limitations and potentials of major intervention approaches. Eur J Clin Nutr 1997;514:16S–24S.
2 Fleming AF: Iron deficiency in the tropics. Clin Haematol 1982;11:365–388.
3 Zlotkin S: Clinical nutrition: 8. The role of nutrition in the prevention of iron deficiency anemia in infants, children and adolescents. CMAJ 2003;168:59–63.

4 Florentino RF, Guirriec RM: Prevalence of nutritional anemia in infancy and childhood with emphasis on developing countries; in Stekel A (ed): Iron Nutrition in Infancy and Childhood. Nestlé Nutrition Workshop Series. Vevey, Nestec/New York, Raven Press, 1984, vol 4, pp 61–74.

5 Zlotkin S: Iron deficiency in Canadian children? Implications and prevention. Can J Pediatr 1992;4:18–23.

6 Dallman PR: Iron deficiency in the weanling: A nutritional problem on the way to resolution. Acta Paediatr Scand 1986;323:59S–67S.

7 Oski FA: Iron deficiency in infancy and childhood. N Engl J Med 1993;329:190–193.

8 Gibson RS, Ferguson EL, Lehrfeld J: Complementary foods for infant feeding in developing countries: Their nutrient adequacy and improvement. Eur J Clin Nutr 1998;52: 764–770.

9 World Health Organization: Iron Deficiency Anaemia Assessment, Prevention and Control: A Guide to Programme Managers. Geneva, WHO, 2001.

10 Gibson RS, Hotz C: Dietary diversification/modification strategies to enhance micronutrient content and bioavailability of diets in developing countries. Br J Nutr 2001;85: 159S–166S.

11 Zlotkin S: Current issues for the prevention and treatment of iron deficiency anemia. Indian Pediatr 2002;39:125–129.

12 Subbulakshmi G, Naik M: Food fortification in developing countries-current status and strategies. J Food Sci Technol 1999;365:371–395.

13 Hotz C, Gibson RS: Assessment of home-based processing methods to reduce the phytate content and phytate/zinc molar ratio of white maize (Zea mays). J Agric Food Chem 2001;49: 692–698.

14 Nestel P, Alnwick D: Iron/Multi-Micronutrient Supplements for Young Children. Summary and Conclusions of Consultation Held at UNICEF Copenhagen, August 19–20, 1996. Washington, International Life Sciences Institute, 1997.

15 Davidsson L: Approaches to improve iron bioavailability from complementary foods. J Nutr 2003;133:1560S–1562S.

16 DeMaeyer EM, Dallman P, Gurney JM, et al: Preventing and Controlling Iron Deficiency Anaemia through Primary Health Care: A Guide for Health Administrators and Programme Managers. Geneva, WHO, 1989.

17 Dallman PR, Siimes MA, Stekel A: Iron deficiency in infancy and childhood. Am J Clin Nutr 1980;33:86–118.

18 Yip R, Ramakrishnan U: Experiences and challenges in developing countries. J Nutr 2002;132: 827S–830S.

19 Darnton-Hill I, Nalubola R: Fortification strategies to meet micronutrient needs: Successes and failures. Proc Nutr Soc 2002;61:231–241.

20 Stoltzfus RJ, Dreyfuss ML: Guidelines for the Use of Iron Supplements to Prevent and Treat Iron Deficiency Anemia. Washington, International Life Sciences Institute, 1998.

21 Yeung DL, Kwan D: Commentary: Experiences and challenges in industrialized countries. J Nutr 2002;132:825S–826S.

22 Ramakrishnan U, Yip R: Experiences and challenges in industrialized countries: Control of iron deficiency in industrialized countries. J Nutr 2002;132:820S–824S.

23 Mehansho H: Eradication of iron deficiency anemia through food fortification: The role of the private sector. J Nutr 2002;132:831S–833S.

24 Nestel P, Briend A, de Benoist B, et al: Complementary food supplements to achieve micronutrient adequacy for infants and young children. J Pediatr Gastroenterol Nutr 2003;36: 316–328.

25 Andrews NC: Disorders of iron metabolism. N Engl J Med 1999;341:1986–1995.

26 Mora JO: Iron supplementation: Overcoming technical and practical barriers. J Nutr 2002; 132:853S–855S.

27 Ciomartan T, Nanu R, Iorgulescu D, et al: Iron supplement trial in Romania; in Nestel P (ed): Proceedings, Iron Interventions for Child Survival. London, USAID and ICH, 1995, pp 89–98.

28 Schauer C, Zlotkin S: Home fortification with micronutrient sprinkles – A new approach for the prevention and treatment of nutritional anemias. Paediatr Child Health 2003; 82:87–90.

29 Viteri FE: Iron supplementation for the control of iron deficiency in populations at risk. Nutr Rev 1997;55:195–209.
30 Zlotkin S, Arthur P, Antwi KY, Yeung G: Treatment of anemia with microencapsulated ferrous fumarate plus ascorbic acid supplied as sprinkles to complementary (weaning) foods. Am J Clin Nutr 2001;74:791–795.
31 Zlotkin S, Arthur P, Schauer C, et al: Home-fortification with iron and zinc sprinkles or iron sprinkles alone successfully treats anemia in infants and young children. J Nutr 2003;133: 1075–1080.
32 Chan M, Zlotkin S, Yin SA, et al: Comparison of dosing frequency and safety of sprinkles on iron status in preschool children in northern China (abstract). International Nutritional Anemia Consultative Group Symposium, Marrakech, 2003. Washington, International Life Sciences Institute Research Foundation, 2003, p 42.
33 Schauer C, Zlotkin S, Nyamsuren M, et al: Process evaluation of the distribution of micro-nutrient sprinkles in over 10,000 Mongolian infants using a non-governmental organization (NGO) program model (abstract). International Nutritional Anemia Consultative Group Symposium, Marrakech, 2003. Washington, International Life Sciences Institute Research Foundation, 2003, p 39.
34 Zlotkin S, Antwi KY, Schauer C, Yeung G: Use of microencapsulated iron(II) fumarate sprin-kles to prevent recurrence of anaemia in infants and young children at high risk. Bull World Health Organ 2003;81:108–115.

Discussion

Dr. Bloem: In Indonesia one of the problems we are facing with the Sprinkles is actually the approval by the government. Is it a drug; is it part of the fortificant? What kind of approvals are actually needed is very complicated and depends on how the product is named. It is an issue for the industries because they want to have the easiest way to get government approval. Could you comment on that?

Dr. Zlotkin: I think no matter what country one is working in, one will have to get regulatory approval from a government organization, and the regulations as to whether or not Sprinkles will be considered a pharmaceutical agent or a food, I think it is quite dependent on the individual country and may in fact differ from country to country. For example in Canada we have registered Sprinkles. In fact we had to register Sprinkles in order to do research with them and they had to be registered as a drug, despite the fact that there are no pharmaceutical agents in them, only minerals and vitamins and a bland excipient. In Canada all vitamin and mineral products have to be registered as drugs. So again to answer your question, no matter where you are working, whether in Indonesia or Canada, one has to go through the process of registration. It can readily be done but really depends on the individual requirements of the particular country.

Dr. Bloem: Do you think that international agencies can help to support this process? If we have global registration or something like that, is it easier to get these approved at the country level?

Dr. Zlotkin: I am not sure I can answer that question because I have limited experience with the regulatory approval process. My feelings are that countries are pretty strict about what one has to do with regard to registering a product in each individual country. Possibly the people from Nestlé who have more experience with the registration of products might be able to comment, but I feel that it has to be done on a country-by-country basis and there is probably no way of getting around it.

Dr. Bhutta: Once Sprinkles are introduced in developing countries one of the social science challenges would be getting mothers and families to accept this as not being a drug. Have you given thought to the possibility of formulating these in a way that they could become part of the food preparation process, rather than something that just gets added at the end? If under circumstances where cereals or other complementary foods are made in household settings, this could be part of the cooking process or part of the addition during the course of preparation rather than something that is sprinkled on top at the end. Are there any technical limitations to that?

Dr. Zlotkin: In terms of the micro-encapsulation process, if one wants to ensure that the soluble form of iron does not come in contact with the food there are multiple methods of encapsulation, some of which will not be impacted by cooking. The problem is that the dissolution properties of the various micro-encapsulated minerals are quite different, depending on what you use to encapsulate your mineral. For example you can use polymers that will be quite inert. The problem will be for iron which is absorbed quite proximal in the small intestine. If in fact the encapsulate did not dissolve in the low pH of the stomach and did not dissolve in the duodenum, there would probably be close to zero iron absorption. So I do see some significant technical issues around developing a product that would be organoleptically acceptable that could be used in a cooking process. However bioavailability would be a problem.

Mr. Parvanta: I understand in Thailand that the premix that comes with instant noodles is being fortified, and it has been done with iron as well. Does this relate to the comment about using it in the preparation of foods? The other question I have is related to the point of not making a medical product. As was discussed in Ottawa recently, the regulatory agencies determine whether something is a pharmaceutical product versus a food product and that is important. But even if it turns out to have a pharmaceutical classification, I think the channel of delivery is going to be very important to eliminate, reduce or minimize this medical approach. But as far as prevention trials are concerned, I wonder if you have considered if the lack of response was related to the mothers sharing the dose among the other children in spite of the supplement dosage being only for one child, the index child, as we have found in Romania? Have you considered this because it may be an issue of parents distributing the product to others?

Dr. Zlotkin: It is interesting you mention the Romanian study because that is probably the only study that has identified a slightly efficacious response to a large scale distribution of iron drops, although it wasn't a very powerful response. Despite the fact that we target children under the age of 2 years because that is the most vulnerable population, there is no question that an older child or a pregnant woman would not be harmed in any way from ingesting Sprinkles. If the cost were right and if the message was that this had to be a family intervention, there is absolutely no reason why it could not be provided to other members of the family. Again I think it makes most sense that we primarily pay attention to the child under 2 years because that is of course the highest risk age group, but there is no reason at all why it could not be given to the entire family.

Mr. Parvanta: The point is that you have to take that into account if you do those trials. You may have to give them a larger supply than you would ordinarily think.

Dr. Pettifor: In many developing countries the problem of associated malnutrition is a key feature of young children and acid production tends to be relatively low in those children, as I understand it. Are there any data to suggest that your micro-encapsulated iron is equally well absorbed in that situation?

Dr. Zlotkin: I totally agree that children with malnutrition may not have normal gastric pH. The only point I can make is that the population that we chose for our labeled bioavailability study was a typical population of children living in central Ghana. They were chosen according to age and their initial hematologic status. We really did feel that this population represented a typical group of infants. Their Z scores were around −1.5 and −2, which was typical in that population. If we had chosen a population whose Z scores were −0.5 or 0, it might have been a healthier population and we might have achieved a different rate of absorption. The important point is that our initial concern was that because we were using a micro-encapsulated form of iron we really didn't know what the bioavailability would be, and because we were using fumarate and because of the controversy around the absorption of fumarate versus sulfate, we didn't have any notion about what absorption would be other than we thought it would be very low. So we were quite reassured by finding that in the population with hemoglobins of <100 g/l the mean absorption was around 9%. Based on this absorption value we could then logically decide on the dose of iron to use for efficacy studies. Based on the percentage absorption we randomized children into 3 different doses of iron as Sprinkles (12.5, 20 and 30 mg doses), compared to an equivalent dose of ferrous sulfate drops. Our intervention was for 2 months and the subjects were all anemic infants. The response to anemia was identical in all 4 groups including the ferrous sulfate group. The 12.5-mg dose group actually did just as well as the 30-mg dose. These data suggest that infants have the ability to upregulate iron absorption when they need it.

Dr. Pettifor: I was thinking particularly from the multi-mineral supplement point of view that it may be considered useful in the management of malnourished children as a hospital treatment instead of providing powders or other forms of micronutrient supplement. In such a situation iron should not be provided in the initial stages.

Dr. Zlotkin: To be very clear, this product has no calories, no protein and no macronutrients. It could be used quite reasonably with a corn soya blend or corn wheat blend, if these types of cereal were used in the rehabilitation of malnourished children.

Dr. Guesry: I agree with everything you say but I would like to make two comments, one related to the fact that it would be either a drug or a food supplement. I think it is linked to the claim that you are going to make, and this is very universal. If you say this product is to treat the disease, which is iron deficiency anemia, then it is a drug. So that is something you have to think about. The other aspect is related to business and cost because I think the most expensive part of the product would be the packaging, the quality control, the shipping and the distribution. In the price you mentioned, I don't think everything was accounted for, so you have to increase it a little bit. One way to reduce all these variable costs would be to try a weekly version of 30 mg/week which would be a very good way to decrease the packaging, quality control, shipping and distribution cost. So I would encourage you to go that way rather than the everyday dose because my rough calculation is that for a family it would be about USD 10, perhaps a little bit more than USD 10/year/baby.

Dr. Zlotkin: Just let me comment. The price included quality control, it did not include shipping, nor did it include distribution which of course is a significant cost, for sure. We envision that Sprinkles will be used for prevention of micronutrient deficiencies. We believe that a 2-month intervention during the first 24 months of life will be adequate. Thus the estimated cost is closer to USD 1 per year, not USD 10 per year. In terms of the once weekly dose versus daily, Beaton [1] did a meta-analysis both for infants and children, women, pregnant women. It seems that a once weekly dose may be efficacious but only in situations where the dose is being given out in a school, in a daycare, or in a crèche where one can be absolutely certain that a responsible person is providing the iron once a week, because with the once-a-week dose, if you have missed 1 dose you have actually missed 2 weeks, and if you have missed 2 doses you have missed 3 weeks. So Beaton's conclusion in the meta-analysis was that there was evidence of efficacy but only when the iron supplement was distributed or given out in a controlled manner.

Dr. Mannar: Given that the whole technology is very much dependent upon the specification of the individual nutrients, especially iron, and also the type of encapsulation and the type of packaging, I think it becomes very critical that all these are very precisely specified. I am just concerned that once you say that this works and countries start tendering for this process and they say we want a powder with so much iron and so much vitamin A, you could easily get someone just mixing these in a crude manner and putting them into small sachets, and you might have quite different bioavailability and other characteristics.

Dr. Zlotkin: I think that is an interesting question. There is nothing to prevent an inferior Sprinkles product from being produced and distributed. I am not sure that this is different from many other products in some developing countries where there is not much quality control. It does bring up another issue I should have mentioned: the technology for putting the micronutrients into the sachet is very simple. Most developing countries have the technology for putting either spices or foods into small sachets. It takes a machine that has the capacity to make and fill a sachet, and again this is not a high tech type of production facility. So part of our long-term plan is to transfer the technology to countries in the developing world so that there would be the facility, for example in Bangladesh, to produce it locally.

Dr. Tolboom: I am worried: Ghana, tropics, malaria of course. Did you look at the malaria outcome in your interventions?

Dr. Zlotkin: Yes, we examined malaria status and parasite load. We also looked at the number of fever episodes. There were no differences between groups. However, I have to emphasize that in these anemic populations we did not have a control group, for ethical reasons.

Dr. Tolboom: Because of the folic acid, I get a little bit of a 'black box feeling', about the effects of supplementation on severity of malarial illness.

Dr. Zlotkin: Since we did not include a control or placebo group, it really is not possible for us to say that the outcome in terms of malaria status or the number of fevers, would have been different in a similar population receiving no intervention. However, we feel quite strongly that since we are dealing with an anemic population we have an obligation not to use a placebo group.

Dr. Bloem: When we started the program about 2.5 years ago, we didn't want to import Sprinkles so we started to think about how we could produce it in Indonesia. We got the funding to do the trial and to look at sustainable approaches to distribute this product. We are almost ready to start, but it took us about 2.5 years to actually bring it to Indonesia which is a quite sophisticated country with a lot of big industries when it comes to this kind of thing. So I would be a little bit cautious when it comes to how you implemented it in a country like Bangladesh when it comes to quality control, when it comes to all these other issues, because it took us a long time.

Dr. Bhutta: Have you considered the possibility of alternative methods of dispensing? Why does it have to be a sachet, is it technically possible to put a multi-dose dispenser of the kind that is used for sugar dispensing? That would save substantial costs and make it somehow or other more acceptable to families as a non-medical food-based intervention.

Dr. Zlotkin: In Pakistan for example, sachets are used for foods and condiments more than medicine. So I don't think that the use of a sachet is necessarily associated with the delivery of pharmaceuticals. Our concern really with iron is to give enough

245

but not too much, so that any dispensing methodology that has the potential to be easily misused by an older child in a family or any one had us extremely worried. In Canada the most common death from poisoning is from iron overdose and toxicity, and it is because young children can get into the iron that their mothers are using and typically the prenatal supplements contain 60 mg iron, so iron toxicity is certainly a real issue that is associated with death. So our great concern was to ensure that (1) the intervention is easy to use, and (2) there is absolutely safety. We have considered other methods of delivery. For example it has been suggested that it might be more acceptable if Sprinkles were sweet. Children would like it more. But again the response to that is that if it is sweet it is more likely to be ingested inappropriately as a treat, and we would again have the problem of potential toxicity. So we feel that the delivery via the sachet is a way to ensure safety. One would have to ingest something like 30 or 40 sachets even to approach toxicity, and because they have a very neutral taste, they are neither sweet nor particularly pleasant tasting but also not unpleasant, we really think that there would not be the incentive for an older child to use them as a treat.

Dr. Gebre-Medhin: Some concerns have been raised and the first is the issue of the medication and the concepts and thoughts of mothers and families that this is no longer a nutrient but a medicine. The second is the risk of it being used in other age groups and, as Dr. Lönnerdal said, landing in the hands of those who don't need it. The third, the one that concerns me most, is the use of this for purposes other than intended. The minute there is a sachet out and some benefits are attributed to it, it may be used for purposes of enhancing one or the other or a third thing in the community. Finally there is the risk of allegations that such sachets cause other problems, in other words families and individuals and groups may very well associate other complications to the addition of this sachet. There is pedagogical problem here that may be very important.

Dr. Zlotkin: Concerning the last question, a component of the social marketing strategy would be to warn parents that, for example, the color of the stool may change when the fortificant is added to food. It is our experience that if you warn parents in advance of a potential change in the infant, and again I am not saying an adverse change because I think coloring the stool dark is not really an adverse change, but if we warn parents that this is likely to occur then the chances of the parents associating it with a negative connotation are less. It is quite possible, and as you well know if an infant in the developing world has 7 or 9 episodes of gastroenteritis per year there is no doubt that a baby is going to have diarrhea at some point while taking Sprinkles. Again I think part of the social marketing strategy would have to include a comment that Sprinkles are not going to prevent every disease in your child and your child is still going to get diarrhea, a cold or an upper respiratory tract infection. Again I think the social marketing strategy has to address those issues. In terms of the medication, families are quite used to adding things to the foods as condiments. We add salt to our food, we add sugar to our food, and in fact sugar is a good example because at least in the Western world we often find sugar in a sachet and most people would not say that by adding sugar to a food you are medicating the process by adding it to a food. So our hope is that it will not be medicalized but that it is being put forward as a food based strategy, not as a supplement but as a home fortificant. Because there is experience with using condiments, it is hoped that it will be recognized as a condiment or a fortificant but not as a medical supplement. It is quite different from the delivery of pills or capsules or even syrups or liquids for young children.

Dr. Gibson: One question I would like to ask you is what was the food vehicle that was used to test iron bioavailability? Was it refined maize porridge?

Dr. Zlotkin: We used the exact recipe that we got from the mothers in the village. It consisted of 80% maize, 10% groundnuts and 10% beans.

Dr. Gibson: I would like to make a comment in relation to a study that I am involved in with a group in Thailand. We have just completed an efficacy trail on a seasoning powder which is sold in sachets with noodles, and certainly in that setting in Thailand it hasn't been perceived as a medicine. An efficacy trial was done in schoolchildren and the results are being analyzed at the moment. The seasoning powder is fortified with iron, vitamin A, iodine and zinc and it was very well accepted.

Dr. Zlotkin: The reason I was slightly hesitant in talking about acceptability is that it is very difficult to assess acceptability in an efficacy study. We had field workers in the village who were reminding the mothers what to use. It wouldn't be fair to say that this was a typical free-living population. The families and children were randomized into a drops group and a Sprinkles group. The same questions were asked of both groups and inevitably the number of parents who complained about the drops was relatively high and inevitably the number of parents who accepted the Sprinkles without any complaints at all was also relatively high. I don't have the final results of our study in Mongolia, so I can't tell you what they are. I have been there twice and I visited the people who are using them, and although they probably said it because it was me asking the question, anecdotally they were extremely well received. The child is very passive in this case and really doesn't know that he is ingesting the micronutrients because the taste or the look of the food to which it has been added doesn't change, so I would expect that with a reasonably good social marketing program we could get families to accept the intervention.

Dr. Gibson: Certainly the seasoning powder in Thailand has been on the market for some time although its efficacy and effectiveness have not been formally tested. It has been used by families over a number of years already.

Mr. Parvanta: Here is a crazy idea for you following the discussion about the cost of transportation and distribution. Recently I heard some news, I don't know if it is true or not, that in Brazil the distributors of Mary Kay cosmetics reach the farthest villages in the deepest parts of the Amazon jungle, and then in the heart of Atlanta in the Coca Cola Museum one of their pieces of promotion is that they also reach the farthest villages of the Amazon. I am wondering if there is some way that we could combine distribution. I think you said that one of the strengths of the Sprinkles is that it is so light, you can carry large amounts and maybe Coca Cola wouldn't mind putting a few on their trucks with no cost, strange idea, but to get it into these deepest villages.

Dr. Tolboom: The lack of controls in your study still keeps bothering me. You said it was unethical to do that, but you could have control villages without any intervention. I mean is the problem so widespread that you could not get control villages, because still I would like to find out what you are doing exactly in terms of malaria morbidity and mortality because I still think it is a relevant point.

Dr. Zlotkin: I don't disagree with your point. I think it is an important question because we are adding iron. Of course bacteria proliferate in the presence of iron, and my understanding from the analysis of the various studies that have looked at the impact of iron supplementation on malaria is that the current recommendation is that if you are treating malaria in an area where iron deficiency is also present that it is quite acceptable to both treat the malaria as well as provide an iron supplement. Again Dr. Lönnerdal made the point that there is a difference between the response to a supplement that is often taken on an empty stomach versus what may be a food-based product where the response may not be identical. But I think the question is very important, it just can't be answered with the design we used.

Dr. Tolboom: But the control village, would you agree with control villages? To have a control village in which you don't intervene? That is what was done in Tanzania, villages where no intervention was used at all.

Dr. Zlotkin: It is not a perfect design but it certainly could be done.

Reference

1 Beaton GH: Iron needs during pregnancy: Do we need to rethink our targets? Am J Clin Nutr 2000;72(suppl):265S–271S.

Pettifor JM, Zlotkin S (eds): Micronutrient Deficiencies during the Weaning Period and the
First Years of Life. Nestlé Nutrition Workshop Series Pediatric Program, vol 54, pp 249–262,
Nestec Ltd., Vevey/S. Karger AG, Basel, © 2004.

Crystal Ball Gazing: Micronutrients for All by 2015

M.G. Venkatesh Mannar

The Micronutrient Initiative, Ottawa, Ont., Canada

In ways that would be unrecognizable to history, we are living in the most exciting of times. Using intuition, imagination, and creative ideas over the millennia of human past, and scientific methodologies especially over the last two centuries, human beings have succeeded in developing methods of agricultural management, disease control among living beings, means of communication, transport, interconnecting the world, looking after the environment, and installing systems of diffusion of knowledge through experience, education and research to effect an overall improvement in the quality of life. Even more than effective improvement, the immense potential for it has been opened up for the future.

Given all of this progress it is tragic that we have allowed something as basic as malnutrition and micronutrient malnutrition to persist in many parts of the world – for at least half a century too long.

It is therefore appropriate that at the end of a symposium in which we have heard from some of the most eminent experts on the subjects of epidemiology, etiology, and the impacts of nutritional deficiency which should never have been allowed to persist for so long, that we reflect on some of the underlying issues and strategies that will enable us to quickly and effectively eliminate the scourge of micronutrient deficiency from the face of the earth.

We have heard that the vitamins and minerals that the human body needs have to be taken in microgram or milligram quantities in daily diets for human well being. In such minute quantities they are essential as constituents of vital enzymes and proteins for the normal processes of growth, development, maintenance and resistance to infection. To call them micronutrients could be in conformity with the minute quantities needed, but it is certainly not in consensus with the nature and extent of the damage. In their absence individuals and families suffer serious consequences expressed as increased mortality, morbidity and disability rates; communities and nations suffer losses in human potential and unaffordable social and economic costs.

The physiological roles of micronutrients have been known for a considerable period of time and were prominent in the early history of nutritional science. Their deficiencies have long since been brought under control in the industrialized world, while they continue to persist in large parts of the developing world. The young, the poor and the female in some cultures are the worst affected, but micronutrient malnutrition is a pervasive phenomenon and its consequences are felt at all stages of the human life cycle [1].

As recently as the 1970s and 1980s in many countries micronutrient malnutrition was considered a symptom to be treated when clinical signs are evident, which was often too late. It was the key research during those decades that clearly exposed both the pervasiveness of the problem and its far-reaching consequences in terms of survival, health, social and economic impacts. It became increasingly evident that clinical signs were only the tip of the iceberg – they concealed a much larger and invisible problem that affected many more people. It was only in 1985 that Prof. Basil Hetzel coined the phrase 'iodine deficiency disorders' to replace the term 'goiter', and in the late 1990s the phrase 'vitamin A deficiency disorders' was proposed by IVACG to refer to the range of disabilities caused by insufficient intake.

The turning point really came at the World Summit for Children in 1990 when 69 heads of state met in New York and approved a plan [2] that included 7 major goals and 26 supporting/sectorial goals of which 3 related to micronutrient malnutrition. Although the micronutrient goals seemingly constituted only a fraction of all the goals, they were the cutting edge, they were amenable to fulfillment in the shortest possible time, and their cost-benefit ratio was highly favorable. They also underscored the unique opportunity we had to provide nutritional well-being as fundamental to sustainable human development on a scale not witnessed before. The summit goals became a mission for the entire UN family, for the aid agencies, for governments and non-governmental organizations. Policy makers realized that in the wider picture technological problems are not nearly as serious as operational ones related to making programs work in communities where deficient people live. Issues of supply and logistics, communications and community participation, partnership building across a wide spectrum of players – public and private – were recognized as equally important to ensure the success and sustainability of efforts to eliminate micronutrient deficiencies in large populations.

The 1990s witnessed a spectacular expansion of the world economy as the technological innovations and dismantling of trade barriers known as globalization gathered strength. These forces have brought tremendous new opportunities but also raised new or greater challenges in terms of economic or political instability. But the massive benefits and opportunities generated by globalization failed to eliminate the micronutrient malnutrition problem.

While there was progress on the nutrition and micronutrient front, it still fell far short of the expectations. Today 70% of the world has access to iodized salt. 50% of the world's under-5 children receive at least one high-dose of vitamin A. But the problem of iron deficiency persists unabated. It affects several billion people and is one of the top 10 preventable risks for disease, disability and death in the world today.

In 2002 world leaders reconvened at the UNGA Special Summit for Children. They reaffirmed their commitment to '... achieve sustainable elimination of iodine deficiency disorders by 2005 and vitamin A deficiency by 2010; reduce by one third the prevalence of anemia, including iron deficiency, by 2010; and accelerate progress towards reduction of other micronutrient deficiencies, through dietary diversification, food fortification and supplementation ...' [3].

Today it has become clear that our goal is beyond simply food security, based on per capita calorie availability. Rather, it is a comprehensive nutrition security, based on an affordable diet of high nutritional quality – a diet whose outcome is judged by mental acuity and economic productivity rather than simple physical survival. This amounts to a dietary quality revolution every bit as profound as the green revolution of the 1960s.

As we look forward, what dramatic action could we take that would really make a difference? How could we move the world towards eliminating the problem within, say, the next decade – within the broader development framework of globalization (in trade, capital flows and environmental issues) and localization (in terms of decentralization of political power to sub-national levels of government and growing urbanization) [4]?

Let us gaze at the crystal ball and see what the future has in store for us in order to eliminate micronutrient malnutrition in terms of: (1) technology; (2) delivery; (3) policy, and (4) social mobilization.

Technology

The task at hand is relatively simple on one level. We need to give all essential micronutrients to everyone on this planet in one form or the other on a permanent, continuous and self-sustaining basis. Strategies have to be appropriate to the need and the use of existing delivery systems and available technologies where they serve the need. In addressing micronutrient malnutrition a combination of interventions involving the promotion of breast-feeding, dietary modification (e.g., improving food availability and micronutrient bioavailability, and increasing food consumption), food fortification and pharmaceutical supplementation will need to be emphasized and implemented in a complementary manner.

They need to go well beyond traditional health and nutrition systems and based upon enabling people and communities so that they will be capable of arranging for and sustaining an adequate intake of micronutrients, independent of external support. Strategies are necessarily to be multi-sectorial and integrated interventions with strong social communications, evaluation and surveillance components.

In the best of worlds the nutrients should come through the food we eat. Perhaps we will get there one day, but we are not there yet. For several reasons – economic, geographic, social, cultural – this has not been a practical solution, and even if this were possible there are issues related to the lack of bioavailable minerals and vitamins from staple diets. This is exacerbated by the fact that commonly consumed foods and beverages (rice, wheat, corn, legumes, tea and coffee) are high in inhibitors and low in enhancers of micronutrient absorption.

Let us look at some of the opportunities that could help eliminate the stealthy scourge of micronutrient malnutrition.

Multiple Micronutrient Interventions. Increasingly the thrust will be in the direction of multiple micronutrient interventions. Addressing more than one deficiency through a single intervention is more effective and efficient than isolated and potentially competitive control of each micronutrient individually. Multiple micronutrient deficiencies, the required technical skills, facilities and information resources frequently overlap and interventions to address several deficiencies could often be delivered through the same system.

Fortified Foods for All. A significant proportion of cereal flours can be fortified with essential vitamins and minerals: wheat flour in the Americas, Europe and Asia, corn flour in Sub-Saharan Africa and Central America, cooking oils and fats, sugar, milk and condiments can become important vehicles through innovative technologies that permit fortification both on a large and a small scale. Salt, the ubiquitous part of our diets, can carry a range of nutrients including iodine, iron, zinc and vitamins as well.

Where Fortified Foods Don't Reach. Here we could use multiple ways to deliver micronutrients to homes to enable mothers to either add them to the cooking pot or to mix them into the food they feed their infants. These are labeled as complementary food supplements [5], are available as water-dispersible or crushable tablets, Sprinkles or spreads that can be added to complementary foods just before feeding infants and young children. They are designed to provide 1–2 recommended daily allowances of vitamins and minerals in a small volume, at a low cost and are easily integrated into existing food practices.

Special Needs. Certain vulnerable groups may need supplements for an indefinite period of time. Safe motherhood programs need to address the multiple deficiencies that women face through improvements in intake, preferably through optimal diets. However, where dietary intake is unable to meet the women's requirements, multiple vitamin and mineral supplements should be considered as an intervention to improve safe motherhood, pregnancy outcome and the health of breast-fed infants and their mothers.

Biofortified Foods. Breakthroughs in plant breeding and nutritional genomics could simplify and hasten the development of nutrient-rich varieties and improve nutrient availability in staple crops such as rice, maize, sweet potato, cassava, common beans and wheat. Advanced biotechnology tools, such as genome mapping and marker-assisted selection could enable us to identify, select, and transfer desirable traits, including those linked to high micronutrient content (iron, zinc and β-carotene), from one variety to another with or without transfer of genes across species [6]. By producing plants that are dense in minerals and vitamins, a process referred to 'biofortification', we could have crop varieties with improved nutritional content in the staple foods people already eat. This can be a feasible means of reaching malnourished populations in relatively remote rural areas, with limited access to health programs through which supplements are channeled or to commercially marketed fortified foods.

The key issue that is yet to be fully resolved is whether we limit our efforts to biofortification through conventional plant breeding or extend it to provide novel traits for breeding that are not available in the existing germplasm (β-carotene in rice endosperm as an example). The expanding ability to manipulate provitamin A carotenoid synthesis (e.g. Golden Rice), vitamin E synthesis and mineral composition in plants can be directly traced to advancements in nutritional genomics and exemplifies the power and potential benefits of the approach.

The argument for genetically modified crops is that breeding is limited to the variations that are generally present in the germplasm but not anything beyond the breeder's germplasm. Furthermore breeding could be time consuming. With biotechnology, it is possible not only to increase the level of the micronutrient but also ensure its bioavailability. For example, the bioavailability of β-carotene could be enhanced by its being engineered into an oil seed like canola, soybean, germ of corn and wheat thus providing the appropriate matrix for absorption of a lipophilic molecule.

We have the two strong positions on this issue. Anti-biotechnolgy activists have tapped into a powerful rhetoric as old as Dr. Frankenstein – add to this modern scientific and regulatory disasters like thalidomide and mad cow disease, plus actors in laboratory coats hawking everything from soap to diet supplements, and you have a profoundly skeptical public. So on one side, we have children in monarch butterfly costumes accompanied by activists with a shaky premise; on the other, a scientist with charts, graphs and a compelling body of evidence. In the age of the 10-second sound bite, who wins? While the public may be unsophisticated in their knowledge, they are extremely sensitive to attempts to manipulate their opinion. The ultimate aim is not propaganda, or even persuasion. It is making sure the correct information is heard, so people can make informed decisions.

Rapid Assessment Techniques. These can enable micronutrient status (iron, vitamin A, zinc, iodine) to be determined from a blood spot sample collected on a filter paper.

Supplement Assimilation. Where people have side effects or difficulties in absorption we have slow release tablets or patches that could be taken weekly or twice a week. We could probably develop a tablet to be taken once every month or once every 6 months.

Delivery

For several decades in the past the primary responsibility for the health and nutritional well-being of the people was viewed as that of the government or the public sector. For too long, nutrition issues were dealt with in isolation by different sectors and organizations. This lack of communication and collaboration across sectors to address problems in a unified manner was in part responsible for the poor nutritional outcomes in many countries.

In the recent past we have seen the roles of government and private industry change dramatically. Food production and consumption patterns are shifting to more centrally processed and packaged food products with increasing attention to food safety, hygiene and quality. The food business is becoming more global with new trade agreements accelerating the worldwide movement of food technology, products and capital. Markets in developing countries are providing unprecedented opportunities to attract private investment and entrepreneurial energy. Publicly funded food and nutrition programs are gaining from past experience and improving in effectiveness. In this new environment governments, food companies, scientific establishments and development agencies are beginning to work together on ensuring adequate nutrition status for all. The public sector is recognizing the need to engage and stimulate the private sector to contribute to the public good and motivate it to do more. In turn the private sector is seeing value in expanding its market through penetration of lower-income groups that are much larger in size but offer slimmer profit margins. The world is going to increasingly see such collaboration in several sectors of human development, and nutrition could be at the forefront of that movement.

The challenge therefore for all of us is to consider how we can channel the capacities of the private sector – and the huge potential for good – in a constructive and responsible manner. Clearly adequate regulations by both governments and international bodies – and public–private partnerships – must be in place to prevent any actions that might in any way detract from the goal of reducing malnutrition. Along with such checks and balances, both government and industry need to devote more energy and ingenuity to build such an alliance that could exploit the potential for common good and ensure a significant corporate contribution to improve the condition of malnourished people.

Governments, businesses and the nonprofit sector can engage in several types of collaborative arrangements for public good. For ease of understanding

I will categorize these [7] as (1) core business engagement (a public private partnership); (2) supportive partnerships, and (3) philanthropy (public private not-for-profit arrangements).

Core Business Engagement

In core business engagement the private sector contributes to the public good through the redesign and marketing of its products and services.

(1) Fortification of staple foods with nutrients is a good example of a collaboration that should be led by the public sector in active consultation with the private sector. It would identify the deficiencies to be addressed, the foods to be fortified, levels of nutrient addition and standards to which they should be fortified. The initiative should also set clear norms for quality assurance, product certification, product promotion, social marketing, monitoring and evaluation.

(2) The production and marketing of industrially produced fortified complementary foods targeted at 6- to 24-month-old infants is another example. Such foods could ensure higher energy density, protein quality and micro-nutrient bioavailability, not to mention the safety and convenience. Government encouragement and guidance could encourage the food-processing sector to produce a nutrient-dense, low-bulk complementary food at affordable prices and a fraction of the price of branded infant foods.

(3) Food companies can also work with governments to produce processed foods for distribution in public institutional feeding programs.

(4) Experience in several South-East Asian countries like Vietnam, Thailand and Indonesia has shown that more and more people are able and willing to purchase nutritional supplements if they are properly developed, fairly priced and encouraged by the government.

(5) Public and private sectors can collaborate to lower the prices of conventional foods such a fish, dairy products and land-based crops of nutritional significance. For instance, corporate experience can be helpful in designing and carrying out projects for more effective processing, storage, transport and distribution.

(6) There is significant potential for donation of genetic information patents held by private corporations to the public domain. This could support the improvement of nutritional quality of a range of cereal and tuber crops.

Supportive Partnerships

In supportive partnerships, the private sector offers services not necessarily central to its business actions: (1) corporate distribution facilities can be used to market low cost foods produced under government programs; (2) skills of private industry can be marshalled to devise education programs that create greater nutrition awareness, and (3) industrial research capabilities and facilities can be made available for government programs.

Philanthropy

In addition to private sector involvement in products from which they expect to benefit financially, there are growing instances of private philanthropic support for nutrition where the donors do not have a direct connection or interest in the food and pharmaceutical industry. Recent examples include support from the UN Foundation created by Ted Turner for a range of preventative health and population programs, support from the Bill and Melinda Gates Foundation for the establishment of the Global Alliance for Improved Nutrition.

Private voluntary organizations such as the Rotary have been key partners in the Universal Child Immunization effort. Lions Clubs have done yeomen service to deliver eye care. More recently at the global level Kiwanis International has adopted the elimination of insulin-dependent diabetes as its worldwide service project and raised in excess of USD 75 million to support the effort. Can we draw these and other organizations to expand their support to nutrition programs?

Policy

We have also realized that addressing micronutrient malnutrition cannot be through stand-alone vertical programs. Also we became much more effective in inserting nutrition into broader health and social development goals rather than waiting for them to be addressed in order to serve the cause of nutrition. We must focus increasingly on 'intersecting' micronutrient programs with major development challenges. These include: HIV/AIDS, malaria, hookworm and reproductive health, and emergency programs. Additionally nutrition should be included on the agenda of important reproductive and child health initiatives; vitamin A deficiency on the agenda of the ophthalmologists, and iron deficiency a priority in early child development, school health and maternal health programs.

Social Mobilization

An effective communications campaign supported by the government should necessarily accompany any major micronutrient effort in order to gain the understanding and support of key sectors from policy makers and legislators to medical professionals, health workers and consumer groups. The communications component should consist of the following.

(1) Presentations to the highest policy-making bodies to ensure continued national commitment and national effort.

(2) Communication with public health professionals, government officials at every level, and private industry and trade to obtain their understanding and support.

(3) Communication research among the consumers to understand the perceptions with respect to the micronutrient deficiency problems and the use of fortified foods.

(4) Dissemination of effective messages through appropriate channels to the target populations in order to educate, persuade and motivate them to accept the new product and to change their behavioral patterns. Subconscious consumer demand for micronutrients needs to be made conscious and directed to appropriate foods and pharmaceuticals. This demand will serve as a 'pull' factor to bring the target groups to distribution points for supplements, to overcome resistance and, if necessary, to induce consumers to pay a little more for a fortified diet [8].

The time is ripe for a rededicated initiative to eliminate the global micronutrient problem. We have new technologies, improved communications, and an expanded public infrastructure through supervised feeding programs. In parallel, by demanding the supplements and fortified foods that they need, consumers enable themselves to achieve their full social, physiological and economic potential. By eliminating micronutrient malnutrition through complementary public–private–civic sector initiatives we could make an enormous difference to the health and well-being of millions of people around the world.

References

1   Ramalingaswami V: Ending Hidden Hunger: Challenges and Opportunities. Proc Policy Conf on Micronutrient Malnutrition, Montreal, 1991.
2   UNICEF: World Declaration on the Survival, Protection and Development of Children and a Plan of Action for the 1990s. New York, UNICEF, 1990.
3   A World Fit for Children. New York, United Nations, 2002.
4   World Bank: Entering the 21st Century: World Development Report 1999/2000. Washington, World Bank, 2000.
5   Nestel P, Briend A, de Benoist B, et al: Complementary food supplements to achieve micronutrient adequacy for infants and young children. J Pediatr Gastroenterol Nutr 2003;36: 316–328.
6   International Food Policy Research Institute: Harnessing Agricultural Technology to Improve the Health of the Poor: 'Biofortified' Crops to Combat Micronutrient Malnutrition. Proposed as a Challenge Program of the CGIAR. Washington, International Food Policy Research Institute, 2002.
7   Venkatesh Mannar MG: Public/Private Partnerships for Improved Nutrition: How Do We Make Them Work for the Public Good? UN Standing Committee on Nutrition Annual Meeting. Chennai, 2003.
8   World Bank: Enriching Lives. Overcoming Vitamin and Mineral Malnutrition in Developing Countries. Washington, World Bank, 1994.

Discussion

Mr. Parvanta: As an example, I just wanted to give a kind of follow-up to a comment that Dr. Zlotkin made on the first day that these programs have to be continuous. In Scandinavia some people are thinking about eliminating fortification of infant foods just because the problem has gone away. In the map that you showed of the world, the former members of the Russian Union and all of those eastern European countries are a big block which has a problem with salt iodization or lack of salt iodization. It is important to remember that apparently in the old days in those countries, in the 1960s and perhaps even in the early 1970s, those programs were in place. But for some reason, perhaps because the problem had been eliminated, the programs were stopped, and now they have just resurfaced again [1]. So this is important for policy makers to realize that it is not over, it will always be there and we have to deal with it.

Dr. Mannar: We have seen cases in countries which had developed good levels of iodization and then slipped, and the problem has recurred very quickly. Within 1 or 2 years cases of iodine deficiency and goiter recur.

Dr. Zlotkin: We have both raised the issue of advocacy, and having Bill Gates on our side certainly does help. This may be a tough question, but as pediatricians, and there are pediatricians here, we have many opportunities to interact with other like individuals. But at the individual level as opposed to a government or a UN level, is there anything that as individuals you think that we professionals can be doing to advocate this particular issue at the individual level?

Dr. Mannar: I think all of you are key advocates. I have just talked to Dr. Mayya and he said that he was going to give a talk at the next meeting of the Indian Pediatric Association in the nutrition section of the program. I said that he should be talking about micronutrients and he agreed that he will. So each of you can go back to your country and do that, and spread it even among your own pediatric and other medical communities, that would certainly be of great help to promote the cause.

Dr. Tolboom: That was a very stimulating presentation. You mentioned that the world leaders in 2002 were recommitting themselves. But if you look at the goals that were formulated in 1990 and those formulated last year (2002), the goals of 1990 were reformulated. That is one of the problems we are dealing with because goals are set and then they have to be reformulated. So if the world leaders commit themselves, at what price is it? How can we hold them to their promises? You showed that vitamin A deficiency is declining, subclinical vitamin A deficiency, but are these lines really linear curves or are they different? The lines look so nice and on the basis of this type of picture we make our global crystal ball gazing which you have been doing. But do you think they are really straight lines or do we have to formulate the goals again in 3 years time? What is your idea, when you look into the future?

Dr. Mannar: Certainly I agree with you that global commitment is only the first step and a lot of work has to follow that. We are doing that with UNICEF, each of these global leaders is going to get a score card next January, 2 years from the time they made the commitment. We (MI) are going to give them a score card on how their country is doing in terms of addressing each of these deficiencies, what is the current coverage and what are the consequences. We are translating that into the functional consequences saying that do you realize that 50,000 children are being born with intellectual impairment; do you realize that so many mothers are dying because of very low levels of iron, and so we want to hit them with that, and UNICEF is of course the major advocate of this approach. We know that some people won't like it because they will get a bad score card, but we believe that they need to know the facts. As you said they made the commitment 2 years ago, and they can easily be forgotten in the midst of competing priorities, and can easily slip off the agenda all together. It is very important to constantly keep renewing and reminding leaders regarding the commitments and progress being made. On the second question I agree with you that it is very simplistic to just draw straight lines, we need to do more precise work for each country and it will obviously not be linear and it could fluctuate both up and down. Each country has to be considered separately.

Dr. Bhutta: This was really inspiring and I agree with almost all the crystal ball gazing that you have done. I want to make two comments that I believe are key in the global quest for addressing micronutrient malnutrition. I think there is a global issue in terms of global advocacy, but perhaps equally if not more important is the issue of national investments. The problem at this point in time of micronutrient deficiency is not only restricted to parts of the world where there is a real link with poverty, but also with areas like south Asia where there is no shortage of resources but there is a tremendous policy gap in terms of main streaming micronutrient malnutrition within the national nutrition programs. I come from a region where there has been a recent investment of 600 million rupees in a liver transplant program. Yet the national micronutrient program is starved for funds. So the point that I would like to make is that a lot of the advocacy really needs to be at a local level with policy makers. In your design of how you will do this, please make sure that they are involved. The second comment is in terms of the challenges that we have. It is nice to see approaches such as agricultural-based approaches to micronutrient malnutrition, and I believe it is one of the global challenges that have come out of the recent call for proposals. But a much bigger challenge in terms of micronutrient malnutrition is really how you get these to deliver within health systems. Although we may have the best program, when it comes to delivering these right down to the grass roots through existing health systems there is a big gap between evidence, research and intervention programs. So one would have very much liked to see an equivalent investment in delivery systems for existing interventions. We may have the best formulation but we still don't know how to get it right down to the grass roots. So I just wanted to flag these as two possible areas of attention.

Dr. Mannar: Absolutely, the work and commitment have to be at the national level, and in terms of dealing with national planners we have to get the attention of not only the ministry of health but other ministries such as education, planning and finance. They have to realize that this is something that they are also responsible for. In many countries, ministries of health tend to be under-funded, the minister is a junior minister and doesn't have the clout to mobilize huge resources. As you said making the decision to invest in something like a health facility is probably important but will benefit only a few people. It needs to be compared with something that would benefit millions of people, and a decision based on costs and benefits needs to be made. We certainly need to integrate micronutrients into sectors outside the health system, e.g. the food sector needs to take an active part in the solution so that at least part of the problem in terms of nutrient intake is addressed outside the health sector. This will also enable the health sector to focus its limited resources on those who cannot afford micronutrient-rich foods or have no access to them. But I agree with you that we need to improve those systems to reach even those people.

Dr. Pettifor: I refer to your comment that in fact we should perhaps do away with micronutrient deficiencies as a vertical program. I am worried about that because I have seen a number of countries trying to remove vertical programs. What happens is that you lose the advocacy, you lose the direction of that particular program that gets incorporated into general health care or whatever it happens to be; in fact the program dies. I would like to make the strong plea that in fact we don't remove the issues of micronutrient problems out of a vertical program, we need the advocacy, we need people who are going to be committed to try and address this problem. When we look at it on the ground and we may need to implement it, then sure we may need to use programs that are already there.

Dr. Mannar: I agree absolutely. I was talking of model integration at the community level in terms of the delivery and you are right, it still has to remain distinct in government policy and programs as well, not something buried under some other project.

Dr. Abrams: I want to make a comment about the gap between pediatricians and nutritionists. I think that they see the problem very differently and don't necessarily all agree on the ideas and approaches that need to be addressed. Pediatricians see a disease model, somebody is anemic and needs to be treated, and don't particularly think that global nutritionists have much to offer. I am certain that global nutritionists don't often think very much of what pediatricians do and their approach of the problem. So here we have a very biased group, pediatricians and nutritionists, which doesn't represent the busy pediatrician throughout the world who is occupied by taking care of lots of disease processes. I think a lot more needs to be done in terms of integrating the pediatrician as the advocate in understanding it, and also make the nutritionist a little bit more aware of what the pediatric world is about.

Dr. Gebre-Medhin: One thing that I would like to ask you about is the fact that within the next two decades the process of urbanization will continue. We are likely to be living more and more in towns, in urban settlement areas, with the result that food supply systems are going to be very different. What are your views on the micronutrient initiative that you have discussed vis-à-vis the classical issues of production of industrially produced breast milk substitutes and industrially produced complementary foods, I mean industrially produced foods for younger children and the rest. You did not link these two together. Are we going to abandon this classical approach that we have had, and how do we talk to governments about the continuation of these classical tested approaches vis-à-vis the micronutrient initiative?

Dr. Mannar: I think urbanization is something which we cannot avoid, it is something that is happening and it is something we have to live with. The question is how do we adapt our strategies in this rapidly changing environment, and I would say that the classical approaches have not been abandoned, and we should continue to push for both dietary promotion and of course expansion of food fortification and supplementation within the new health systems that are now coming up in urban centers, and work within that.

Dr. Gebre-Medhin: As was mentioned, my point is that we encourage governments and big organizations to take a stand. We push them to make declarations of different types. Earlier we talked about the necessity of supplying the increasing urban population with something for the first 6 months. Thereafter complementation issues are not being addressed adequately yet. Now we are shifting the emphasis in the area of micronutrients, perhaps partly to the detriment of other investments. This is really the problem.

Dr. Mannar: I hope not, I hope they can be complementary to all the other health nutritional interventions that we are doing, and I am hoping that micronutrients can in fact, through their quick impact and success, have an impact on addressing broader nutritional problems as well.

Mr. Parvanta: Just a comment, and I wonder if you might be able to share your thoughts on this? I refer to the importance of sharing the stories of special successes with the partners who may not know that they are part of the partnership. We forget that they are partners especially with the private sector for example. How can the surveillance information be shared, as you mentioned the idea of monitoring and surveillance? As scientists or academics we tend to publish the results of scientific research, monitoring it in scientific journals and that is where it stays. I don't know how much of that information gets passed into the sectors that we are working with. I want to ask the colleagues from Nestlé for example, if you have an idea about how we might go as a public agency? What do you think are options for us to share; in what format to share such information with the food industry such as yours, for example, in various parts of the world?

Dr. Guesry: Every morning our managers at the top level receive nutritional information coming from at least 20 scientific journals.

Dr. Mannar: I would add that in this era of high-speed communication we should be able to very rapidly synthesize information and then transmit it as widely as possible or make it available. This is perhaps the role of institutions like ours (MI) and CDC.

Dr. Hurrell: I would like to talk about biofortification, you mentioned that it is a strategy of the future, but your crystal ball was only gazing to the next 10–15 years. I would argue that it is going to take a lot longer than 10–15 years to get into biofortification. Plant breeding can only perhaps double or triple the level of iron or zinc in some of the staple crops, and this isn't really high enough, so we have to go to genetically modified organisms (GMOs), and we have to convince people that they have to accept GMOs. So how would you propose that we go about this?

Dr. Mannar: That relates to the broader issue of the safety and acceptance of GMOs. This is an ongoing debate which is reaching some kind of resolution. People tell me that the nutritional enrichment of crops could be one way in which you can demonstrate the necessity and the importance of GMOs, and it could in some way take off the negative perception that people have of genetically modified foods. But I agree with you, this is going to take anywhere from 10 to 20 years for us to see commercial products with significantly higher iron and zinc. I think you are going to see a marginally high iron and zinc content fairly soon in the next 5–8 years, but in order to meet the full requirement you are right, probably 20 years.

Dr. Barclay: Coming back to what industry could do, perhaps you could describe the program that was set up in the Philippines to encourage the food industry to move towards voluntary fortification?

Dr. Mannar: The Philippine Government has a fairly innovative program which is a seal of approval for any food that contains micronutrients at a specific level which they defined [2]. It is a way to get foods fortified as much as possible. But I don't know if it really addresses the problem of reaching the most vulnerable groups. There were cases of even hot dogs being fortified just to get the seal. I think the idea is good but the government has to aggressively promote it to reach some of the widely consumed lower priced staple foods as well.

Dr. Barclay: In this context, one of the projects we had in this program in the Philippines was the fortification of instant noodles, quite an inexpensive and widely consumed food product. We fortified instant noodles with calcium, iron, zinc and some vitamins; these products began to lose market share and this was thought to be due to fortification. In fact when we compared the competitors' product versus our own, we discovered that our product was inferior in terms of taste and consumer preference; it had nothing to do with the fortification. So coming back to what we are saying about quality, the products have to deliver a certain overall quality and the nutritional message alone will never be enough to ensure that the products are consumed by the target population. I would also like to ask Mr. Parvanta, what sort of information sharing do you have in mind in terms of collaboration between private and public sectors?

Mr. Parvanta: One of the ideas I had was more along the lines of a lot of national flour millers in that kind of sector, but I suppose it could even be national food processors or complementary food producers, a kind of the smaller operation that may not have as sophisticated scientists and people like that who receive scientific information as they would in Nestlé. So I was thinking that there might be some options whether they have newsletters or other kinds of simple information, whether it could be E-mails, I don't know if that is an option, but some way of summarizing some of the key pieces of information. But as far as I am concerned from the CDC perspective in United States, if we were to share that information within the United State companies, I would like to acknowledge the fact that not only the situation changed but also the role of the industry in that. So it is a way to acknowledge their participation and collaboration and contribution, and to keep them motivated like that. Do you think that is even sensible to do?

Dr. Guesry: I am really sorry but honestly I don't believe that the solution of food fortification and the solution of these micronutrient deficiencies is a scientific issue. I think we know everything we need to solve it. The problem is political and financial, and we have very little influence on this aspect. So it is not because instead of 20, 30 people receive pieces of information that it will change anything. They know what they need to know. We were speaking of the commitment of the opinion leaders and politicians, and since the half-life of politicians is about 4 years, they don't care about their commitments. So I am not as optimistic as you are. In spite of knowing for 20 years or more what we have to do, we still do not progress very rapidly.

References

1 Partnership for Sustained Elimination of Iodine Deficiency. US Update, Nov 2000.
2 Sangkap Pinoy Information Brochure. Department of Health, Government of Philippines, Manila.

Pettifor JM, Zlotkin S (eds): Micronutrient Deficiencies during the Weaning Period and the First Years of Life. Nestlé Nutrition Workshop Series Pediatric Program, vol 54, pp 263–268, Nestec Ltd., Vevey/S. Karger AG, Basel, © 2004.

Conclusions

Dr. Zlotkin: We started talking about epidemiology, went on to understanding physiology and impact, and ended I think very appropriately with looking at how we can deal with this issue. So we have appropriately gone full circle. For the last few minutes there is really nothing specific prepared. I thought I would ask the audience if they had any questions for any of the speakers, I think this would be the time to do that. Depending on the number of questions I thought it might be an interesting way to close by offering each of the speakers a final word. It is always difficult to write your thoughts before you have heard the other people speak. If anyone has the desire to make a couple of final comments, we are the experts in our individual areas and you have a willing audience here. Are there any questions for any of the speakers of the last 3 days?

Dr. Specker: A question that has been going through my mind is whether it would be useful to have people directly address the vulnerability of the breast-fed baby. In the course of the 3-day workshop any number of times we have talked about the importance of breast-feeding but there are real issues about the micronutrient status of the breast-fed baby under certain conditions, and it seems as though it has been articulated in bits and pieces but not necessarily as a synthesis of what is known about that.

Dr. Zlotkin: I actually think that it is a very interesting question. Not a simple question to answer without giving it a lot of thought because like most things certainly breast milk is a complex biological fluid which has complex immunologic properties, important and complex social properties in terms of bonding, and complex and important nutritional properties. If we think of the nutritional properties it is a nutritionally complete food, with the possible exceptions of vitamin D if you happen to live in Canada or Mongolia, with the possible exceptions of iron if you happen to be born prematurely or born to a mother with poor iron status. It is an important topic but not a topic without controversy and emotion. I think that the general statement that we have to live with is a WHO statement. Whether we agree or disagree with it, we have to live with it because at least in the short-term we can't change it. I think that we should in fact plan around the boundaries in terms of our attitude toward the developing world. We have to live with the statement that breast milk is recommended exclusively for the first 6 months. We all know that this recommendation is not followed and many of us may feel that there are problems with this but despite how we feel as an organization we have to live within these boundaries. I asked Dr. Lönnerdal why is mammalian milk such a poor source of iron and the answer is not perfectly straightforward. Dr. Lönnerdal, do you want to comment on that?

Dr. Lönnerdal: I can only reiterate what I said that it is remarkable that anemic women in southern India have identical iron content in their milk as Finnish women

Conclusions

taking 120 mg of supplemental iron/day. That means that the body has invented a very delicate mechanism in order to regulate this very tightly and to me it seems to be the reason. So it may not be that iron is too low, there are other things that we should be more concerned about. Since I have been given the opportunity I would like to go back to a discussion I had with Dr. Bhutta during the break. One of the things we have discussed very little here is education. Whatever we do should come with proper education. They have done a study just having education as an intervention without micronutrients and had a very significant effect on micronutrient status, which I think is highly relevant for discussion. When it comes to breast-feeding, we can take the example that many cultures have discarded colostrum for a long time. Everybody knows that this is disadvantageous for the newborn child. The only way to overcome that is education and say that there are very valuable components in colostrum. A similar thing could be done about exclusive breast-feeding. I don't think that the problem is that breast milk is of poor quality, the problem is early weaning at 1 or 2 months, but this is still a relatively recent development. Take farmers for example, they would never put a newborn cow on a straw diet. Similarly we are all mammals and there is a certain time when we should most likely be on milk. That message has not been carried out and education can do a lot of good. That doesn't negate any of the other things we are talking about, but education should come integrated with all these things rather than just dietary interventions.

Dr. Neufeld: I agree completely with that, and in practice the message of breast-feeding until 6 months is completely meaningless unless the patient is told how to do that, unless very concrete advice is given on what happens if there are physiological problems, what happens when the mother goes back to work. Perhaps some companies need to develop an effective low-cost breast pump which could be very useful to women in developing countries. Right now anything that is actually worthwhile tends to be very costly and people don't have access to that. There is a whole series of things that could be brought into education and practical solutions that we just don't do and without that, 6 months is just some number that the scientists have come up with, it is not real to the world. But with some concrete recommendations it could be.

Mr. Parvanta: I agree completely in the concept, the issue, the importance of education. I would like to just mention one specific point related to that: we need to involve professionals who know how to develop an education method or messages in a good way, especially behavioral scientists and communication specialist because often we target the wrong audience. Often women are not the ones who decide what the baby should eat, in many societies grandmothers decide or the mother may not immediately have the say. So education is important, but beyond education we have really to consider the audience to receive that education in order to make the kind of societal changes that need to take place. There are examples of successes of these kinds relating to infant feeding practices.

Dr. Castillo-Durán: I think that in research there are many international collaborative efforts. Many of the results come from privileged groups in collaborative efforts, but when we cross from research to intervention I think we must sometimes separately analyze in different ways in countries. The poorer people may need different strategies and not extrapolation from one to the other kinds of groups. Some approaches that I showed in my presentation tried to divide into different kinds of countries. Maybe the conclusions for the 2 or 3 varying groups could be different for the interventions and not extrapolated from the solution for the very underprivileged group to the more developed countries.

Mr. Parvanta: I would like to take the opportunity to come back to Dr. Guesry. At CDC we would like to get some feedback on how best we can engage the industry globally and also in relation to what you said with regard to political will. You are absolutely right, there is a lack of political will. In a different food fortification effort that Dr. Venkatesh referred to, the flour fortification initiative which is headed by MI and CDC and other partners, the idea was that we would engage the flour industry, the flour and grain industry around the world to take on the cause as something that is their responsibility and something good for them to do. In 12 months we have really moved very far, and they have taken on major responsibilities. But one of things that is important is the political will. Our contacts at the government level of countries is through the ministries of health, so that is where our leverage is and that is where we can influence political decisions. Industry on the other hand has other contacts within the government or the public sector. So my question is how do you think we as public agencies should engage the commercial baby food industry in various parts of the world to help them to take on the cause in a more global way, and to let them take on some responsibility coming from their side of the equation rather from our side of the equation alone?

Dr. Guesry: I think we have already covered this issue earlier today when we spoke about the Codex Alimentarius Recommendation which is a guideline for the whole world industry for infant products: breast milk substitutes, follow-up formula, growing up milk, and baby cereals, and these recommendations are very clear and there are norms for food fortification. But I understand that these recommendations from the Codex Alimentarius are not mandatory in every country. By the way in Europe it has been translated into mandatory recommendations by the European Committee of Nutrition, so in Europe there is no other choice than to put on the market products which are enriched. Although I am not so much in favor of imposing things, I suspect that it would probably be faster and more efficient to contact the ministers of health to recommend implementing this Codex Alimentarius Recommendation in their own countries. That would be quite fast and efficient.

Dr. Horton: I would like to take a somewhat different tack on Dr. Specker's initial question, the difference between the short run and the long run and the quick fix and the underlying solution. The problems with breast milk for babies with very low birth weight born to mothers with very low iron stores to start with brings up the problem of the quick fix. To some degree micronutrient fortification is a medium term quick fix for us being able to do longer-term things with the quality and the variety of the diet, and the baby of less than 6 months shows us the problem of a quick fix. I think a long-run fix on that is you have to do something with the status of women and the nutritional status of women, and there is no quick fix for that. This is something Dr. Lozoff and I were separately discussing as we pondered on Dr. Bloehm's very interesting presentation which was both encouraging and discouraging. On the one hand he said all these health interventions that Indonesia has been undertaking, all these projects the non-governmental organizations have been undertaking, didn't do much in the face of enormous economic disruption and negative economic growth. My view is that it is not possible to do that in a context where people's real incomes declined by 40% and we should not expect micronutrient fortification to be able to succeed in the face of that. On the other hand we should not give up either. Perhaps there are things that can be done with these more limited programs. The thing that is encouraging about micronutrients, that is less encouraging about macronutrients (energy and protein), is you can do things, there is a possibility to achieve the millennium goals, but I think it would be much harder to achieve millennium goals that are described in the nature of stunting and underweight for children.

Dr. Parampalli Maiya: We are not supposed to give multivitamin drops to babies born in hospital. So supplementations including vitamins and these micronutrients are drawn if these babies continue to be exclusively breast-fed for 6 months. I heard from the different presentations that subclinical micronutrient deficiencies do occur before the age of 6 months. So when we withdraw this supplementation from these babies are we going to have trouble with these babies? My second question is, I heard that vitamin D deficiency does occur before the age of 6 months if the mothers are vegetarian and they exclusively breast-feed their babies. Vegetarianism is very common in our country and I feel that such exclusively breast-fed babies should be given vitamin D supplementation also. The third thing is, this morning we touched upon oral rehydration and zinc fortification. It is very well known now that a lot of zinc is lost in diarrheal stools. Probably this is one of those things which could go through the pharmaceutical industries without going through the politicians, supplementing or fortifying the oral rehydration solutions with zinc.

Dr. Abrams: I think the first question was, is there any consistency between the rules for the baby from the hospital and current guidelines to give vitamin D supplementation in infants, and as I understand nothing should be given in the newborn nursery other than breast milk. But the American Academy of Pediatrics recommendations don't suggest that vitamin D needs to be given before 2 months of age because there is really not much need in any of these circumstances before that. Now I could imagine that there could be a small conflict between a hospital that is really trying to admit 2- or 3-month-old babies and trying to keep breast-feeding going. We are talking about supplements, not vitamin drops, and I can tell you that although there is some opposition to the vitamin D recommendation in general, it is not that strong.

Dr. Specker: As far as the vegetarian mother is concerned I don't think the vitamin D requirements are any higher and, as long as the infant and mother are outside, they are going to be getting the all the vitamin D that is necessary. The reason for the high rate of vitamin D deficiency among some vegetarian mothers has also to do with the clothing customs of certain vegetarian groups and their lack of sunlight exposure. There should be no reason why the vitamin D requirements are any greater in vegetarians than non-vegetarians.

Dr. Pettifor: I think there is some evidence that low-calcium diets, seen often in vegetarian diets, may in fact increase the catabolism of vitamin D. There were some studies done looking at the effect of low calcium diets on the turnover of 25-hydroxyvitamin D and vitamin D itself [1]. It reduces the half life of 25-hydroxyvitamin D from about 17 or 21 to about 10 days, when an individual is put on a low-calcium diet. So there is some evidence.

Dr. Specker: But I would argue that those mothers would have to be marginally vitamin D-deficient.

Dr. Pettifor: I think the issue is that an individual may be marginally vitamin D-deficient for instance in an urban environment, particularly an Indian environment for instance where clothing is fairly extensive, where houses are very close together, the mothers don't get out very often, they may well be marginally vitamin D-deficient. On top of that there is a low-calcium diet that is associated with vegetarianism, then vitamin D deficiency may well be precipitated. So I think what one must do in individual countries is to assess the vitamin D status of mothers to discover whether or not there is a need for vitamin D supplementation during pregnancy or during lactation in fact. It may not be necessary and obviously each country will be different, so to take the American Academy of Pediatrics recommendation and say that is a global international policy, is probably inappropriate. We haven't answered the third question which was related to the need for zinc in oral rehydration fluid. Was that the issue? Vitamin A, was it?

Dr. Guesry: It was zinc but also vitamin A.

Dr. Pettifor: Would somebody like to answer this question: why isn't vitamin A and/or zinc put into an oral rehydration solution? Now the comment that was made this morning was that the duration of time that oral rehydration is given is short and therefore the effect would be marginal. I don't know what the effect on cost would be.

Dr. Barclay: There are studies showing that administration of zinc during acute diarrhea does shorten the duration of diarrhea [2].

Dr. Castillo-Durán: There is evidence that supplementation during acute diarrhea decreases the duration and the risk of complications due to diarrhea, but in relation to the zinc content of oral rehydration solution, I don't know if we can use the amount needed to increase the zinc status because the amount that the children drink would be greater. Most the children drink about 500–700 ml/day during 2 or 3 days, and it is difficult to increase the amount to increase zinc status.

Dr. Ribeiro: The experience with using oral rehydration solution for any other additional purpose besides prevention and/or dehydration treatment has not been successful. The possibility of misunderstanding is quite high. In the past, the addition of some caloric content to the oral rehydration solution led mothers to keep using the oral rehydration solution as a food later on. So I don't think it is a good idea to put zinc into oral rehydration solutions.

Mr. Parvanta: On the same issue of vitamin D and a follow-up from Dr. Pettifor's comment about using US-based recommendations or Canadian-based Academy of Pediatrics recommendations and adapting those to the other settings. Dr. Specker, in your presentation you mentioned that the American Academy of Pediatrics made a recommendation about infants not being exposed to sunlight. Could you explain what that exactly means?

Dr. Specker: The American Academy of Pediatrics is going along with dermatologists who do not recommend sunlight for infants. That is why the meeting of the CDC was called because if you can make adequate vitamin D through sunlight exposure then vitamin D should not necessarily be a problem, but the American Academy of Dermatologists recommends no sunlight exposure for infants.

Dr. Abrams: The American Academy of Pediatrics agreed with the American Academy of Dermatology that children should have effective sun block when they are out in the sun.

Dr. Specker: Because of those recommendations they are now saying you cannot depend upon sunlight exposure in infants for vitamin D synthesis. We can't encourage sunlight exposure for production of vitamin D, but at the same time turn around and say they shouldn't be exposed, so that is the reason for the change in the recommendation.

Mr. Parvanta: So to follow-up what would your advice be to other countries vis-à-vis that recommendation?

Dr. Specker: I think moderation is great.

Mr. Parvanta: Basically you are suggesting that not everybody adopt that type of recommendation.

Dr. Specker: I personally would not recommend that.

Mr. Parvanta: I think it is dangerous in dark-skinned individuals. In those individuals skin cancer is not that common.

Mr. Specker: I think 10 min of sunlight exposure a day in even a fair-skinned infant does not represent a significant cancer risk. But the dermatologists may disagree with that. My concern actually with that recommendation is not just so much with vitamin D, but if parents are now told that children should have minimal exposure to sunlight, what is that going to do to obesity rates? It is also a big issue because in all of our studies on factors affecting physical activity in children, one of the biggest predictors is time outside, and now there are recommendations that children should not go outside, and I am not so sure that it is a healthy recommendation.

Dr. Zlotkin: I would like to thank the Nestlé Company. They gave Dr. Pettifor and I absolute carte blanche in inviting whom we wanted into this meeting; we had absolute carte blanche in determining what the program would be, and what they did was the hard part of making it all happen. So on your behalf I would like to thank the Nestlé Company for giving us the opportunity to get together and have a free and open discussion about what I think is an interesting and important topic. Thank you.

Conclusions

References

1   Clements MR, Johnson L, Fraser DR: A new mechanism for induced vitamin D deficiency in calcium deprivation. Nature 1987;325:62–65.
2   Bhutta ZA, Bird SM, Black RE, et al: Therapeutic effects of oral zinc in acute and persistent diarrhea in children in developing countries: Pooled analysis of randomized controlled trials. Am J Clin Nutr 2000;72:1516–1522.

Subject Index

Anthropometry, undernutrition studies 106, 107

Appetite, micronutrient intake effect, weaning period 84, 99, 100

Ascorbic acid-iron interactions 71, 72, 80

Bone
  calcium/phosphorus status
    linear growth relationship 160
    mineralization studies 160–163
    overview 159, 160
  copper effects 168
  density measurements 153–155
  developmental parameters 153
  early diet effects, long-term bone health 163, 164, 169
  exercise effects 166, 167
  micronutrient supplementation studies 170, 171
  vitamin D status
    linear growth relationship 156, 157, 164
    mineralization studies 157–159
    overview 155, 156
  zinc effects 166, 167

Breast milk
  adequacy during 1st year of life, complementary food rationale 83, 84, 203, 213, 263, 264
  iron content 263, 264
  vitamin D content 23, 32, 156, 266

Calcium
  bone effects
    linear growth relationship 160
    mineralization studies 160–163
    overview 159, 160
  deficiency
    phytic acid/dietary calcium bioavailability 27, 33, 34
    prevalence 27, 28, 34
    rickets 26, 27, 29, 30, 34
  dietary sources 26
  excretion 30
  recommended dietary intakes 25, 26
  stable isotope studies
    absorption, cystic fibrosis 54, 55
    calcium-41 features 65
  supplementation, pregnancy 33

Calcium-iron interactions 19, 20, 228–230

β-Carotene
  bioavailability, weaning period 91
  immune function studies 151, 152

Complementary foods
  calcium content 99
  dietary diversity 87
  dietary inadequacies, micronutrient deficiencies 93–96
  fortification
    affordability 209–211
    barriers
      overview 204

Complementary foods (continued)
  fortification (continued)
    barriers (continued)
      production side barriers 215,
        216, 232
      reaching the most needy 216,
        217
    efficacy trials, developing countries
      220, 221
    food industry globalism 210
    Nutrisano case study, Mexico
      efficacy, infant micronutrient
        status improvement 219
      iron bioavailability/stability/
        acceptability 219, 222, 223,
        226, 227
      nutrient content 222
      Oportunidades program 219, 231
      weaning practices 228, 229
    perceptions 204, 205
    program development 205–210, 223
    rationale 203, 214, 215
    research prospects 224
    targeted fortification
      developed countries 218,
        229–231
      developing countries 218, 219,
        231, 232
    universal versus targeted
      fortification 217
  iron-calcium interactions 228–230
  micronutrients
    bioavailability 87–91
    inadequacies 214
  nutritional adequacy evaluation,
    comparison with World Health
    Organization recommendations
    91–93
  recommendations 96, 97, 203, 224
Copper
  bone effects 168
  deficiency
    features 43
    prevalence 43
Copper-iron interactions 70, 71, 78
C-reactive protein (CRP), infection
  marker 182–184

Delivery, micronutrient deficiency
  eradication
  core business engagement 255
  overview 254, 255
  philanthropy 256
  supportive partnerships 255
Diarrhea
  micronutrient losses 177, 179, 181
  oral rehydration solutions 181, 182
  zinc supplementation 267
Dietary diversity, micronutrient intake
  effect, weaning period 86, 87

Economic impact, micronutrient
  deficiencies
  folate deficiency 190–192
  iodine deficiency 192, 193
  iron deficiency 193–196, 201
  mechanisms
    cognition 189
    morbidity 189, 199
    mortality 189, 190, 198, 199, 202
    productivity 188, 189
  overview 187, 188
  policy implications 196
  research prospects 197
  study design 198, 200
Energy density, micronutrient intake
  effect, weaning period 85, 99, 100
Exercise, bone effects 166, 167

Famine
  causes 106
  frequency 106
Feeding frequency, micronutrient intake
  effect, weaning period 85
Folate deficiency, economic impact
  190–192
Food variety, micronutrient intake
  effect, weaning period 85

Gastric pH, malnutrition effects 243,
  244

Helminthiasis, micronutrient status 183
Hemoglobin
  infant/toddler levels 16, 17
  undernutrition surveillance 112

Immune function
  adaptive versus innate immunity 139
  infants 139
  micronutrient effects, see Iron;
    Vitamin A; Zinc
  micronutrient studies, historical,
    background 138, 139

Infection, *see also* Immune function;
    specific diseases
    biomarkers 182–184
    impact, micronutrient status
        indicators 175–177
    mechanisms, micronutrient status
        effects 174, 175
    micronutrient deficiency
        pathogenesis/mechanisms 177, 178
    micronutrient supplementation
        recommendations 178, 179,
        183–185
Iodine
    deficiency
        economic impact 192, 193
        epidemiology, iron/vitamin A
            deficiencies 2, 4, 5, 15, 17
        features 46
        goiter 46
        micronutrient studies, history 250
        scoring 37, 38
    immune function studies 146
Iodine-iron interactions
    cross-sectional studies 9
    intervention studies 10, 11
    mechanisms 9, 10
    overview 8, 9, 74, 75
Iron
    absorption, infants 226, 227, 231, 243,
        244
    bioavailability/deficiency 1, 2, 87–89
    deficiency, *see also* Iron deficiency
        anemia
        developmental study design
            131–133, 135
        disease association 40, 177
        economic impact 193–196, 201
        epidemiology, iodine/vitamin A
            deficiencies 2, 4, 5, 15, 17
        mental development 120, 121, 130,
            131
        motor development 122
        risk factors 233
        scoring 37, 38
        sensory development 123
        sleep/wake cycle effects 123
        social/emotional development 121,
            122, 135
        spontaneous motor activity effects
            122, 123
        undernourished infants/toddlers
            123, 124

    dietary requirements 233
    immune function studies
        controlled studies 145
        deficiency effects 144, 146
        historical perspective 138, 139
        supplementation effects 146
    Nutrisano bioavailability,
        stability/acceptability 219, 222,
        223, 226, 227
    stable isotope studies, absorption,
        fortified foods 54, 62, 63
    status assessment 119
    supplementation
        anemia prevention 235, 236
        effects on malaria 151, 245, 248
        home fortification, *see* Sprinkles
        iron drops/syrup 236
    weanling intake 102, 103
Iron-ascorbic acid interactions 71, 72, 80
Iron-calcium interactions 19, 20,
    228–230
Iron-copper interactions 70, 71, 78
Iron deficiency anemia (IDA)
    etiology 240
    prevalence 1, 15, 38
    prevention, infants
        dietary diversification/modification
            234, 235
        home fortification, *see* Sprinkles
        iron supplementation 235, 236
        targeted iron fortification 235
    vitamin A status effects 2, 3
Iron-iodine interactions
    cross-sectional studies 9
    intervention studies 10, 11
    mechanisms 9, 10
    overview 8, 9, 74, 75
Iron-riboflavin interactions 74
Iron-vitamin A interactions
    intervention studies 8
    iron absorption 6, 7
    iron metabolism 3, 6
    overview 72, 73
Iron-zinc interactions 49, 50, 67–70,
    78–80
Isotope micronutrient research
    body pools 64, 65
    calcium absorption, cystic fibrosis
        54, 55
    calcium-41 features 65
    costs/funding 59, 61, 62, 65
    erythrocyte iron incorporation 62

Isotope micronutrient research
(continued)
  intrinsic versus extrinsic labels 64
  iron/zinc absorption, fortified foods
    54, 62, 63
  isotope purchasing guidelines 57,
    58, 60
  magnesium metabolism kinetics
    55–57
  safety 57, 61
  sample collection 61, 66
  steady state considerations 63
  study design 58, 59
  zinc, body compartments 176, 177,
    180, 181

Kwashiorkor, definition 106

Lead, confounding factor, micronutrient
  deficiency studies 133, 134

Magnesium, stable isotope studies,
  metabolism kinetics 55–57
Malaria, iron supplementation effects
  151, 245, 248
Marasmus, definition 106
Meat, iron/zinc absorption enhancement,
  weanlings 89, 101, 102
Minimal change nephrotic syndrome,
  zinc, prevention 149, 150

Non-government organizations (NGOs),
  micronutrient fortification 117, 118
Nutrisano, see Complementary foods

Oral rehydration solutions
  diarrhea treatment 181, 182
  micronutrient supplementation 266,
    267

Phosphorus
  bone effects
    linear growth relationship 160
    mineralization studies 160–163
    overview 159, 160
  deficiency, rickets 32, 33
Phytic acid
  calcium absorption effects 27,
    33, 34
  iron absorption effects 87, 88, 90
  zinc absorption effects 38, 50, 87,
    88, 90

Pneumonia, zinc deficiency/
  supplementation effects 42, 48, 49
Policy, micronutrient deficiency
  eradication
  barriers 261, 262
  global commitment 258
  overview 256
  relapse, goiter 258
Polyphenols, iron absorption effects
  88, 89
Probiotics supplementation, infection
  185
Protein-energy malnutrition
  definition 107
  zinc deficiency 39

Retinol-binding protein (RBP),
  endotoxin effects 176
Riboflavin-iron interactions 74
Rice
  genetic engineering 116, 117
  price relationship, undernutrition
    110, 111, 114, 115
Rickets
  calcium deficiency 26, 27, 34
  phosphorus deficiency 32, 33
  treatment 168, 170, 171
  vitamin D deficiency 29–32, 156

Selenium
  deficiency
    biomarkers 52
    developed countries 45
    developing countries 44, 45
  food composition 43, 44
  immune function studies 151
  recommended dietary intake 44
Shigellosis, micronutrient losses 177
Social mobilization, micronutrient
  deficiency eradication
  advocacy 258
  overview 251, 256, 257
Sprinkles
  acceptability 238, 246, 247
  advantages 237
  controls, studies 248
  costs 244, 245, 247, 248
  delivery 237, 246
  Ghana trials 237, 238, 240
  government approval 242
  iron
    bioavailability 239

deficiency anemia treatment 240
    formulation 237, 243
    Mongolia study 238, 239
    Thailand study 247
Stable isotopes, *see* Isotope
    micronutrient research
Sunlight exposure
    infants 267
    vitamin D metabolism 21, 22, 155

Tannins, iron absorption effects 88, 89
Technology, micronutrient deficiency
    eradication
    biofortified foods 253, 261
    communications 261
    fortified foods for all 252
    home supplements 252
    multiple micronutrient interventions
        252
    overview 251, 252
    rapid assessment techniques 253
    special needs 252
    supplement assimilation 254

Undernutrition
    causes 108, 109
    definitions 108
    rice price relationship 110, 111, 114,
        115
UNGA Special Summit for Children,
    goals 251
United Nations Millenium Declaration
    105
Urbanization, micronutrient deficiency
    implications 260

Vegetarians, vitamin D deficiency,
    breast-fed infants 266
Vitamin A
    bioavailability, weaning period 91
    deficiency
        disease association 40
        epidemiology, iodine/iron
            deficiencies 2, 4, 5, 15, 17
        micronutrient studies, history 250
        scoring 37, 38, 150
    immune function studies
        controlled studies 142, 143
        deficiency effects 140, 141
        historical perspective 138
        prospects, study 146, 147
        supplementation effects 141

infectious disease, supplementation
    recommendations 178, 179
Vitamin A-iron interactions
    interventions 8
    iron absorption 6, 7
    iron metabolism 3, 6
    overview 72, 73
Vitamin A-zinc interactions 73
Vitamin D
    bioavailability, weaning period 91
    bone effects
        linear growth relationship 156,
            157, 164
        mineralization studies 157–159
        overview 155, 156
    breast milk content
        adequacy 23, 32, 156
        vegetarian mothers 266
    cutaneous synthesis, factors affecting
        22, 23, 32
    deficiency
        epidemiology 24, 25
        infants/young children 24
        rickets 29–32, 156
    dietary sources, infants/young
        children 23
    forms 21, 22
    immune function studies 146
    infant sunlight exposure 267
    metabolism 21, 22, 155
    placental transfer 30, 31
    recommended dietary intakes 26
    status assessment 23, 155
    storage 30, 31
Vitamin E
    bioavailability, weaning period 91
    immune function studies 152
Vitamin K, bioavailability, weaning
    period 91

Weaning, *see* Complementary foods
Women, Infants, and Children's
    Supplemental Nutrition Program
    (WIC), overview/approved foods 205,
    245

Zinc
    bone effects 166, 167
    deficiency
        developed countries 42, 43
        developmental study design 126
        diagnosis 37, 38, 49, 52

Subject Index

Zinc (continued)
  deficiency (continued)
    disease association 39, 40
    growth retardation 39, 41
    infectious diseases 41, 51, 177
    mechanisms, developmental
      effects 127
    mental development 125
    motor development 126
    pathogenesis 173, 174
    pneumonia 48, 49
    prevalence 38, 39
    protein-energy malnutrition 39
    social/emotional development
      125, 126
    spontaneous motor activity effects
      126
  immune function studies
    controlled studies 145
    deficiency effects 141, 144
    historical perspective 138
    prospects, study 146, 147

    supplementation effects 144
  infectious diseases, supplementation
    recommendations 178, 179, 183,
    184
  minimal change nephrotic syndrome
    prevention 149, 150
  phytic acid effects, absorption 38,
    50, 87
  plasma levels, coincidental infections
    175, 176
  stable isotope studies
    absorption, fortified foods 54,
      62, 63
    body compartments 176, 177, 180,
      181
  status assessment 125
  supplementation
    diarrhea 267
    diarrhea/pneumonia prevention 42
Zinc-iron interactions 49, 50, 67–70,
  78–80
Zinc-vitamin A interactions 73